Winning the Battle Against Prostate Cancer

Winning the Battle Against Prostate Cancer

GET THE TREATMENT THAT IS RIGHT FOR YOU

Second Edition

Gerald Chodak, MD

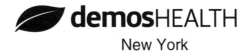

New York

Visit our website at www.demoshealth.com

ISBN: 978-1-936303-54-0
e-book ISBN: 978-1-61705-185-2

Acquisitions Editor: Julia Pastore
Compositor: Exeter Premedia Services Private Ltd.

Library of Congress Cataloging-in-Publication Data
Chodak, Gerald W., 1950–
  Winning the battle against prostate cancer : get the treatment that is right for you / Gerald Chodak, MD.—Second edition.
      p. ; cm
  Includes bibliographical references and index.
  ISBN 978-1-936303-54-0—ISBN 978-1-61705-185-2 (e-book)
  1. Prostate–Cancer–Popular works.   I. Title.
  RC280.P7C545 2013
  616.99'463—dc23
                                                            2013020150

Printed in the United States of America by Edwards Brothers.
13 14 15 16 17 / 5 4 3 2 1

FOR ALL MEN WITH PROSTATE CANCER OR
YET TO BE DIAGNOSED WITH IT,
HOPING THOSE NEEDING TREATMENT GET CURED
AND ALL THE REST ARE NOT HARMED.

Contents

II How to Treat Clinically Localized Prostate Cancer

III Managing Locally Advanced Prostate Cancer

Foreword

Dr. Chodak has made a valuable contribution in writing this comprehensive book and his revised edition updates this important resource. I am pleased to see this revised edition because we live in a time of rapid new developments in treating prostate cancer. This book is a much-needed tool for men, their friends, family, and others, as they battle this deadly, under-recognized disease and attempt to live with pride and a winning, positive attitude. I know from the thousands of men and women I see that this book provides useful information with regards to the fight.

Prostate cancer took the life of my wife Margaret's father when she was a young mother and her younger sister was still in high school, and it places our family at risk now and in the future. As America and the world ages, more men are at risk of prostate cancer than ever before. It is the next most diagnosed cancer in men after skin cancer. It is diagnosed at a similar or higher level than breast cancer is in women. This fact is becoming more recognized and *Winning the Battle Against Prostate Cancer* will provide information to millions of men, as well as those who care about and love them, who need to know their risk and what they can do about it.

As Dr. Chodak points out, being empowered and learning to cope comes through knowledge and hope. Us TOO was founded on that principle 20 years ago, and today thousands of volunteers continue to help support each other, learn, and together make their voices heard. Dr. Chodak is one of the well-informed good guys in the battle against prostate cancer with a long history of contributions. His book provides a comprehensive view of a complex and often controversial disease and he continues to be an active leader who shows sensitivity and a commitment to patients being active in their own care and finding the latest information necessary to fight on.

My personal "Thank you" goes out to him.

Thomas N. Kirk
President/CEO
Us TOO International
Prostate Cancer Education and Support Network
Downers Grove, Illinois

Acknowledgments

For this second edition of *Winning the Battle Against Prostate Cancer* I have many people to thank and acknowledge.

First, I dedicate this book to my mother Roslyn Oestreich Chodak, who died unexpectedly in February 2013. She was a source of inspiration for living life to the fullest and I was fortunate to have her in my life for so many years.

To my agent Bob Silverstein, who succumbed to an illness in the fall of 2012, I am thankful for all his past advice and support, may he rest in peace!

To my wife, Robin, for providing her support, her love, and her editing prowess throughout this project. I am truly a lucky man to have such a wonderful partner in my life.

To Beth Barry who in her new role at Demos has given me the opportunity to write this second edition so soon after the first one was published.

Lastly, to men with prostate cancer who will benefit from the many advancements in the management of this challenging disease. I hope that this book will help guide them down the right path for their treatment.

Introduction

If you or a loved one has been diagnosed with prostate cancer, many emotions and questions probably are going through your head. You might be scared, anxious, and uncertain about what to do and what may happen. If you're the patient, you may want answers to questions such as:

- How dangerous is my cancer?

- Can I be cured?

- Which is the best treatment for me?

- How much will the treatment affect my quality of life?

- Will my cancer recur?

- Who can I trust to give me the best advice?

Winning the Battle Against Prostate Cancer will help you by giving you answers to these questions and letting you know what other questions you should be asking.

For many men, learning about prostate cancer can be overwhelming and confusing. There are so many opinions on what to do and way too much information to read. In the beginning of April 2013, surfing the Internet with the words "prostate cancer information and treatment" had over 70 million hits! Unfortunately, many of them contained outdated information. In addition, advertisements in newspapers and magazines, and those on television and even roadside billboards are constantly promoting different treatments by using incomplete or biased information. One of the major reasons for writing this second edition is that even more options are now available due to the approval of new therapies and drugs by the U.S. Food and Drug Administration (FDA) in the last three years. These are important changes that can significantly improve men's survival and quality of life. Also, many important studies that started 10 or more years ago have been completed and the results are now available. None of the books published before 2012 have this information. Unfortunately, you cannot count on all doctors to give this new information because too many of them also are not keeping up to date. One of the major strengths of this second edition of *Winning the Battle Against Prostate Cancer* is that it provides the most accurate and up to date information available.

Also, as your learning process proceeds, you will soon find out that prostate cancer is unlike most other cancers in several ways:

- The majority of other cancers are almost always life threatening and must be treated aggressively, but many men with prostate cancer are not in danger and may never need treatment.

- Other cancers have few treatment options but there are many ways to treat prostate cancer.

- Most doctors agree on how to manage other cancers but they very rarely agree on how to manage prostate cancer.

The last point can make it hard for you to get the right treatment. After all, aren't you supposed to trust your doctor to give you the best advice? You might want to know why that isn't always true. One reason is because of the different ways doctors are trained and another is because of their personal biases. For example:

- Surgeons are more likely to recommend surgery while radiation therapists more likely will recommend radiation, even though there is no proof either one is better.

- Surgeons who perform an open prostatectomy say it is the best method while those using a robot believe all surgeries should be done that way. Here again, neither option is clearly better.

- Urologists who purchased radiation equipment are recommending radiation at their centers when other treatments may be a better option or at least as good, though less profitable for the doctor.

- Doctors who treat men with proton radiation, stereotactic radiation, or high-intensity focused ultrasound are recommending those treatments even though there still is no information about their long-term cure rates. This limitation is rarely being explained to patients.

Winning the Battle Against Prostate Cancer will make you aware of these possible biases, so you can avoid getting a treatment that may not be the right one for you. This book avoids potential biases because it strictly follows the principles of *evidence-based medicine* or *EBM*. It means that a therapy will be *recommended* only when high quality scientific studies have demonstrated it is the best option. If such studies do not exist, this book will help you understand the pros and cons and risks and benefits of *all* the treatments available without a bias toward any one of them.

Another important feature of this new edition is its added ability to help you play a role in deciding what is done. Today, many men are not content to let the doctor make all the decisions even though they are the ones with the medical training. The reason is that patients are the ones who have to live with the effects of treatment, not the doctors. Also, the goals and concerns of doctors and patients may not be the same. Some men prefer to preserve their quality of life rather than live as long as possible and others want the opposite. This is a very personal decision and it means your treatment must be tailored to meet *your needs and goals* based on your age, health, type of prostate cancer, and quality of life. Many doctors do not take this into consideration when advising you. The key is to be adequately informed so you can work with your doctor to find the treatment that is right for you. To play an active role in this decision, *you need to know what you need to know*, which means asking the right questions. *Winning the Battle Against Prostate Cancer* will provide the questions to ask in a way that should be acceptable to most doctors. Once you get those questions answered you will be able to help make the decision.

Asking the right questions is also important in knowing what you can do on your own to improve your chances of surviving this disease. Today, men spend large amounts of money on "alternative" therapies in the hope of improving their overall health or treating their prostate cancer. That includes paying for herbs, vitamins, supplements, and other holistic treatments. Unfortunately, good studies have been rarely done and unless you ask the right questions or learn important facts about them, you might be wasting your time and money. In some cases, it is also possible that these alternative therapies could make you worse or keep you from getting better by interfering with standard treatments. *Winning the Battle Against Prostate Cancer* will provide you with an up-to-date assessment of all these unconventional therapies so you can make educated decisions about ways to help yourself.

As you begin to read and learn about this disease, take your time and don't panic. There is no need to rush into a treatment. Your prostate cancer did not develop yesterday or last month and in most cases it does not need to be treated tomorrow or even within the next several weeks or months. Learn about all the options available, don't be afraid to ask questions and use *Winning the Battle Against Prostate Cancer* to help you get the best result possible.

Unlike the first edition, which provided information about prevention and detection of prostate cancer, this second edition is primarily intended for the man who has already been diagnosed with the disease. If you do not have prostate cancer and want to know what you might do to prevent it or you have concerns about whether you should get tested for it, you can visit my free video website at www.prostat evideos.com. It also will tell you how you can arrange for a consultation to help you get the treatment that is best for you.

I

WHAT YOU NEED TO KNOW BEFORE CHOOSING YOUR TREATMENT

The Male Anatomy: How It All Fits Together

Before you learn about your treatment options, you may benefit from an increased awareness of your anatomy and the role of each organ in your general health.

The Prostate Gland

The prostate sits in your lower pelvis, tucked behind your pubic bone and just beneath your bladder. It surrounds the *urethra*, which is the tube that carries urine from your bladder out through the tip of the penis. Directly behind the prostate is the rectum. Very little tissue separates these two organs, which is why the rectum can be injured when the prostate is being treated. Located between the prostate and rectum are the two *pelvic nerves*, which enable erections to occur. They also can be easily damaged during any treatment directed at the prostate. At the top of the prostate, just behind the bladder, are the two seminal vesicles.

The normal adult prostate is approximately the size of a walnut and weighs about 20 grams. It has five regions or *lobes*. Prostate cancer most commonly grows in the *posterior lobe*, which is closest to the rectum. This makes it possible for your doctor to examine the prostate by placing a gloved finger inside the rectum and pushing toward the front of your body. Surrounding the prostate is a very thin layer of tissue called the *capsule*. It serves as a barrier separating the prostate from the surrounding organs. Prostate cancer may grow into or through the capsule. If cancer extends through the capsule, it is no longer considered "localized."

The prostate gland usually increases in size as men get older, which can cause the following urinary symptoms:

- Slowing of the stream

- Difficulty starting and stopping urination

- Needing to urinate during the night

- Frequent urination

- An inability to empty the bladder

- Dribbling

These symptoms may also occur in a man who has prostate cancer.

The Urinary Bladder

Urine is made in your kidneys and passes down to your bladder through a tube called the ureter. Most people are born with two kidneys, one on the right and the other on the left, so there are two ureters. As your bladder fills with urine, it enlarges and eventually you will begin to feel some discomfort in your lower abdomen. This is a signal that your bladder is getting full and it is time to urinate. A normal bladder can hold about 300 to 400 milliliters before causing severe discomfort. That is about 10 to 13 ounces. The maximum capacity is about 400 to 600 milliliters unless the bladder has been damaged.

The reason urine stays in the bladder is because of two muscles called the external and internal urinary sphincters. They are located in your lower pelvis. The internal sphincter is located at the bottom of the bladder where it connects to the prostate. The external sphincter is located beneath the prostate. The external urinary sphincter is a striated muscle, like the muscles in your arms and legs. Striated muscles are under your voluntary control, which means you have the ability to tighten or relax them. The external sphincter can be strengthened by exercises, which can help decrease urinary leakage following some of the treatments for prostate cancer. The internal urinary sphincter is a *smooth* muscle, like the muscles in your heart. Smooth muscles work on their own, meaning you have no voluntary control over them.

The external urinary sphincter normally is contracted, which prevents urine from leaking out. As your bladder fills, it sends a signal to your brain that causes the internal sphincter to relax. In response, you voluntarily tighten your external sphincter so that urine does not leak out until you decide you want to urinate. At that time, you relax your external sphincter and your bladder contracts, which forces the urine to exit from your body. These muscles may be injured by the treatments for prostate cancer.

The Seminal Vesicles

These are two small glands measuring about five centimeters in length that are located near the top of the prostate behind the bladder. The seminal vesicles play a vital role in fertility by making fluid that helps to nourish sperm cells. When you have an orgasm, the fluid from each seminal vesicle is delivered down a tube called the *ejaculatory duct* and then it passes into the urethra and out the tip of the penis.

The seminal vesicles are not needed for any other bodily function besides fertility. They are removed along with the prostate during a radical prostatectomy. The only consequence is that you will have a *dry orgasm*, which means that no fluid will come out of the tip of the penis.

The Testicles

These are two egg-shaped glands located in the scrotal sac beneath the penis. The testicles have two major functions. They are responsible for making sperm cells that will fertilize a woman's egg and they produce a hormone called testosterone. Hormones are chemicals produced in certain organs that affect other parts of your body. Testosterone is responsible for your male characteristics such as hair growth, muscle development, your sex drive, and the growth of the prostate gland. Since this hormone also helps prostate cancer cells grow, one of the treatments is to remove the testicles, which is called surgical castration. Medical treatments are also available that can stop the testicles from producing testosterone.

When a man has an orgasm, the sperm from each testicle is released into long, thin, muscular tubes called the vas deferens. The end of each vas deferens joins with a seminal vesicle to form the ejaculatory duct. The two ducts pass through the prostate gland and join with the urethra. Following an orgasm, the sperm and seminal fluid are forced down the two ejaculatory ducts and then out through the tip of the penis. Men who no longer want to have children can have a vasectomy during which each vas deferens is divided. Both vas deferens tubes are also cut when the entire prostate is removed, which makes a man unable to father a child during sexual intercourse.

The Penis

This organ is responsible for sexual intercourse, and although it needs little explanation, several facts about it may not be known. It is made up of three columns of tissue. The two columns located on the sides of the penis are called the corpus cavernosum, and the third one, called the corpus spongiosum, is located in between them. The tip of the penis is called the glans and the remainder is called the shaft. The corpus cavernosum and spongiosum are filled with blood vessels. When a man becomes sexually aroused, signals are sent from the brain to the penis from the pelvic nerves, which causes more blood to flow into and less blood to leave the penis. This causes an erection. Following an orgasm, the blood is drained out through veins in the penis and the erection goes away.

The treatments for prostate cancer can affect the nerves and the blood vessels resulting in a decreased ability to get an erection. One of the major advances in treating men who have decreased erections has been the development of drugs that increase the blood flow into the penis.

Lymph Nodes

Lymph nodes are small glands scattered throughout the body that help fight infection. Prostate cancer can spread into the lymph nodes near the prostate by entering lymphatic channels located in the gland or they can spread to lymph nodes in other parts of the body by first entering blood vessels.

Now that you understand the basics about your anatomy you should find it easier to understand what happens during the different treatments for your prostate cancer.

Staging Your Prostate Cancer

Clinical and Pathological Stage

Now that you have been diagnosed with prostate cancer, you probably want to know how your doctor will determine which treatment is best for you. It depends in part on where the tumor is located, which is called the **tumor stage**. Before making any recommendations, doctors want to know if all the cancer cells are contained inside the prostate (called *localized prostate cancer*) or if some have spread to other locations (called *locally advanced* if cells are found outside the prostate capsule and **metastasized** if they have spread to other parts of the body). They do this by combining information from the digital rectal examination (DRE) and other tests that they may order. Doing so enables them to assign you a *clinical stage*, depending on where they think the cancer is located. Despite improvements available in the staging tests, the clinical stage they assign to you is not always correct. In some cases, cancer may be present in different locations but it may be so small that the tests can't detect it. In this case the test may give you a *false-negative* result. At other times, staging tests overestimate your cancer and tell you it has spread when it really hasn't. These are called *false-positive* results. The only way to know the exact location of the cancer in your body, called the *pathological tumor stage*, is to do an autopsy, which of course is not feasible. So your doctor will tell you the best options for treating your cancer based on your clinical stage, which is determined using the following tests.

The Digital Rectal Examination (DRE)

The easiest staging test is the DRE, which is performed by the doctor inserting a gloved, lubricated index finger into the rectum and pressing it against the rectal wall. A normal prostate gland feels smooth, with no lumps, bumps, or hardness. During the examination, the doctor also checks for symmetry; whether it feels the same on the left side of the gland as on the right. Another important determination is whether cancer is growing through the outer covering or capsule of the prostate. Based on this examination, the doctor will assign a clinical stage to your prostate cancer.

Staging Transrectal Prostate Ultrasound

Everyone who has been diagnosed with prostate cancer is familiar with transrectal ultrasound because almost every biopsy is performed using this procedure. Its main value is to help direct the prostate biopsy needle into specific locations in the prostate gland. Prostate cancer usually appears as a dark spot on the ultrasound scan. Doctors can also measure blood flow in the prostate by doing a *color Doppler ultrasound*, which some doctors believe can increase the ability to identify the locations of the cancer.

Ultrasound can also be used to stage the cancer in the following ways. Doctors look at the outer surface (prostate capsule) for distortion, which could mean cancer is outside the gland. Unfortunately, a mere look at the surface of the prostate gives many false-positive and false-negative results. One well-done study conducted in 1997 found that the ultrasound performed without additional biopsies was not much better than the DRE in deciding which cancer was outside the gland.

A better way to use prostate ultrasound to stage the disease is to direct a biopsy needle into any areas that look suspicious for cancer growing through the capsule. Ink is placed on the side that is nearest to the capsule. If cancer cells are seen touching the ink, it means the cancer is outside the gland. Doctors also can tell if cancer is growing into the seminal vesicles by taking a biopsy of any abnormal areas seen on the scan. However, the test is only helpful if it confirms extracapsular cancer because there is no guarantee that a negative biopsy is correct.

Although most doctors use transrectal ultrasound to perform a prostate biopsy, few use it to stage the tumor. Some doctors, however, also anticipate that cancer is present when they perform the intial biopsy. In some cases they may take additional samples to find out whether the cancer is confined inside the prostate or has grown through the wall or into the seminal vesicles. If your doctor does use this method, then the necessary biopsies were taken at the same time your cancer was detected. If staging biopsies were not done and you go for a second opinion, then some doctors may recommend doing another ultrasound with more biopsies to stage the cancer.

If another scan is advised for staging, the technique is the same as your first one in terms of the preparation, and anesthesia should be used to limit your discomfort during the biopsies. It is a good idea to discuss pain control if a different doctor will be doing the test, to make sure your discomfort will be minimized.

Who Should Have a Staging Transrectal Ultrasound?

The men most likely to benefit from a staging transrectal ultrasound are those with a high risk for extracapsular disease and/or cancer in the seminal vesicles. That includes anyone with a prostate-specific antigen (PSA) value over 20 ng/ml and those men suspected of having cancer outside the prostate based on the DRE examination.

Although everyone reading this book is likely to be aware of their PSA and what it is used for, some information is worth providing. PSA is a protein produced in the prostate by normal cells and cancer cells. In men with prostate cancer, the more cancer they have, the higher will be the PSA. Some noncancer conditions can raise the PSA including a prostate infection or inflammation in the prostate and prostate trauma. A staging transrectal ultrasound is not worth doing on men with low-risk or intermediate-risk prostate cancer, which includes those with a PSA less than 20 ng/ml, a normal prostate examination, and a Gleason score (a grading system for tumors; see p. 13 for more detail) less than 8.

The Bone Scan

The most common test used for staging prostate cancer is the technetium-99 bone scan because bones are the most common site for metastatic prostate cancer. It is performed by first injecting a small amount of a radioactive drug called technetium into a vein. It circulates through the bloodstream and then throughout the entire body. Abnormal bones take up the radioactivity and the remainder passes out of the body in the urine. There is little danger from the small amount of radioactivity used for the test.

The bone scan is done with the patient lying on his back on a table for one to two hours while a *gamma counter* takes pictures. Any bones that have taken up the technetium will show up as a dark spot. The test causes no pain except for the discomfort of lying on a hard table. Less than 1% of men get an allergic reaction to the injected material. When the test is completed, the patient can immediately resume his normal activities.

An abnormal bone scan does not mean that a man definitely has cancer in the bones. Some non-cancerous conditions also can result in a "positive" bone scan. These include:

- Bone fractures

- Arthritis

- Bone island (non-cancerous growth of bone)

- Paget's disease (excessive breakdown and formation of bone)

If the bone scan is abnormal, additional tests are done to find out the cause, but sometimes they are unable to determine if cancer is present. About 3% of men have a false positive scan, meaning that for every 100 men with a suspicion of cancer in the bones, the suspicion will prove true in only 97. The scan also can give a false negative result in about 3% of men, meaning the test was negative but cancer still was present.

Who Should Have a Bone Scan?

The use of the bone scan as a staging test for prostate cancer has changed over the last 10 years because of the PSA test. In the 1980s and 1990s, most doctors would order a bone scan on *every* man diagnosed with the disease. However, after the PSA test was developed, studies found prostate cancer had spread to the bones in only 3 out of 1000 men when the PSA was less than 20 ng/ml. Yet, more than four times as many men had an abnormal scan from a noncancerous cause. As a result, many doctors stopped doing a bone scan on everyone and only ordering them for some patients. Now, most experts recommend *not* doing a bone scan if the PSA is less than 10 ng/ml, unless a man is having pain in one or more bones. Some doctors combine the DRE and the Gleason score on the prostate biopsy with the PSA result to select patients for this test. This enables them to assign patients into a low-risk, intermediate-risk, or high-risk category as defined below:

- *Low risk:* The prostate examination shows no cancer or only a lump on one side of the gland; the Gleason score is less than 7 and the PSA is less than 10 ng/ml.

- *Intermediate risk:* Prostate examination shows cancer occupying more than half of one-side of the prostate but not outside the gland; the Gleason score is less than 8 and the PSA is between 10 and 20 ng/ml.

- *High risk:* The PSA is over 20 ng/ml or the Gleason score is between 8 and 10, or the tumor can be felt on both sides of the gland.

A bone scan is omitted for the low-risk and intermediate-risk patient provided they have no bone pain. Some doctors recommend a bone scan for all high-risk patients and others limit it to those with a PSA over 10 ng/ml if the Gleason score is 8–10. Around the United States, many doctors order a bone scan for all their patients because they want to establish a baseline to compare with future scans or they are concerned about missing even a single patient with bone metastases. This is no longer a very sensible approach. If your doctor does want you to have a bone scan when you have either low-risk or intermediate-risk cancer, you should consider asking him or her to explain their reasons.

PET/CT Scan

An alternative and potentially better way to scan the bones is called the *sodium fluoride PET/CT* bone scan. PET stands for *positive emission tomography* and CT for *computed tomography*. A CT scan is performed at the same time as the PET scan to further increase the accuracy of the PET scan. Radioactive material is first injected into a vein. About 30 to 60 minutes later, the patient lies on a table and is moved into the scanner. About one hour is needed for the machine to take the pictures. After the test, the patient can go home and resume all activities. Drinking lots of water helps to get rid of the radiation from the body. The PET scan has some advantages over the technetium scan. More radioactive material is taken up in the bones and it is cleared more rapidly from the body. Also, sometimes not enough technetium has been available to do a bone scan but that has not been a problem with sodium fluoride.

Although few comparisons have been done, the limited information available suggests that the PET/CT scan may do a much better job than the technetium scan in finding bone metastases. Even so, at the present time, PET/CT has not replaced the technetium bone scan as the best test for finding bone metastases, but that could change in the near future.

The CT Scan

A test that has greatly helped doctors care for patients is the *computed tomography*, or *CT scan*. It takes a series of x-rays spaced small distances apart and uses a computer to create a three-dimensional picture. A CT scan is done to look for cancer in the lymph nodes, but it also may tell whether cancer has spread into the area around the prostate. A weakness of the test is that it cannot detect small amounts of cancer.

The CT scan requires that the bowels must be cleansed. A bowel-cleansing product such as GoLYTELY® is used most commonly but others are available. It is taken until only clear fluid appears in the toilet during a bowel movement. Before the test begins, special dye is put into the rectum and some is injected into a vein in the arm. The person lies on a table for about one hour while the pictures are taken.

Who Should Have a CT Scan?

Similar to the bone scan, the CT scan also was done in most men with prostate cancer before the PSA became available. Now, most doctors do not order this test unless the PSA is over 20 ng/ml. Below that level, the odds of a CT scan finding cancer in the lymph nodes are less than 1%. Even above that level, small cancers in the lymph nodes are often missed. For men who will be treated by any form of radiation, a CT scan or magnetic resonance imaging (MRI) will be done regardless of the PSA because the information is needed to plan where to deliver the treatments. If you decide to have a different treatment other than radiation and have a low PSA, a CT scan is not worth doing.

Magnetic Resonance Imaging (MRI)

Another test used by some physicians is the MRI test. Like the CT scan, the goal of this test is to see whether cancer has spread to the area near your prostate or into the surrounding lymph nodes. The MRI uses a strong magnetic field to give detailed images of your body. A unit called tesla (T) defines the strength of the magnet. Older machines were 1.0 T or 1.5 T and more recently machines with 3.0 T coils are being used. An MRI differs from a CT scan in two ways. The MRI does not use x-rays and no preparation is needed before the test is done. Normally you lie on a table that moves into a tunnel that is part of the machine and then pictures are taken. Newer machines called Open MRI are being used, which do not require the patient to be placed into a tunnel. Both methods usually are completed in less than one hour. So far, the stronger machines have not demonstrated better accuracy. Some doctors now are doing an *endorectal* MRI instead of an abdominal MRI to determine whether cancer is growing outside the prostate into the surrounding tissues. A special probe is placed in the rectum to perform this test.

Who Should Have an MRI?

Most men do not need an MRI for two reasons. First, the odds of having cancer in the lymph nodes are very low when the PSA is under 20 ng/ml. Second, the test gives incorrect information in about 25% to 30% of cases; many false-positive and false-negative results occur. For that reason, selecting a treatment based on this test often results in the wrong choice. Although the accuracy of the endorectal MRI is improving, it still is not good enough to warrant routine use. The bottom line is that MRI will not really help determine which is the best treatment for you. For that reason, you should not have it until the test becomes more accurate.

The ProstaScint® Scan

This test uses antibodies and a small amount of radioactive material; these are injected into a vein, and they then attach to a protein on the surface of prostate cancer cells. The ProstaScint scan has the ability to find prostate cancer cells anywhere in the body. The test is done in two parts. First, you will go to the hospital to receive an injection of the antibodies. There is a very small risk of an allergic reaction to the injection. Four days later you must return to the hospital to have the scan done. No food should be eaten for eight hours before the scan. On the day of the test, you will be advised to take an enema to clean the bowel. Then you are placed on a table and pictures are taken with a special camera. Often, a CT scan also will be performed, which helps improve the accuracy of the test.

Who Should Have a ProstaScint Scan?

Although its accuracy has improved, not many doctors use this test for staging a newly diagnosed prostate cancer because it also gives too many false-positive and false-negative results. It may be more useful when the PSA is rising after a radical prostatectomy, but at this time, its value in managing prostate cancer is low.

What Is a Ploidy Analysis?

When doctors look under the microscope at a biopsy, they cannot be sure whether the cancer will grow slowly or quickly. A test that may be useful is called a *ploidy analysis*. It measures the amount of genetic material, called DNA, that is contained in the cells. *Diploid* cells have a normal amount of DNA and *aneuploid* cells have more DNA than normal. Weak studies suggest that aneuploid tumors are more likely to recur after treatment than diploid tumors. For that reason, some doctors recommend a more aggressive treatment if an aneuploid tumor is found.

If you do want this test done, it does not require you to do anything. It can be done using the original biopsy specimen you had when your cancer was first diagnosed. Since not all laboratories perform a ploidy analysis, your biopsy material may have to be sent to a special lab. The test is done by cutting additional material from the biopsy specimen and staining it with certain chemicals. It is then put through a machine that measures the amount of DNA in the cells.

Who Should Have a Ploidy Analysis?

This study was more popular several years ago but now is rarely used for several reasons. First, no study has shown a benefit from treating aneuploid tumors differently than treating diploid tumors. Also, like the other tests discussed above, ploidy analysis has too many false-positive and false-negative results. The bottom line is this test will not really help you get the best treatment.

Summary of Staging Tests

A summary of the various staging tests is provided below.

Test	Information Provided by Test	Optimal Patients for Test
Digital rectal examination	Determines whether cancer has spread outside the capsule or into the seminal vesicles	Everyone
Staging transrectal ultrasound	Determines whether cancer has spread outside the capsule or into the seminal vesicles	PSA over 20 ng/ml Extracapsular disease suspected on digital rectal examination
Bone scan	Determines whether prostate cancer has spread to the bones	Presence of bone pain PSA greater than 20 ng/ml PSA greater than 10 ng/ml and Gleason 8–10 or T2c disease
PET/CT scan	Determines whether bone metastases are present	Not yet ready for routine use
CT scan	Determines whether cancer has spread to the seminal vesicles, lymph nodes, or other abdominal organs	Needed before radiation therapy PSA greater than 20 ng/ml
MRI	Determines whether cancer is growing outside the capsule or into seminal vesicles	Test not needed but can be done instead of CT scan if radiation is planned PSA greater than 20 ng/ml
ProstaScint scan	Determines whether cancer is in lymph nodes	Test not needed
Ploidy analysis	Predicts odds that tumor will spread	Test not needed

You should now have a good understanding of the tools doctors use to determine if the cancer has spread outside the prostate. Before learning about the different treatments, the next chapter will explain what doctors learn from your physical exam and your biopsy results.

What Is Your Tumor Stage and Grade?

Now that you understand the different tests used to stage prostate cancer, the next question is, how dangerous is your cancer? This information is critical for deciding which treatment is the right one for your specific case. Two ways this can be determined is from the *tumor stage* and *tumor grade*. The tumor stage represents the location of the cancer; Is it entirely in the prostate or has it spread outside the gland, into the seminal vesicles, the lymph nodes, the bones, or other organs? The tumor grade describes how the cancer cells look under a microscope. It is a measure of how fast a cancer might grow or spread.

Tumor Stage

Doctors use different methods to define the tumor stage. The *TNM Staging System* and *Whitmore–Jewett System* are used most often in the United States. In the TNM system, T stands for the extent of cancer within the prostate gland, N is for the presence of cancer in the lymph nodes, and M is for metastases or the presence of cancer in other parts of the body. The following tables show a description of all the tumor stages for both staging systems.

Table 3.1 Stages of Cancer in the Prostate Gland

Clinical T Stage	Whitmore–Jewett	Description
TX		Prostate gland cannot be assessed.
T0		No evidence of cancer in the prostate.
T1	A	Cancer is located inside the prostate. The DRE is normal and not seen on radiological tests.
T1a	A1	Cancer is found in less than 5% of the tissue removed during an operation to improve urination. The DRE is normal.
T1b	A2	Cancer is found in more than 5% of the tissue removed during an operation to improve urination. The DRE is normal.
T1c	B0	Cancer is found on a prostate biopsy and the DRE is normal.
T2	B	DRE shows cancer inside the prostate.
T2a	B1	DRE shows cancer in less than 50% of one side of the prostate.
T2b	B1	DRE shows cancer in more than 50% of one side of the prostate.
T2c	B2	DRE shows cancer on both sides of the prostate.
T3	C	DRE shows cancer outside the prostate.
T3a	C1	DRE shows cancer outside the prostate on right or left side.

Table 3.1 Stages of Cancer in the Prostate Gland (continued)

Clinical T Stage	Whitmore–Jewett	Description
T3b	C2	DRE shows cancer outside the prostate on both right and left sides.
T3c	C3	DRE shows cancer into one or both seminal vesicles.
T4a	C	DRE shows cancer in the bladder, the rectum, or the muscle that prevents urine from leaking.
T4b	C	DRE shows cancer in the pelvic wall or pelvic muscles.

The N stages for the lymph nodes are shown in the next table.

Table 3.2 Lymph Node Stages

N Stage	Whitmore–Jewett	Description
NX	D0	The status of the lymph nodes is not known. Stage D0 means PSA is rising but no metastases are found.
N0		Cancer is not in the lymph nodes.
N1	D1	Cancer is present in one lymph node less than 2 cm in diameter.
N2	D1	Cancer is in one lymph node between 2 and 5 cm in diameter. Cancer is in more than one lymph node less than 5 cm in diameter.
N3	D1	Cancer in lymph nodes is greater than 5 cm in diameter.

The last table shows the M stages that represent tumor in other parts of the body. This is determined from the bone scan, CT scan, MRI, x-rays, or biopsies.

Table 3.3 Stages for Metastatic Disease

M Stage	Substage	Description
MX		The status of metastases is unknown.
M0		No evidence of metastases.
M1	D2	Cancer has metastasized to other organs.
M1a		Cancer has spread into lymph nodes above the division of the aorta.
M1b		Cancer has spread into the bones.
M1c		Cancer has spread into other organs either with or without spread into the bones.

Clinical Versus Pathological Stage

In the previous chapter, the difference between clinical and pathological stage was explained. When doctors write the stage of the disease, sometimes they place a small "c" or a small "p" in front of the assigned stage to represent whether it is the clinical or pathological stage.

For example, if a doctor feels a tumor during the prostate examination, thinks it has not spread outside the gland, and the scans or ultrasound tests do not show it has spread, then the patient is said to have stage cT2. However, if the prostate is removed and all the cancer cells are contained inside the gland, then the patient is said to have pT2 disease.

Tumor Grade

You have probably learned by now that not all prostate cancers act in the same way; some of them grow very slowly and are very unlikely to cause a man any harm, but others are very aggressive and may cause a man's death. Doctors have gained some ability to determine how dangerous each cancer might be by looking under a microscope at the cancer cells from the prostate biopsy. The least dangerous cancer cells almost look like normal cells and are considered *low grade*. As cells become increasingly abnormal in appearance they also become more dangerous to the patient and are given a higher tumor grade.

Two grading systems are in use today. The *Gleason Grading System* is used almost exclusively in the United States, but some European countries use the *World Health Organization (WHO) grading system*. The Gleason score is named after Dr. John Gleason, a pathologist. After looking at many biopsies, he divided the cells into five grades, which he numbered from 1 to 5. The cells looking least abnormal were scored Gleason grade 1 and the worst-looking cells were scored Gleason grade 5. Dr. Gleason noticed that many biopsies showed more than one type of cancer cell. To account for this he gave each patient a *Gleason score* consisting of two numbers. The first number was for the most common type of cancer cell in each biopsy core and the second number was for the second most common type. These two numbers were added together. If a man's biopsy only showed one type of cell, the Gleason grade is doubled to get the Gleason score. Using this system, the lowest Gleason score is $1+1=2$ and the highest score is $5+5=10$. More than 60% of all new cases of prostate cancer have a Gleason score of $3+3$.

The Gleason grading system has its strengths and weaknesses. The strengths are:

- It can be used to help select the most appropriate treatment.

- It can help estimate a patient's response to some treatments.

- It can be used to estimate the chances that some cancer cells have spread outside the prostate wall into the seminal vesicles or into the lymph nodes.

- Not all Gleason scores of 7 are the same; a Gleason 3+4 is not as dangerous as a Gleason 4+3.

The weaknesses of this grading system are:

- About 20% to 30% of men are given a different Gleason score when the entire prostate is removed compared with the score assigned when the biopsy was done.

- It is very subjective and can vary depending on the doctor reading the biopsy. Two pathologists reading the same biopsy will give different Gleason scores in about 20% to 30% of the cases. Even the same pathologist will give a different score 20% of the time if asked to re-read a biopsy.

- Some men have three types of cancer cells in their biopsy, but the Gleason score only counts the two that are most common. If the least common cell has a higher Gleason grade, then the Gleason score assigned to this patient will underestimate the aggressiveness of the cancer.

- After a man has radiation to the prostate the Gleason score is more difficult to define.

Despite these weaknesses, the Gleason Grading System is a very valuable asset for helping doctors counsel men about the best treatment option.

Because of the variability among pathologists, doctors sometimes will have a man's biopsy re-read by a pathologist specializing in reading prostate biopsies. Two that are known for their expertise are Bostwick Laboratories (www.bostwicklaboratories.com/home) and Dr. Jonathan Epstein at Johns Hopkins Hospital (jepstein@jhmi .edu). If you would like to get a second opinion of your Gleason score, you or your doctor can contact either of these places.

The WHO grading system uses only three grades, *WHO grade 1, 2, or 3*. With only three grades, it is not as good as the Gleason system either for predicting the true tumor stage or the outcomes after different treatments.

Predicting Your Pathological Stage

Since the clinical stage often is not the true pathological stage, many men want some idea about their true stage before they get treated. Two methods are commonly used to do this and the results can help you decide which treatment would be most suitable. They all use the findings from your biopsy, your physical examination, and the PSA.

Doctors at Johns Hopkins Hospital created the Partin Tables, which show the odds the cancer is growing outside the prostate, into the seminal vesicles, and into the lymph nodes. They have done several updates, with the latest one reported in 2012. Two examples using these tables are shown below. The first one shows the results for Mr. Jones, a 65-year-old man who had a normal DRE. He underwent a prostate biopsy because his PSA was 5.5 ng/ml. Twelve samples were removed of which three showed Gleason 3+3 cancer. Neither a bone scan nor a CT scan was done because he had a low risk for the cancer spreading to the lymph nodes or bones. Based on this information his clinical stage is cT1C, NX, MX. Using the Partin tables, what are the odds that his clinical stage is really his true pathologic stage?

Table 3.4

True Location of Cancer	Odds for This Patient
All cancer is inside prostate gland	83%–86%
Some cancer growing outside the prostate	13%–16%
Cancer is growing into seminal vesicles	0%–1%
Cancer has spread to lymph nodes	0%

As you can see, this patient has a very high chance his prostate cancer is contained inside the prostate capsule and a very low chance that cancer is in his seminal vesicles or lymph nodes. If this man is considering having his prostate removed he has a high chance he would be cured by surgery alone without needing additional treatment. Also, there is no reason to remove the lymph nodes because there is almost no chance they contain cancer.

The second table shows the results for Mr. Smith who also was 65. He had an abnormal DRE that was staged cT2b. His PSA was 18 ng/ml and the biopsy showed cancer on 6 of the 12 samples, each with a Gleason score of 4+4.

Table 3.5

True Location of Cancer	Odds for This Patient
All cancer is inside prostate gland	8%–16%
Some cancer growing outside the prostate	28%–51%
Cancer is growing into seminal vesicles	18%–42%
Cancer has spread to lymph nodes	9%–32%

According to the Partin Tables, this patient has a high chance his stage is really T3 and a moderate chance he has N+ disease. His chance of being cured by surgery is much lower than Mr. Jones. If this patient does decide to have surgery, removing the lymph nodes should be done.

Although some doctors will use these tables when counseling you, many do not. It is worth looking at them as you begin thinking about your treatment options because they can help you get the right treatment for your individual case. If your doctor does not use these tables, you can access them yourself at no charge using the website: http://urology.jhu.edu/prostate/partintables.php. The information you will need to determine your true pathological stage can be obtained by asking the doctor for your Gleason score, physical examination findings, and the most recent PSA result.

The second method being used to predict your true stage is called the *Kattan Nomogram*. It is also available for free at http://nomograms.mskcc.org/Prostate/PreTreatment.aspx. It requires the PSA result, the clinical stage from the DRE, and details about the Gleason score including the number of cores of tissue obtained during your biopsy and the number showing cancer. The results for Mr. Jones using this method are shown in the next table.

Table 3.6

True Location of Cancer	Odds for This Patient
All cancer is inside prostate gland	87%
Some cancer growing outside the prostate	9%
Cancer is growing into seminal vesicles	1%
Cancer has spread to lymph nodes	1.4%

The results are very similar to those obtained with the Partin Tables, with only a slightly higher chance that cancer might be in the lymph nodes. In addition to predicting the pathological stage, the Kattan nomogram also gives patients some idea of the odds that the cancer will not recur and will not cause a man's death. If Mr. Jones has his prostate removed, his chance of cancer recurring in the next 10 years is 4% and the chance the cancer will cause his death is only 1% in the next 15 years.

The Kattan nomogram predicts a more severe situation than the Partin tables for Mr. Smith.

Table 3.7

True Location of Cancer	Odds for This Patient
All cancer is inside prostate gland	18%
Some cancer growing outside the prostate	77%
Cancer is growing into seminal vesicles	55%
Cancer has spread to lymph nodes	14%

He has a 55% chance his cancer is stage pT3 and a 14% chance of being N+. The reason for the worst prediction is partly because it includes more information from the biopsy rather than only the Gleason score.

It is worth using these two prediction methods when thinking about which treatment you want to pursue because they provide a realistic estimate of where the cancer is located and that will greatly influence the chances for success with the different treatment options. In chapter 5 you will learn about two new gene tests that are being used in addition to the Gleason score and Kattan Nomogram for helping men decide what to do.

Understanding Medical Studies Used to Evaluate Different Treatments

Before helping you learn about all the treatment options for this disease, you need some understanding of how doctors know whether a treatment is effective in preventing you from being harmed. They do this by conducting a clinical study. Several types of medical studies can be performed, but unfortunately not all of them provide reliable results. This is very important to understand because very often the media will report results from studies that are not well done without making it clear that the conclusions may be incorrect. *You cannot assume that a study is good simply because it gets published in a medical journal or quoted in the media.* Without understanding what makes a study good or bad, you run the risk of not getting the treatment that is right for you. The reason is that too many doctors use weak studies to support their recommendations for a particular treatment. This chapter provides you with an explanation of the different types of studies along with their strengths and weaknesses. Understanding what makes a study good or bad will increase your ability to help your doctor select the best treatment for your case.

Let's begin with a list of studies and an explanation of how each one is done. The options include:

- The Prospective, Randomized, Controlled Study

- The Cohort Study

- The Retrospective Study

- The Epidemiological Study

- The Meta-Analysis

The Prospective, Randomized, Controlled Study

This is the "gold standard" of clinical studies because it provides the most objective and reliable information possible. A *prospective, randomized, controlled study really is the only way to prove that one treatment is as good as, or better, or worse than another treatment.*

This study design can be explained as follows. *Prospective* means the study was designed before anyone was treated. *Randomized* means that the study compared more than one type of treatment and neither the patient nor the doctor was able to choose which one to receive. Sometimes two treatments will be compared and in other cases a treatment is compared with a placebo, which is an inactive treatment that should have absolutely no effect on a disease. Usually a computer decides the treatment that each patient will receive. Randomly assigning people to their treatment rather than having them or their doctor choose the treatment *reduces* the chance that the results will be biased or incorrect.

Controlled means patients can be enrolled into the study only if they meet certain requirements. In other words, not everyone with the disease being studied is eligible. For example, a study might want to test a new treatment for men with prostate cancer that has spread into the bones. Only patients with a bone scan showing metastases can join. Anyone who does not meet this requirement will be excluded. Controlled studies also require that each patient must undergo the same tests at the same time interval as the other patients in the study. If, for example, a controlled study is done to compare surgery with external radiation, each patient in the radiation group would be given the same amount of radiation using the same technique. The goal is for the different treatment groups to be as identical as possible so that any differences in the outcome can only be explained by differences in the effectiveness of the treatments being used. All new drugs must be tested in this way to gain approval from the U.S. Food and Drug Administration (FDA).

Although the most reliable results are provided by randomized, controlled studies, they do have some limitations. They are very expensive to do and usually take many years to complete. For these reasons, they have not been done very often, particularly for prostate cancer. Without a randomized, controlled trial, doctors must counsel patients using studies that give less reliable results.

The Cohort Study

A cohort study differs from a randomized study in that all the individuals get the same treatment. This type of study can be either prospective or retrospective, which means that the patients have already been treated and someone is now retrieving the records to find out what happened. It has the advantages of being easier to do and is far less expensive than a prospective, randomized, controlled study. That is partly why it is done so often. Unfortunately, cohort studies suffer from serious limitations. First, the patients included often are not very similar. They may have a wide range of tumor stages and tumor grades. Also, the ages and overall health of the participants may vary. This creates a problem when two cohort studies of different treatments are compared with each other. If one shows better results, it could be because it included many men who have less dangerous cancers or who are in better health than those included in the other study, rather than because the treatment was really better.

An example of the problem with these studies is shown in the following table. One cohort included men treated by a radical prostatectomy and the other one included men treated by external radiation.

Table 4.1

Patient Characteristics	Cohort 1: Radical Prostatectomy	Cohort 2: External Radiation
Mean age	65	71
Gleason score 6 (%)	80%	65%
Gleason score 8–10 (%)	5%	15%
Mean prostate-specific antigen (ng/ml)	5.5	7.5
10-year survival rate (%)	69%	60%

The cohort study of men having their prostate removed showed a higher 10-year survival rate (69%) compared with the cohort study of men having radiation (60%). The doctors who did the surgery study might conclude that surgery is a more effective treatment, but is that really valid? The answer is definitely no. One reason is that the two groups are very different from each other. The men having radiation were older, had a higher prostate-specific antigen (PSA), and a higher percentage had more aggressive cancers. Comparing these two cohorts is like trying to compare apples to oranges. Even if radiation were as effective as surgery, one would not expect the survival results of these two cohorts to be the same. That is just one of the problems with trying to compare results from cohort studies; the participants may have many obvious and not so obvious differences.

Another problem is that even when the men in two cohort studies do have very similar characteristics, valid conclusions still are not possible because men were able to choose their own treatment. This creates biases in unknown ways that also may affect the results. The bottom line is that cohort studies cannot be used to make valid claims about whether one treatment is as good as or better or worse than another treatment. This problem can only be avoided by doing a randomized study.

The Retrospective Study

This type of study has the advantage that it is the easiest one to do because all of the patients were treated sometime in the past. Rather than have to wait many years after treatment has been completed before results become available, retrospective studies provide immediate information. All that is required is for the records to be reviewed to gather the necessary information, which is then fed into a computer. A retrospective study can either look at a single treatment and compare it with other studies or record the results on more than one type of treatment and compare them to one another. Despite the ease of doing this type of study, it has the same weaknesses as the cohort study: patients undergoing different treatments may not have similar tumor characteristics and a bias can occur because the patients chose their treatment. Also, some men may have to be excluded because information is missing, which can further bias the results. Lastly, the information contained in the charts sometimes is incorrect and doctors cannot tell when that has occurred. Therefore, the results of retrospective studies also cannot be used to make reliable conclusions. Patients should be aware that many doctors rely on retrospective studies to justify their recommendations for certain treatments without informing men about the weaknesses of that type of study.

The Epidemiological Study

This last type of study also is a retrospective look at what happened to a group of individuals treated in the past. Information is collected from the medical records and then fed into a computer. The data are analyzed to see whether any associations can be made between a person's health and what happened to him or her. For example, a doctor may do an epidemiological study of men with localized prostate cancer who all were treated in the past by external radiation to see whether any factors may have contributed to their survival. They may collect information about the tumor grade, the patients' ages, PSA level, amount of vitamin C intake, and their intake of a cholesterol-lowering drug and body weight.

When the results are analyzed, the study may find that the longer men were taking a cholesterol-lowering drug, the higher was their survival. The study would then conclude that taking a cholesterol-lowering drug may improve a man's chances of surviving prostate cancer following radiation therapy. Is this a valid conclusion? The answer is *maybe*, but this study design does not prove whether it is definitely true. There can be many other explanations for why some men did better than others who have not taken the drug.

The real value of an epidemiologic study is that it can generate an idea for doing a well-done randomized, controlled study in the future. In this case, the results would support doing a study in men receiving radiation, randomizing them to receive a cholesterol-lowering drug or a placebo. Only then would it be possible to conclude whether taking the drug was beneficial.

Epidemiological studies are also much easier to do than prospective, randomized, controlled studies and they are often mentioned in the media. The problem is that the results are made to appear reliable while the weaknesses of the study design are rarely reported. For these reasons you should be very cautious when making decisions based on epidemiological studies.

The Meta-Analysis

Unlike the studies explained so far, a meta-analysis is different. It is not a formal study that enrolls patients. Instead, it is a way of combining the results of several studies that have already been performed. The reason a meta-analysis is done is to increase the confidence of the conclusions that resulted from each of those individual studies. For example, suppose four studies were performed comparing surgery and radiation. One enrolled 100 men, the second and third each enrolled 150 men, and the last one enrolled 200 men. None of them showed that one of the treatments definitely was better than the other. However, by doing a meta-analysis that combined the 600 men from all four studies, one of the treatments could show a significantly better survival rate. Without doing this type of analysis, this conclusion would not be possible. The question is whether a meta-analysis using multiple studies can substitute for one large randomized study. The answer is no. Even a well-done meta-analysis using several small studies cannot reliably predict the results of a single large study. Increasing the number of patients or the number of studies does not eliminate all the biases that can provide misleading results. In other words, sometimes a meta-analysis can result in the wrong conclusion about the effectiveness of a treatment.

The Bottom Line on Medical Studies

The main message here is that the outcomes reported following different treatments may come from well-designed medical studies but often they are based on studies that are not well designed. The better the study design, the more you can trust the results. As you learn about the different treatments in this book you will be told what kind of study was done when describing the results. You also will be made aware of any factors that could bias the results. This is intended to provide you with the best information possible to help you decide which treatment is right for you.

Understanding How Medical Studies Report Results

When you start comparing different treatments, you also need to be aware of the different ways the results can be reported. In some cases, the information used by doctors may be misleading, even if it is from a randomized study. This is best explained with some examples.

Suppose you want to know the odds of your being alive 10 years after undergoing radioactive seed implantation. The doctor tells you about a study involving 100 men who received this treatment in 1999, of which 70 were still alive in 2009. That means the 10-year survival rate is 70% (70/100). This information would give you an excellent idea of what to expect if you had this treatment, assuming you also have a similar type of tumor. Ideally, all studies would report their results based on the same duration of follow-up. Unfortunately, this is seldom the case.

Most studies do something different because a number of years are required to accumulate enough patients who get the same treatment. That means they will have been followed for different times after their treatment was completed when the results are reported. For example, suppose a study reports on 100 men who had a radical prostatectomy, of which:

- 10 were treated 10 years ago.
- 20 were treated 7 years ago.
- 50 were treated 4 years ago.
- 20 were treated 2 years ago.

When doctors decide to report their 10-year results on all these men, they cannot give an exact result because only 10 were followed the full 10 years. But they can use a technique called the *Kaplan–Meier statistical method to estimate* the 10-year survival rate for the entire group. In this case, the estimated 10-year survival might be 70%. Along with giving an estimated survival, the Kaplan–Meier method also provides a range for the true result. In this case, the range for the 10-year survival might be between 60% and 80%. This means the true 10-year survival could be as low as 60%, as high as 80%, or anywhere in between. Until all the men have been followed the full 10 years, the results cannot be more precise. Obviously, studies that have a wide range for the true result are not very helpful. Studies that include more patients or have a longer follow-up will have a more narrow range for the true result. Although this is very important to understand, your doctor is very unlikely to explain it to you when you are told these results. If you ask, "What are my odds of being alive in 10 years with this treatment?" You will be told "about 70%." The problem with that answer is it can be misleading. You *should be told,* "We think the 10-year survival rate is 70%, but it could be as low as 60% or as high as 80%."

Now, suppose you want to know how radical prostatectomy compares with seed implantation. The doctor tells you about another cohort study of men treated by seed implantation. It estimated the 10-year survival at 69% with a range for the true result between 58% and 82%. You want to know whether the two treatments have a similar effect. The correct answer is, "They appear to give similar results but we cannot be sure; surgery might be better or it might be worse than the seed implantation." Since the ranges for the two treatments overlap each other (60%–80% and 58%–82%, respectively), one cannot be sure whether they are equally effective or one is better. That the two treatments do not *appear* to differ is the only conclusion that can be made.

Now, suppose two cohort studies are compared and the ranges for the true result do not overlap. For example, study 1 has an estimated survival of 68% with a range from 65% to 72% and study 2 has an estimated survival of 76% with a range from 74% to 78%. Are these treatments different? The answer is probably yes, because the best possible result for treatment 1 is 72% and the worst possible result for treatment 2 is 74%. Of course that assumes that the characteristics of the the patients in both studies was almost identical. You should be wary if your doctor uses estimated results from cohort or retrospective studies to tell you that one treatment is better than another.

Another problem with many of the studies being published in medical journals is that they involve small numbers of patients with short follow-up, for example only three to five years, yet they still report the estimated results at 10 years. In those cases, the ranges for the true results usually are very large, which means the study has tremendous uncertainty. You may be wondering, why do medical journals publish weak studies? The reason is they have to fill their pages and good articles are in short supply. Keep this in mind as you learn about the results of different studies.

Understanding the Outcomes of Clinical Studies

The next thing to understand is the different types of results that are presented in prostate cancer studies. The possibilities include:

- *Biochemical Failure Rate:* The percentage of men with a rising PSA

- *Treatment-Free Survival:* The percentage of men not getting additional treatment

- *Metastasis-Free Survival:* The percentage of men not developing any metastatic disease

- *Disease-Specific Survival:* The percentage of men not dying from prostate cancer

- *Overall Survival:* The percentage of men still alive

The most reliable result is overall survival but obviously it takes the longest time to get this information. Because prostate cancer often is a slow growing cancer, at least 10 or 15 years is needed to know how men will do from a treatment. Five-year results, although often reported, are simply not good enough since many men will live 10 years or longer even if they don't get treated.

When studies do not have long-term survival results, they will report the results for one of the other outcomes. The most common one is the *biochemical failure rate,* which is the chance that the PSA rises above a certain level. It is important for you to know that biochemical failure is not an adequate predictor of long-term survival results. Also, the FDA has never approved a treatment based only on studies reporting the biochemical failure rate. Treatments that have similar biochemical failure rates at five or seven years do not always have similar survival rates at 10 and 15 years. The same is true for the other outcomes. For these reasons you should be cautious if your doctor recommends a treatment based on anything other than long-term survival.

This does not mean it is wrong to choose a treatment that lacks information about the 10- or 15-year survival. But you should understand that it is more of a gamble, like playing "blind poker," because you have no idea whether it will give you as good a survival as other treatments that do have long-term results. Perhaps you find something appealing about a newer treatment and are willing to accept the uncertainty of not knowing the long-term results. In that case, you are making an informed decision and have chosen to live with the uncertainty. The most important message here is you should be aware of what happens to other men who received each treatment.

What Is Evidence-Based Medicine (EBM)?

A growing practice around the United States is the use of evidence-based medicine, or EBM. A simple definition is "assessing the quality of medical studies that are used to counsel people about the best treatment for their disease." Ideally, you will get counseled about treating your tumor based on this principle. If so, your doctor only will recommend a treatment when prospective, randomized, controlled studies show it is as good as or better than the other options. What happens if randomized studies are not available? In that case, no treatment should be recommended. Instead, you should be told about the possible risks and benefits of all the reasonable options. If a doctor is going to recommend a treatment without support from a randomized study, you should be informed that it is only his or her personal opinion and well-done studies have not proven it is best. This awareness will help you decide which treatment is right for you.

With this information as a foundation, the pros and cons of each treatment will now be provided. This book is not intended to promote any particular treatment. Rather, the goal is to enable you to make an informed choice based on the best and most reliable information available.

How Dangerous Is Your Cancer? Using Tumor Grade and Stage to Assess Your Risk

In the past several years, doctors have become increasingly aware that a large percentage of the prostate cancers being diagnosed are not life-threatening. In fact, many will grow so slowly that they never will need to be treated. Of course, some are dangerous and definitely will need to be treated aggressively. How do you know which kind of cancer you have? Although more work is needed, progress has been made in identifying the ones that do and don't need aggressive treatment.

What Is a Low-, Intermediate-, and High-Risk Tumor?

For many years, doctors used the Gleason score to separate men with cancer into three risk groups—those with a Gleason score of 2–4, 5–7, or 8–10. Although it proved somewhat helpful for the Gleason 2–4 and 8–10 cancers, eventually doctors realized that it was not so helpful for the majority of newly diagnosed cancers, which fell into the Gleason 5–7 category.

However, the discovery of the prostate-specific antigen (PSA) test gave doctors another tool to identify dangerous cancers. It was combined with the clinical stage from the prostate examination and the Gleason score to arrive at the *D'Amico risk stratification*, which divides cancers into *low-, intermediate-* and *high-risk* groups. The higher the risk group, the greater the odds that the cancer eventually will spread and cause harm if not treated aggressively. The following table shows the characteristics of each group.

Table 5.1

Risk Group	PSA (ng/ml)	Clinical Stage	Gleason Score
Low risk	Less than 10	T1c or T2a	Less than 7
Intermediate risk	Between 10–20	T2b	7
High risk	Over 20	T2c or T3	8–10

The low-risk cancers must have all three of these factors: a PSA under 10 ng/ml, a stage of T1 or T2a, and a Gleason score less than 6. The intermediate cancers must either have a PSA between 10 and 20 ng/ml and a Gleason score of 7, or a clinical stage of T2b. Lastly, a man is considered having a high-risk cancer if the PSA is over 20 ng/ml, the Gleason score is 8–10, or the stage is T2c or T3.

The second method being used is called the Cancer of the Prostate Risk Assessment (CAPRA) score. It combines a patient's age, his PSA, clinical stage, Gleason score, and the percentage of the biopsy cores that contain cancer. The lowest score is 0 and the highest score is 10. As the score increases, a man has an increased chance that his cancer will recur within five years of undergoing a radical prostatectomy (RP).

You can get the necessary information to determine your risk group from your biopsy report, which states the primary and secondary Gleason patterns. The primary pattern represents the most common Gleason grade seen on the biopsy and is mentioned first in the report. The secondary pattern is the second most common tumor grade and is mentioned second in the report. Some biopsy reports will tell you what percent of the cores show cancer. If they don't, you can easily figure it out based on the number showing cancer and the total number of cores reported. You then can calculate your CAPRA score using the table below:

Table 5.2

	Patient Information	Points
Age at diagnosis (years)	Under 50	0
	50 or older	1
PSA at diagnosis (ng/ml)	Less than or equal to 6	0
	Between 6.1 and 10	1
	Between 10.1 and 20	2
	Between 20.1 and 30	3
	More than 30	4
Gleason score of the biopsy (primary/secondary)	No pattern 4 or 5	0
	Secondary pattern 4 or 5	1
	Primary pattern 4 or 5	3
Clinical stage (T-stage)	T1 or T2	0
	T3a	1
Percent of biopsy cores involved with cancer (positive for cancer)	Less than 34%	0
	At least 34% or more	1

After you add up your points, you can then look at the next table to find your estimated three- and five-year risk of having your PSA rise after undergoing an RP.

Table 5.3

CAPRA Score	3-Year Risk for Biochemical Recurrence after RP	5-Year Risk for Biochemical Recurrence after RP
0–1	88%–95%	80%–91%
2	79%–88%	68%–80%
3	70%–81%	57%–71%
4	65%–79%	51%–69%
5	56%–75%	40%–63%
6	33%–58%	17%–41%
More than 6	23%–48%	10%–32%

Unfortunately, the CAPRA score is only moderately helpful for counseling patients, mainly because the range of results for each one-point increase in the score is very wide. Thus, a 60-year-old man with a PSA of 6.5 ng/ml, a T1c cancer, a Gleason 3 primary pattern, and a Gleason 4 secondary pattern with more than a third of his cores showing cancer, has a CAPRA score of 4. If he undergoes an RP, he has a chance of not being cured falling between 51% and 69%. What should he do? More importantly, what would *you* do if that was your score? Is surgery the wrong treatment for this man or should he take the gamble that he has between a 30% and 50% chance he will be cured by the operation? Clearly, there is no right or wrong answer. It all depends on the individual; some will think the risk is acceptable and choose surgery, while others will want a different treatment. This will be reviewed again as the different treatments are discussed. Your take-away message from this chapter is that some cancers are more dangerous than others, and before you get treated you should be fully aware of the risk posed by your cancer. This will increase your chance of getting the right treatment.

Gene Tests to Assess Tumor Aggressiveness

As stated earlier, more doctors now recognize that a large percentage of prostate cancers are not life threatening and can be treated conservatively. Although the Gleason score, the clinical stage, and the CAPRA score offer some help in selecting out the low-risk cancers, better ways to select patients are needed. Two tests are now available that may offer additional help. They are called the Prolaris test (Myriad Pharmaceuticals) and the Oncotype DX Genomic Prostate Score (Genomic Health). They both test for the presence of a number of genes that are associated with tumor growth and progression. Both of them are performed on the biopsy that was done to make your diagnosis of prostate cancer and both provide a number that correlates with the aggressiveness or danger posed by a man's tumor. Although both are commercially available, they are expensive and coverage by insurance companies is unclear.

The Oncotype test provides information about whether the patient has a high-risk prostate cancer but it provides no information about the outcome following conservative or aggressive treatment. Without that information, its value is difficult to assess.

The Prolaris test has undergone more extensive evaluation. It evaluates 31 genes associated with tumor growth and combines that information with the PSA and Gleason score. The test provides a cell cycle progression number or CCP, which is combined with the Gleason score and PSA to provide a combined score that ranges from 0 to 8. The higher the number, the greater are the chances that a man will die from prostate cancer with conservative treatment at 10 years. Several problems exist at present with using this test. First, about 10% of men have inadequate material to enable the test to be performed. Second, the test would only be appropriate for men with low-risk disease who are considering conservative management. If they had a high combined score that would mean conservative therapy would be a risky course to follow. The problem is that much of the information about men managed conservatively came from a group who had severe urinary symptoms that were treated by surgically removing some of the prostate. Presently, little information is available from a group of men without symptoms who were diagnosed by a screening PSA. Another problem is little is known about how the test will be used in clinical practice. For example, if a man has low risk disease based on his PSA, Gleason score, and DRE, his chance of dying from prostate cancer in 10 years is less than 10%. If he has the Prolaris test and it shows his risk is actually 12% or 15%, will it alter his decision regarding therapy? Will he go from choosing conservative therapy to a more aggressive treatment based on his combined value? Without some information about this decision process, the costly test may have very little effect on most men's decision. Hopefully, more information will be forthcoming to answer these questions so that men can decide if the test is right for them.

II

How to Treat Clinically Localized Prostate Cancer

Beginning the Process of Choosing Your Therapy

By now, you should have a good understanding of your tumor stage and grade, the risk posed by your cancer, and the medical studies that are used to help you understand the potential benefits of each treatment. The focus of the next several chapters is to help you understand the advantages and disadvantages of every treatment available for clinically localized prostate cancer, cancer that has not moved outside the prostate gland. This disease has more potential choices than any other disease. With so many options, your first reaction might be to feel overwhelmed. Fortunately, you do not have to make a decision immediately. Your prostate cancer did not develop yesterday; most likely it has been in your body for several years. Also, it is highly unlikely to get worse in the next few weeks or months while you learn about each option.

One of the challenges you will face in making an informed decision is the abundance of bias and misinformation. Although many doctors have strong opinions about which treatment is best, the truth is that no one knows for sure because optimal studies have not been done. This statement is based on a report by the Agency for Healthcare Research and Quality, or AHRQ, which is part of the U.S. Department of Health and Human Services. Its mission is to improve the quality, safety, efficiency, and effectiveness of health care for all Americans. In 2008, they published a critical analysis of the treatment of localized prostate cancer and made the following conclusions:

> "No one therapy can be considered the preferred treatment for localized prostate cancer due to limitations in the body of evidence as well as the likely tradeoffs an individual patient must make between estimated treatment effectiveness, necessity, and adverse effects. All treatment options result in adverse effects (primarily urinary, bowel, and sexual), although the severity and frequency may vary between treatments. Even if differences in therapeutic effectiveness exist, differences in adverse effects, convenience, and costs are likely to be important factors in individual patient decision-making. *Data from nonrandomized trials are inadequate to reliably assess comparative effectiveness and adverse effects. Additional randomized controlled trials (RCTs) are needed* [emphasis added]."

Although this report is now five years old, nothing done since then would change the conclusion. Keep this in mind as you do your research on the different options, and be wary if a doctor strongly advises that you have a particular treatment. As you learned in chapter 4, comparing treatments based studies that are not prospective and randomized may not give you correct information. One thing you can do that will help you make a good decision is to ask your doctor the right questions. You might want to write down this list or highlight this page and take it with you when your doctor is going to discuss your options.

Questions for Your Doctor

- Which treatments are appropriate for my age, health, tumor stage, Gleason score, and PSA?

- What are the chances that each treatment will get rid of my cancer?

- What are the chances my cancer will recur?

- What are the chances I will need additional treatment?

- What are all the complications or side effects, and how often does each one occur in men with a similar age and health as mine?

- Are the complication rates you are telling me specific to your experience or were they obtained from some prostate cancer expert?

- Was the information obtained from valid written surveys or are you estimating the results?

- How long does each complication typically last and can it be permanent?

- If a complication does occur, how is it treated and how often does it go away?

- How will my quality of life be affected by each complication?

- What percentage of your patients that had erections before each treatment is able to have intercourse without any aids 12 to 18 months after the treatment?

- How many patients use aids such as a medication or a pump to achieve an erection?

- What percentage of your patients has the same urinary control one year after treatment compared with their control prior to any treatment?

Unless you get answers to these questions, you will be playing an imaginary game called "blind poker." The rules are quite simple. The dealer gives you five cards and also takes five. Now you must place your bet, but instead of risking money you will be risking your health and quality of life. Not getting the answers to these questions would be the same as not being able to see the cards you are holding. You would be making a decision as if you're "blind." How much would you be willing to bet without a clue about your odds of winning and losing? Clearly, if you knew you were holding four aces in the card game, you would think the odds of winning were very high. In that case you would be willing to place a very large bet. However, if your hand were very poor, you would most likely fold rather than risk losing.

Deciding on a treatment for prostate cancer sometimes may feel as if you're playing a game with similar rules. You are told about the treatment options and possible side effects, but too often a doctor does not tell you the odds of "winning" and "losing." You aren't told *how often* a treatment will cure you (you win), or cause complications that reduce your quality of life (you lose). Only by getting the questions answered can you decide whether the benefits of a treatment are worth the risks.

Another reason the answers are so important is because this disease does not behave the same in each patient; some prostate cancers are life-threatening but many are not. That is why *treatment must be individualized*. The choice made by some men may not be the right choice for you. One thing to remember is that each treatment comes as a "package" that includes both good and bad results. To get the potential benefits of a treatment you must be willing to accept the risks, which are the odds of getting side effects and the odds the cancer will recur and need additional treatment. You may find that the specific side effects and how often they occur following some treatments are acceptable, while others are not. The key is to make sure you get enough information to make your decision.

You are strongly encouraged to ask your doctor these questions. They are not intended to challenge the physician but you do have every right to know the answers so you can be part of choosing your treatment. Although it is understandable that asking these questions may make you feel uncomfortable, you run the risk of getting the wrong treatment if you don't ask.

Don't be surprised to find out that your doctor cannot answer all these questions, particularly about the side effects. Sadly, most of them do not keep track of their own results so they either estimate them or tell you what "prostate cancer specialists" report. One factor that definitely affects the results is the experience of the physician. Studies show that surgeons who perform a small number of radical prostatectomies annually had more complications than more experienced doctors. Although written surveys are the most accurate way to obtain information about side effects, few doctors use them. Instead, they make an estimate, which is very inaccurate.

Suppose you ask for a doctor's results and are told they can only be estimated? Does that mean you should get a different doctor? Not necessarily, but it certainly should be considered if you hope to do everything possible to get the best result. It is you, not your doctor, who will have to live with the consequences of your treatment, so why not do everything you can do to get the best results? If your doctor feels insulted by your asking for a second opinion, that is not your concern. Doctors who specialize in treating men with prostate cancer can be found in most major cities. If you live in a small community, making a trip to a larger city to get to an expert is definitely worth considering. The next several chapters will will help you understand all your options.

Watchful Waiting

The term *watchful waiting* describes a treatment in which no therapy is given to your prostate gland and no attempt is made to cure the cancer. Instead, you are treated only if the cancer causes symptoms or if it spreads to other parts of your body. There are two reasons this therapy may be right for you. One is the cancer may pose very little danger because it will grow very slowly. That means you are far more likely to die from something other than prostate cancer. A second reason is that it allows you to avoid experiencing any of the side effects that may occur when the prostate gland is treated. By not doing anything to the prostate gland, you are able to maintain your current quality of life until it changes due to aging or because the cancer does progress. For example, surgery can cause immediate impotence and urinary incontinence that may last for the rest of your life. With watchful waiting, impotence may never occur or it may not happen until you are much older.

Of course, watchful waiting does have risks. By not treating your cancer when it is still inside the prostate, you might miss out on a chance to be cured. If your cancer grows and spreads, it can cause many problems that also may affect your quality of life and possibly shorten your survival.

What Are the Outcomes with Watchful Waiting?

The thought of having prostate cancer and not trying to cure it might scare most people. One reason is the mistaken belief that all cancers are equally dangerous. Fortunately, this is not the case with prostate cancer. In fact, now doctors are finding that a large percentage of newly diagnosed prostate cancers are not dangerous. Before you can decide whether watchful waiting is acceptable, you need to be aware of the results that can occur with this approach. Two randomized studies now are available that provide helpful information about what may happen. One was done in the United States, and the other was done in Scandinavia (Sweden and Finland). Both of them compared this option with radical prostatectomy, the surgical removal of the entire prostate along with both seminal vesicles and a portion of both *vas deferens*.

The average age in the U.S. study was 67 years and the average prostate-specific antigen (PSA) was 7.8 ng/ml. About 50% of the men had a normal prostate examination and were diagnosed based on a PSA test. Men in the watchful waiting group could receive hormone therapy and chemotherapy if their cancer progressed but not any treatment solely aimed at the prostate gland. The 12-year results are shown in the next table.

Table 7.1 Results at 12 Years in a U.S. Randomized Study Comparing Watchful Waiting and Radical Prostatectomy

	Radical Prostatectomy	Watchful Waiting	Net Difference
Overall survival	59%	56%	2.9%
Prostate cancer mortality	5.8%	8.4%	2.6%
Metastatic disease	4.7%	10.6%	5.9%

At 12 years, the overall survival was about 59% for men having surgery compared with 56% in men on watchful waiting. The actual difference was 2.9%. Death from prostate cancer occurred in 5.8% of men undergoing surgery compared with 8.4% of men treated by watchful waiting for a difference of 2.6%. Surgery also resulted in a 5.9% lower risk of getting bone metastases at 12 years (10.6% vs. 4.7%). These results mean that:

1. About 33 men have to undergo surgery so that one man can avoid dying in 12 years.

2. Nearly 40 must undergo surgery to prevent one from dying of prostate cancer in that time.

3. For every 16 men undergoing surgery, one avoided bone metastases after 12 years.

In other words, the benefits of radical prostatectomy appear to be very small during this time.

The authors further analyzed the results looking at patients with specific characteristics as shown in the next table. These results must be interpreted with caution, however, because each group is based on a small number of patients. Even so, they can provide you with some idea of your potential risk if you fit into one of these groups.

In the United States, the majority of newly diagnosed cancers currently have low-risk disease, defined as a PSA less than 10 ng/ml; a Gleason score of 6 or less; and a clinical stage of T1a, T1b, T1c, or T2a. According to this study, at 12 years overall survival for men treated with watchful waiting was not significantly worse than those treated with radical prostatectomy. A similar finding was observed for men with a PSA under 10 ng/ml regardless of their clinical stage or Gleason score. The greatest risk with watchful waiting occurred in men with a PSA over 10 ng/ml at diagnosis, a Gleason score over 6, or high-risk disease. Men treated by radical prostatectomy who were thought to have intermediate-risk cancer (a PSA between 10 and

Table 7.2 Overall Survival for Subgroups at 12 Years

Risk Factor	Radical Prostatectomy	Watchful Waiting	Actual Difference (Surgery Minus Watchful Waiting)
PSA less than 10 ng/ml	59.2%	61.8%	−2.6%
PSA greater than 10 ng/ml	58.7%	45.6%	13.1%
Gleason score less than 7	64.3%	62.2%	2%
Gleason score greater than 6	54.6%	48.6%	6%
Low-risk disease	64.9%	67.2 %	−2.4%
Intermediate-risk disease	60.6%	54.7%	6%
High-risk disease	48.7%	43.5%	5.2%
Age under 65	68%	68.7%	−0.7%
Age 65 and older	54.5%	49.1%	−5.4%
Caucasian	57.8%	55%	2.8%
African-American	60.4%	57.8%	2.5%

20 ng/ml or a Gleason score of 7 or T2b) according to the pathologist at each hospital appeared to have a 5% lower chance of dying from prostate cancer. However, that benefit disappeared when a single pathologist re-read all the biopsies. In other words, some of the

Gleason scores originally were misread. For men with high-risk prostate cancer (either a PSA over 20 ng/ml, stage cT2B, or a Gleason score 8–10), surgery appeared to offer a 10% higher survival.

In the men with low-risk prostate cancer, 1% of the men undergoing surgery compared with 4.6% of those undergoing watchful waiting developed bone metastases. In the intermediate-risk patients, the difference in bone metastases was 2.8% and for high-risk patients, the difference increased to 12.5%. In other words, men with low-risk disease had little benefit from surgery, but the benefit increased as the aggressiveness of the tumor increased.

Comparing the Side Effects of Watchful Waiting and Radical Prostatectomy

Another important part of this study was the self-assessment of urinary, sexual, and bowel functions two years after beginning the study (Table 7.3).

Table 7.3

Patient-Reported Side Effects	Surgery	Watchful Waiting
Urinary incontinence – A lot of problems with dribbling – Lose large amounts of urine but not all day – Have no control of urine – Wear a catheter	17.1%	6.3%
Erectile dysfunction – Unable to have an erection – Erection inadequate for intercourse	88.1%	44.1%

Although no difference was seen in problems with bowel function, urinary and sexual functioning was significantly worse for men undergoing surgery. These results must be interpreted cautiously for two reasons. First, more than 50% did not undergo nerve-sparing radical prostatectomy. More men are likely to have their sexual function preserved when nerve-sparing surgery is performed. Second, some of the men assigned to watchful waiting actually declined and had surgery while more than 22% of those assigned to get surgery declined. Thus, the true odds of developing these side effects will probably differ from those reported in the study.

Although the study was well designed, the real benefit from surgery may have been underestimated because of the number of men who did not undergo their assigned treatment. You might wonder why the results weren't analyzed according to the treatment men *did receive* rather than the treatment they were *randomized to receive*. The simple answer is it would violate the following principle of statistics; *randomized studies must analyze the results according to the treatment group to which they are assigned, whether or not patients comply*. The authors did re-analyze the results and believe that the noncompliance did not significantly alter the results.

Another randomized study done in Scandinavia began several years before the U.S. study and has longer follow-up. The authors reported the results at 15 years. The average age was 65 years and the average PSA was 13 ng/ml. A recent update shows the following results:

Table 7.4 15-Year Results of Scandinavian Study

Outcome after 15 Years	Watchful Waiting	Surgery	Difference in Survival
Alive	47.3%	53.9%	6.6%
Died from prostate cancer	20.7%	14.6%	6.1%
Treated with hormone therapy	63.4%	39.6%	23.8%
Developed metastatic disease	33.4%	21.7%	11.7%

In contrast to the U.S. study, this study did show that radical prostatectomy significantly reduced the risk of dying from prostate cancer. At 15 years, surgery prevented 6.6% of the men from dying of any cause, 6.1% from dying from prostate cancer, and 11.7% from developing metastatic disease. This means 15 men had to undergo surgery to prevent one from dying from prostate cancer in 15 years. Also, metastatic disease was prevented in one out of every nine men undergoing surgery.

This study also reported the chance of developing problems due to enlargement of the tumor in the prostate gland. This is called local progression of the disease. By 12 years, it occurred in 22% of men having surgery compared with 46% of men on watchful waiting. That means surgery prevented local progression in almost one out of every four men.

The authors also reported results for several subgroups. First, the men's age had a big impact on the results. In contrast to the U.S. study, in the Scandinavian study those under 65 treated by surgery had an 18% lower chance of dying from prostate cancer in 12 years compared with the watchful waiting group. This means surgery helped almost one out of every seven men in the younger age group. They also had a better overall survival and a lower risk of developing metastases. For men over 65, however, surgery did not improve overall survival, prostate cancer survival, or the chance of developing metastases.

In men with low-risk disease, which they defined as having a PSA under 10 ng/ml and a Gleason score under 7, men undergoing surgery had a 13% higher survival and an 11% lower risk of developing metastases. Of note, this is not the same group of patients as the low-risk group reported in the U.S. study, for which no benefit was seen.

The authors also reported the percentage of men getting major complications one year after surgery. The rates for impotence and incontinence are much higher than reported in the United States. The authors point out that the surgeons were not very experienced, so men should not expect these same risks if operated on by more experienced U.S. surgeons.

Table 7.5 Surgical Complications of Scandinavian Study

	Radical Prostatectomy
Impotence	58%
Incontinence	32%
Urinary obstruction	2%
Pulmonary embolus	1.4%
Deep venous thrombosis	1%

Although this study was well designed, it too has some weaknesses. Similar to the U.S. study, some men assigned to get watchful waiting chose instead to have surgery and some men assigned to get surgery refused to do it. The percentage of men not complying with their assigned treatment was similar in both the U.S. and Scandinavian studies. Again, this could have reduced the benefit from surgery but also underestimated the side effects.

After reading about these two studies, you may find yourself quite confused because one study shows surgery is significantly better than watchful waiting and the other shows almost the complete opposite. The obvious question is what it means for your particular case. You should know that the studies differed in several important ways. First, almost no African Americans participated in the Scandinavian trial. Also, it had:

- A much smaller percentage of men diagnosed by the PSA test.

- Nearly twice the percentage of men with a PSA over 20 ng/ml at entry.

- A higher average PSA in the entire population.

- A greater percentage of men with clinical stage T2b disease.

- A higher percentage of men with a Gleason 7 cancer.

- A much higher percentage of men who were diagnosed due to symptoms.

- Almost twice as many men undergoing surgery had cancer at the margin of the prostate gland.

- Nearly twice the death rate from prostate cancer at 12 years.

These differences mean that the Scandinavian study enrolled more men with an aggressive or more advanced cancer. Also, the results of the U.S. study are more appropriate for men diagnosed in the United States because more than 60% are found following a screening PSA. Still, the bottom line from the two studies may be that if you have a low-risk cancer, you may not gain very much from aggressive therapy; at least, not within the first 12 years of your diagnosis. With further follow-up, things may change. Men with higher risk cancers may have more to lose by choosing watchful waiting.

Useful information about watchful waiting is available from one other study. Although it was retrospective, it does include men with a normal rectal examination who were diagnosed by PSA (clinical stage T1c). They were part of the SEER (Surveillance, Epidemiology and End Results) national cancer registry. Table 7.6 shows the chance of dying from prostate cancer 10 years after diagnosis.

This study also shows that men over age 65 with a Gleason score of 5, 6, or 7 have a low risk of dying from prostate cancer in 10 years. For those diagnosed by PSA, which is stage T1c, it happened to only 2% of men between the ages of 65 and 69. If they were over 80, only 6% died of their disease. The results provide added confidence about the accuracy of the results seen with watchful waiting in the U.S. randomized study.

Table 7.6 Percentage of Men on Watchful Waiting Who Died from Prostate Cancer in 10 Years

Clinical Tumor Stage When Diagnosed	Gleason Score	Age 65–69 at Diagnosis	Age 70–74 at Diagnosis	Age 75–79 at Diagnosis	Over age 80 at Diagnosis
T1a or T1b	5, 6, or 7	Not enough men	3%	4%	6%
T1c	5, 6, or 7	2%	3%	6%	6%
T2	5, 6, or 7	7%	6%	8%	10%
T1a or T1b	8, 9, or 10	28%	25%	28%	29%
T1c	8, 9, or 10	9%	20%	17%	16%
T2	8, 9, or 10	29%	18%	22%	20%

This study has the following weaknesses:

- It was retrospective. This means there could be a bias in how men ended up with this therapy; they could have been less healthy and some of the information could have been recorded incorrectly.

- It does not show what happens after 10 years. A longer follow-up may result in more cancer deaths.

- It combined the results for Gleason scores of 5, 6, and 7. A Gleason score of 7 is more dangerous than a Gleason of 5 or 6. This means combining all three together will underestimate the risk of dying for men with a Gleason 7 cancer but overestimate the risk for those with a Gleason score of 5 or 6. Unfortunately, without re-reviewing the biopsies, the results for men with each specific Gleason score cannot be determined.

- Men under age 65 were not included, so younger men diagnosed with prostate cancer cannot assume they would get the same results from watchful waiting.

- The group with T1c tumors was contaminated since nearly one-quarter of them eventually had either surgery or radiation. This could have made the results look better, which means the risk of dying may be underestimated.

Despite these problems, this study does provide older men with more information about what to expect from watchful waiting.

How Does Watchful Waiting Affect Your Quality of Life?

Each treatment can have negative effects on a man's quality of life. The Scandinavian randomized study assessed how often this occurred. Written surveys asking about sexual and urinary functions were mailed to nearly one-half of the men and were completed about four years after the study began. The results are shown in the next two tables. The first one shows the results for sexual function and the second one the results for urinary function.

These tables show several key differences between the two groups. A positive difference means the effect was more common in the watchful waiting group and a negative difference means it was more common in the surgery group. Compared with the watchful waiting group, a significantly higher percentage of men treated with surgery are:

- Unable to achieve erections good enough for intercourse.

- Unable to have an orgasm.

- Unable to maintain an erection in at least 1 out of 5 attempts.

Table 7.7 Effect of Watchful Waiting or Surgery on Sexual Function in Scandinavian Study

Survey Question	Watchful Waiting Group	Surgery Group	Difference
1. Erections seldom or never good enough for intercourse	45%	80%	−35%
2. Unable to maintain erections in more than 1 of every 5 attempts	30%	55%	−25%
3. No orgasm in past 6 months	31%	62%	−31%

Table 7.8 Effect of Watchful Waiting or Surgery on Urinary Function in Scandinavian Study

Survey Question	Watchful Waiting Group	Surgery Group	Difference
1. Urinary stream weak more than 1 of every 5 times	44%	28%	16%
2. Urinating at least twice per night	57%	44%	13%
3. Leaking urine at least once per week	21%	49%	−28%
4. Moderate or severe distress from urinary leakage	9%	29%	−20%
5. Regular use of some protective aid for leakage	10%	43%	−33%

- More likely to leak urine at least once per week.

- Moderately or severely distressed by their leakage.

The trade-off is that more men treated with watchful waiting:

- Have local progression of their cancer.

- Get up at least twice per night to urinate.

- Have a slow or weak urine stream.

This study also has some weaknesses.

- No baseline survey was done. Without that information, it is not possible to know if the sexual or urinary difficulties developed because men got older or they already were present when the study began. One thing is clear. Both problems may occur in some men as they get older, but impotence and incontinence are much more likely to occur following surgery.

- Only one-half of the men in the study were sent the survey. There is no way to know whether the same results would occur in the men who were omitted.

- Surveys were completed by about 90% of the men who were sent one. It is not known how the results would be affected if the remaining 10% had answered the survey.

- Some men did not answer all the questions for unknown reasons.

- Twenty percent of the men assigned to have surgery did not get it. They were still counted as if they had surgery. That may have underestimated the side effects in the surgery group.

- Six percent of the men in the watchful waiting group had surgery. They still were counted as if they had watchful waiting.

That may have overestimated the side effects in the watchful waiting group.

- It is not known how many men had nerve-sparing surgery. A man will not have erections unless his nerves are preserved. Some of the men with stage T2 disease most likely had one or both nerves removed to avoid leaving cancer behind. This would increase their chances of having problems getting erections. Since few of the men were diagnosed by PSA, men with a newly diagnosed cancer resulting from their PSA test may expect a lower risk of this complication. Also, some men may have received androgen deprivation therapy (ADT), which also reduces erections.

Although this study reported short-term side effects, it did not include any longer-term quality-of-life results for the men who developed metastatic disease. When that occurs, men can develop several problems from the primary treatment, ADT, as shown in the table. They also are further explained in chapter 14.

Who Is a Good Candidate for Watchful Waiting?

Watchful waiting may be a very appropriate treatment for some men. The best candidates include men who:

- Are above 75 years.

- Have a major illness such as bad heart disease.

- Have a life expectancy of less than 10 years.

- Have low-risk disease, which means having a Gleason score of 6, a PSA under 10 ng/ml, and a T1 or T2 cancer based on the digital rectal examination (DRE).

- Are more concerned about their quality of life now rather than how long they may live.

Table 7.9 Side Effects of ADT

Side Effect	Frequency and Extent
Hot flashes	21%–73%
Decreased sex drive	40%–60%
Problems with sexual function	50%
Decreased muscle mass (average loss)	1%–4%
Weight gain (average increase in weight in 75% of patients)	3%
Osteoporosis (thinning of the bones; per year)	2%–3%
Bone fractures	6%–9%
Increased lipid levels: Cholesterol Triglycerides Low-density lipoproteins	8% 27% 9%
Decreased cognitive function (thinking, calculating, memory)	Progresses over time
Anemia (decreased blood count)	90% of men have 10% drop 13% of men have 25% drop
Fatigue	2%–18%
Breast enlargement (gynecomastia)	10%–25%

Watchful waiting probably is a bad choice for a man who has a Gleason score of 8, 9, or 10 even if his life expectancy is only five years. Those tumors are highly likely to progress and cause harm. Also, this would not be a good treatment if you are a very anxious person who will constantly worry about what is happening to your cancer if you don't do something about it.

Monitoring Men on Watchful Waiting

Before the PSA was available, men were checked using the DRE and an annual bone scan. Today, most men on watchful waiting will have a DRE and PSA test done every 6 or 12 months. The bone scan does not need to be performed until the PSA is above 10 ng/ml or bone pain occurs because bone metastases are very uncommon at lower levels.

Many doctors use the *PSA doubling time* as a basis for deciding when to do a bone scan. The doubling time is a measure of how long it takes for the PSA to double in value. Good studies show that more than two-thirds of men being diagnosed today have a PSA doubling time of more than four years. Since these tumors progress very slowly, doing a bone scan makes little sense unless the doubling time is closer to two years or less. If you want to know your PSA doubling time, two free tools are available for calculating it: http://kevin.phys.unm.edu/psa/, www.mskcc.org/applications /nomograms/Prostate/PsaDoublingTime.aspx

Suppose you have a bone scan and it is negative? When should it be done again? Most doctors will make the decision based on how fast the PSA rises.

The Bottom Line on Watchful Waiting

Watchful waiting is the most conservative treatment for localized prostate cancer. It will result in the lowest chance of altering your quality of life right now and preserve it for many years. If your cancer was diagnosed as a result of a PSA test and you have low-risk disease, or a PSA under 10 ng/ml, surgery may only reduce your risk of dying in the next 12 years by about 3% to 6%. That amount could increase with more years of follow-up, which poses a dilemma for men who have a long life expectancy when they are diagnosed with prostate cancer. There is no way to know what will happen to those men with longer follow-up. If you do have a more aggressive cancer, the risk of being harmed with watchful waiting increases and the odds of benefitting from surgery increase.

You may be wondering how watchful waiting compares with other treatments. Unfortunately, without proper studies, a valid comparison cannot be stated accurately. Some studies are in progress, which should provide answers in the next few years. Hopefully you now have a better idea of the risk posed by your cancer and what can happen if you choose watchful waiting. This information should also be helpful as you now learn about active surveillance in the next chapter.

Active Surveillance: A Safer Approach than Watchful Waiting

It should be clear from the previous chapter that many men with prostate cancer only have a small risk of dying from this disease or benefitting from surgery within 12 to 15 years of their diagnosis. However, even a small risk is a gamble that you may not be able to or willing to accept. Also, the prospect of spending a part of every day wondering whether prostate cancer cells are spreading in your body may cause too much anxiety for you or your life partner to accept. Fortunately, you now have another option called *active surveillance* or *delayed therapy*.

What Is Active Surveillance?

Active surveillance begins the same as watchful waiting with no treatment to the prostate following the diagnosis. Men are monitored at regular intervals by having a digital rectal examination (DRE), a blood test for prostate-specific antigen (PSA), and repeat prostate biopsies. But unlike watchful waiting in which no attempt is made to treat the cancer in the prostate, active surveillance takes a delayed approach to curing the disease. This occurs if, and only if, the cancer shows signs of getting worse.

Active surveillance has advantages and disadvantages. The main advantage is that it gives you a chance to avoid experiencing side effects that may occur from all the local treatments. It offers you a way to maintain your current quality of life at least until it changes due to aging. This means having the same sexual function, urinary control, and bowel function that existed before your cancer was detected.

Active surveillance does have some disadvantages. The main one is that doctors cannot be absolutely sure when your cancer is becoming dangerous. If that does occur, the possibility exists that it may be more difficult to cure compared with treating it when it was first detected. While you are being monitored, some cancer cells may spread to other parts of the body, called metastases, and currently there is no cure for that stage of the disease. In other words, by delaying treatment you could end up with a worse outcome and possibly a shorter life expectancy.

Another disadvantage is active surveillance has not been in use for very long. The oldest study has survival results projected for only up to 10 years. Doctors do not yet know what will happen to men on active surveillance beyond that time. This makes it a harder choice for men with a longer life expectancy.

What Are the Results with Active Surveillance?

More results with active surveillance have been reported in recent years, but none are from a randomized study. The group with the longest follow-up is from a prospective cohort study that began in Sweden as part of a large randomized screening study. Men between the ages of 50 and 64 were randomized to get screened with a PSA test or have no intervention. Of those diagnosed with prostate cancer, 439 were placed on active surveillance. One-half of the men were under age 65 and one-half were followed for more than 6 years. The longest follow-up was 15 years. The following table shows the number of men in the study with each type of tumor.

Table 8.1

Risk Group	Tumor Properties	Number in Study
Very low risk	PSA under 10 ng/ml Gleason score less than 7 Stage T1c disease PSA density (PSA level divided by prostate volume) no greater than 0.15 Fewer than 3 biopsy cores showing cancer	224 (51%)
Low risk	PSA less than 10 ng/ml Gleason less than 7 Stage T1c	117 (27%)
Intermediate risk	PSA 10–20 ng/ml or Gleason 7 or T2b	92 (21%)
High risk	PSA over 20 ng/ml or Gleason 8–10 or T2c or T3	6 (1%)

Thus far, 63% of the men remain on active surveillance and 37% have been treated by surgery or radiation or hormone therapy. At 10 years, only one man had died from prostate cancer, 59 (13.5%) had died from some other cause, and 202 (46%) have not had definite treatment. One other man has also developed metastatic disease. Both the man who died and the one with metastatic disease had an intermediate-risk cancer.

An important part of this study is that it provides some information about what happens to men who start on active surveillance but then get treatment because their disease was thought to have progressed. Thus far, only 2% of the men with very-low-risk disease and 6% with low-risk disease have developed a rising PSA after undergoing radical prostatectomy or radiation therapy. Although the follow-up of these men is limited to only 6 years, the results mean that the risk from delaying treatment appears to be very low for men in the very-low-risk or low-risk disease category. The authors concluded that, "active surveillance should be an option for avoiding overtreatment." A longer follow-up is needed from this study before men can be reassured that active surveillance is a safe long-term treatment.

The second cohort study began in Canada in 1995. It enrolled 450 men, of which more than one-half were under age 71. Eighty-one percent of the group had low-risk prostate cancer and the remainder had intermediate-risk disease. About one-half of the group has been followed for almost 7 years but some have been followed for up to 13 years.

All the men had a PSA measured every three months for two years and every six months thereafter. A second biopsy was done between six and twelve months after diagnosis and additional biopsies were done every three to four years until age 80. Treatment was recommended for any one of the following reasons.

- The PSA level doubled in less than two years (eventually changed to less than three years).

- The Gleason score increased.

- The tumor felt larger on digital rectal examination.

The results from this study are shown in the following table.

Table 8.2 Estimated Results of Active Surveillance

Outcome	Total at 5 Years	Total at 10 Years
Overall survival	90% (range 87%–93%)	68% (range 62%–74%)
Died from prostate cancer	0.3%	2.8%
Stayed on active surveillance	72%	62%
PSA progression after surgery or radiation in men stopping active surveillance	53%	Not available

The estimated survival at 10 years is 68%, but it really could be as low as 62% or as high as 74%. There is no way to be more exact at this time. The overall survival was similar for men remaining on active surveillance compared with those who stopped surveillance and had surgery or radiation. So far, more than 60% of the men still remain on active surveillance while 30% stopped it and were treated by surgery or radiation. Only 3% have died from prostate cancer and 13% had a rise in PSA within 10 years of their diagnosis.

Another finding from this study is the odds of dying from some other cause compared with the risk of dying from prostate cancer. Men under 70 were almost nine times more likely to die of something other than prostate cancer. It happened about 33 times more often for men over that age. The take-away message from these two studies is that the average man with low-risk disease will be better off with active surveillance unless he has an excellent chance of living into his 80s or 90s.

There are many other reports on active surveillance, but the number of men in each of them is smaller and the follow-up time is shorter than these two studies. Additional updates will likely appear in the next several years, which will add to our understanding of the effects of this treatment. Even better, a randomized study called the START (Surveillance Treatment Against Radical Therapy) trial has begun that will compare active surveillance to either radical prostatectomy or radiation therapy. Results are not expected, however, for at least 10 years. Until then, combining the results from the two studies shown above with the results on watchful waiting from the previous chapter does provide you with a good idea of what you can expect with active surveillance. So far it appears that most men with low-risk disease will do well without having immediate surgery or radiation for the first 12 years after diagnosis.

Who Is a Good Candidate for Active Surveillance?

Let's begin by talking about which patients are not good candidates for active surveillance. This would include men with high-risk disease, which means they have either a Gleason 8–10 on the biopsy, a PSA over 20 ng/ml, or a clinical stage T2c cancer. A high percentage of these tumors will grow quickly, spread to other organs and cause death from prostate cancer. For that reason, delaying treatment even for one or two years is a bad idea for anyone hoping to minimize his risk of suffering from this disease.

The best men for active surveillance are those with low-risk disease. These men have a very small chance, if any, of benefitting from surgery or radiation in the next 12 years. This risk is even lower for men with very-low-risk disease. In addition to having a PSA less than 10 ng/ml, a Gleason score less than 7, and stage T1c or T2a disease, they also must have:

- Cancer cells found on less than three biopsy cores.

- Cancer cells found in less than 50% of any one core.

- A PSA doubling time greater than three years.

A PSA density below 0.15 ng/ml per gram. (*The PSA density is determined by dividing the PSA level by the size of the prostate as determined from a prostate ultrasound.*)

Men falling into this group should be very cautious about proceeding with aggressive therapy without first carefully discussing the active surveillance results with their doctor.

Men with intermediate-risk disease have the greatest uncertainty from active surveillance. Not enough of them have been followed long enough to know the long-term effect with this option. However, based on the study cited in the last chapter comparing radical prostatectomy with watchful waiting, the potential benefit of surgery for men in this group appears small at 12 years. Active surveillance may be very acceptable to some men over 70 or those with a short life expectancy. However, younger men with a much longer life expectancy may not be willing to take the risk until a longer follow-up is available. The genetic tests discussed in chapter 5 may offer some men additional information for making this decision.

Follow-Up Care for Men on Active Surveillance

Since active surveillance is relatively new, the "best" way to check someone managed this way is still being worked out. No consensus exists at this time, but usually a PSA and digital examination are being performed every three to six months. Some doctors recommend a repeat biopsy within a year of the initial diagnosis to make sure that a more aggressive cancer is not present. Repeat biopsies then are done at various intervals. Some doctors do it every one or two years and then again at five years, but no consensus exists. At least 12 cores should be removed for each biopsy. Some doctors are doing saturation biopsies, taking 20 to 40 samples, but that approach has not been shown to be better.

When Should Active Surveillance Stop?

Thus far, the factors used most often for stopping active surveillance and proceeding with some other treatment include:

- A worsening of the Gleason score or

- An increase in the amount of cancer seen on a repeat prostate biopsy, or

- An increase in the size of the tumor felt on a prostate examination.

Although most doctors studying active surveillance have used changes in PSA to decide when to stop active surveillance, this approach may lead many men to undergo therapy prematurely. Researchers conducting the Canadian study on active surveillance discussed earlier in this chapter did another study looking at the effect of changes in the PSA on changes in treatment. It is based on 315 men who remained on active surveillance at the time of the report. None of them had died of prostate cancer or developed metastatic disease. The percent of men who would have met each threshold for treatment is shown in the next table.

Table 8.3

PSA Threshold	Percent Meeting Threshold Who Would Have Been Told to Stop Active Surveillance and Have Treatment
PSA rising above 10 ng/ml	38%
PSA rising above 20 ng/ml	14%
PSA doubling in less than two years	37%–39%
PSA doubling in less than three years	48%–50%
PSA velocity greater than 2 ng/ml/year	84%
PSA velocity at one year greater than 2 ng/ml	51%

As you can see, as few as 14%, but as many as 84%, would have been told to undergo treatment using one of the PSA indicators. These results provide good support for not using changes in PSA by itself to stop active surveillance. Until something better comes along, the prostate biopsy and the digital rectal examination may be the most important measures to use for recommending to stop active surveillance and to get the cancer treated.

A word of caution is also needed about stopping active surveillance based on the prostate biopsy results. Earlier you were told that many men thought to have a Gleason 3+3=6 cancer on their biopsy turn out to have Gleason 3+4 disease when their prostate is removed. This does not mean their cancer has gotten worse while they were waiting for surgery. Instead, it does mean that the biopsy sometimes underestimates the true Gleason score.

Now, when you look at what happens to men with a Gleason 3+3=6 cancer, their long-term survival is almost the same whether they have surgery or watchful waiting. This must mean that many men with Gleason 3+4 disease on their biopsy will do just as well with conservative therapy as men with Gleason 3+3=6 disease. For that reason, if you choose active surveillance and your initial biopsy shows Gleason 3+3=6 but a later biopsy shows Gleason 3+4=7, you still may consider staying on active surveillance, especially if the PSA is remaining stable. For those men who have both a rise in the PSA and an increase to Gleason 3+4=7 on the biopsy, active surveillance probably should be stopped until more information becomes available that shows it is safe to stay on this treatment.

Unconventional Treatments for Men on Active Surveillance

One of the main reasons men stop active surveillance is that they have trouble coping with a rise in their PSA. If this could be delayed or prevented, more men might remain on this treatment. One recent study has generated considerable excitement. A randomized study was done in the United Kingdom comparing a mixture of extracts from green tea, pomegranate seeds, broccoli and turmeric to a placebo in men on active surveillance. The product is called Pomi-T®. Men took the pills for six months and at the end of that time, more of those on the active pill had a drop in their PSA and fewer of them had a rise in their PSA. If larger studies with longer follow-up provide additional support for the use of these or other agents, then active surveillance may be easier to accept for some men.

What Do Doctor Groups Say about Active Surveillance?

The number of doctor groups talking about active surveillance has been increasing in recent years. In 2011, the American Urological

Association (AUA), which is the governing body for urologists in the United States, updated their guidelines for managing prostate cancer with the following statement:

> "The AUA strongly supports the option of active surveillance, in lieu of immediate treatment, for certain men found to have prostate cancer."

The National Comprehensive Cancer Network is a group of doctors selected from major cancer centers in the United States. In 2010 they made the following statements:

> "Men with 'low risk' prostate cancer who have a life expectancy of less than 10 years should be offered and recommended active surveillance."

> "Men with 'very low risk' prostate cancer and a life expectancy of less than 20 years *should only be treated with active surveillance.*"

A consensus statement by the American Cancer Society stated:

> "Be sure to explore all treatment options, including active surveillance. In some cases of prostate cancer 'no treatment' may turn out to be the best treatment."

A Consensus conference sponsored by the National Cancer Institute in 2011 concluded:

> "Active surveillance has emerged as a viable option that should be offered to patients with low-risk prostate cancer."

You should be aware that this advice is based on the best information available at this time but not on a randomized controlled study. Clearly more data are needed to better help men make a choice about their prostate cancer.

The Bottom Line on Active Surveillance

Contrary to initial fears, active surveillance with delayed treatment has not resulted in a high risk of death from prostate cancer in

12 years. It has enabled more than 60% of selected men to avoid a treatment that so far would have been unnecessary. It offers a way to increase the odds that local therapy to the prostate gland really is needed. Although active surveillance carries some risk that the cancer might be incurable by the time it is treated, so far that risk appears low; dying from prostate cancer or having it spread to other organs in 12 years does not happen very often. Clearly, a longer follow-up is needed to help younger men decide about this option. Also, until randomized studies report their results, no one can say whether active surveillance is as good as, or better or worse than getting therapy right away. For now, you may find this approach to be an appealing alternative to immediate treatment or watchful waiting. Only you can decide whether the risks are worth the benefits. At the very least, your doctor should provide you with a balanced discussion of active surveillance as one of the options for managing localized prostate cancer.

Surgical Treatment

What Is a Radical Prostatectomy?

Of all the treatments available for localized prostate cancer, *radical prostatectomy* has been in use for the longest time and has the longest follow-up information. For that reason, many doctors call it the "gold standard" for treating this disease. It is called a "radical" prostatectomy because the entire prostate is removed along with both seminal vesicles and a portion of both *vas deferntia* (see chapter 1).

The operation has changed since it was first performed, making it safer with fewer side effects. The most important advance was the discovery of how to remove the entire prostate without injuring the two *pelvic nerves* that enable men to have erections. This is called a *nerve-sparing radical prostatectomy*, which can be performed on most newly diagnosed patients. Another change has been the development of two minimally invasive methods for doing the operation that offers the potential for several benefits. Minimally invasive means the operation is performed through a much smaller cut in the skin and it uses a camera to enlarge the surgical field. All four of the surgical methods in use today will be described later in this chapter.

What Are the Advantages and Disadvantages of Radical Prostatectomy?

The advantage of removing the prostate is that it *may* immediately remove all the cancer in your body, meaning you *may* never have a problem from prostate cancer in the future. In other words, you *may* be cured. Perhaps you are wondering why the word "may" is used in the last sentence. The reason is radical prostatectomy does not cure everyone because cancer cells sometimes have spread outside the prostate before a man gets diagnosed. Removing the prostate cannot remove those cells. Over time, they continue to grow, causing symptoms and possibly death from prostate cancer. Another disadvantage of radical prostatectomy is that it may cause side effects or complications that affect a man's quality of life.

What Are the Results of Radical Prostatectomy?

Only two well-done studies of this operation have been performed and both were reviewed in chapter 7. One study showed a small but significantly better survival rate and a lower rate of developing metastases by 15 years compared with watchful waiting (Scandinavian study). For every 15 men undergoing surgery, one prostate cancer death was prevented. So far, the other study has not shown any significant improvement in survival at 12 years (U.S. study). The difference in survival was less than 3%. However, it did show that surgery reduced the risk of developing metastases in about one out of every eight men with high-risk disease compared with watchful waiting. Although these studies have some weaknesses, they are the best information available about this treatment in all the medical journals.

Does surgery cure more patients than external radiation or seed implantation? The answer is unknown at this time because randomized studies comparing these treatments have not been performed. As discussed in chapter 4, valid conclusions cannot be made from nonrandomized studies. The best that can be said is the 10-year results of radical prostatectomy appear to be similar to external radiation and brachytherapy. Comparing radical prostatectomy to cryotherapy, proton beam radiation, or high-intensity focused ultrasound is difficult because only surgery has long-term survival rates.

Many people reading these last two statements may wonder why it differs from so many articles and websites making claims that one treatment is superior. There are several reasons. First, many of them do not follow the principles of evidence-based medicine that requires the use of well-done studies to make conclusions about how treatments compare with one another. Second, many of them are promoting a particular therapy because that is the treatment they offer and their compensation increases when more patients are treated. Unfortunately, no referees exist to cry "foul" when misleading or inaccurate information is used to make recommendations. The bottom line for you as a patient is to be cautious as you gather information and be prepared to ask the questions that were included in chapter 6.

Does Lowering Testosterone Improve the Results of Surgery?

As some men undergoing radical prostatectomy have cancer cells growing outside the prostate, doctors have questioned whether anything could be done before surgery to kill those cells; that way the prostatectomy could more easily get rid of the cancer. One option was to lower the male hormone called *testosterone* for several months because that is known to kill prostate cancer cells. This treatment is called *androgen deprivation therapy (ADT)* (see chapters 14 and 26–27 for additional information). Several good-quality studies have tested this idea in men scheduled for surgery, but the therapy has failed to improve survival or lower the chance of recurrence. Therefore, *ADT before radical prostatectomy offers no benefit and should not be done.* Even if your surgery is delayed for several months, it should not be used while you wait to get treated. In fact, some reports found that it can make the operation more difficult and cause more blood loss. Despite these studies, however, some doctors still do it. If your doctor wants you to get this treatment, you should consider getting a second opinion.

Who Is a Good Candidate for Radical Prostatectomy?

Most doctors believe that any man with localized prostate cancer who is likely to live at least 10 or 15 years is a good candidate for this treatment. That means men with a serious illness or those who are a poor surgical risk should consider a different option. The reason for putting those numbers on life expectancy is that most prostate cancers diagnosed today will not grow very fast. Even if left untreated, they will not cause problems for at least 10 years as was explained in chapter 7. The exception is men with a Gleason score above 7 because those cancers can grow more quickly and can be more dangerous. About 20% of men with a Gleason score of 8–10 will die from their disease within five years of diagnosis if they are not treated aggressively. For that reason, they only need a life expectancy greater than five years to potentially benefit from radical prostatectomy.

The Pros and Cons of Different Surgical Methods

The original method of removing the prostate is called the *radical retropubic prostatectomy* (RRP). Three other methods that are in use today are the *radical perineal prostatectomy* (RPP), the *laparoscopic radical prostatectomy* (LRP), and the *robot-assisted laparoscopic radical prostatectomy* (RALP). The nerves controlling erections can be spared using any of the four methods.

Radical Retropubic Prostatectomy

This method is performed through a cut made in the skin extending from below the belly button to the pubic bone. The operation usually can be completed in about two to four hours and patients remain in the hospital for one or two nights.

The advantages of this method are that it allows the doctor to feel the prostate, the surrounding tissues, and the pelvic lymph nodes. This helps the surgeon decide whether the pelvic nerves can be preserved and whether the pelvic lymph nodes should be removed, which is called a *pelvic lymphadenectomy*. The disadvantages of the retropubic approach are that the patient has more blood loss, a greater chance of needing a blood transfusion, a slightly longer time in the hospital, and a longer time until exercise can be resumed compared with the other three methods.

Radical Perineal Prostatectomy

The perineal approach is done through an incision made in the skin underneath the scrotum in front of the rectum. It is the least commonly performed radical prostatectomy in the United States because few doctors have been trained to do it. This is unfortunate because it has the advantage of less blood loss, fewer blood transfusions, a shorter hospital stay, and more rapid recovery than the retropubic approach. The operation usually is completed in about one to three hours and most men stay in the hospital for one night.

Similar to the retropubic approach, the surgeon can feel the prostate to determine whether the pelvic nerves can be preserved. However, a disadvantage of the perineal operation is the surgeon cannot feel the pelvic lymph nodes or remove them. That would require a second operation. For that reason, the perineal approach is best for men who have a very low chance that cancer has spread to the lymph nodes and do not need them removed. Another advantage is it has the lowest cost of the four methods, which might be important if you have a very large insurance deductible or no insurance at all and have to pay for your treatment out of your pocket.

Laparoscopic Radical Prostatectomy

The laparoscopic approach was the first minimally invasive method for removing the prostate. It became popular after 2000, but the development of a robotic instrument led to a decline in its use. This operation usually takes about two to four hours to complete, although occasionally it may take much longer. Patients usually are sent home after one night in the hospital.

The laparoscopic method has the same advantages as the perineal approach including low blood loss, an infrequent need for a blood transfusion, a short time spent in the hospital, and a quicker time to resume all normal activities. Unlike the perineal approach, however, the pelvic lymph nodes can be removed using the laparoscopic method, although the doctor cannot feel them to determine whether they should be removed. Another disadvantage is the inability to feel the prostate. This means that the surgeon must decide whether to do a nerve-sparing operation based on the preoperative tests. The laparoscopic approach also has a slightly higher risk of injuring the bladder, bowel, or a blood vessel. Lastly, this operation requires that surgeons have considerable experience to get good results with few complications. For that reason, be sure to ask *exactly* how many your surgeon has performed. If the total is under 50 or 100, your risk for getting a complication may be higher and the duration of your surgery may be longer compared to it being done by a more experienced surgeon. In that case, you might consider seeing a surgeon who has performed many more of these operations.

Robot-Assisted Laparoscopic Radical Prostatectomy (RALP)

Beginning in approximately 2001, a robotic instrument called the DaVinci was developed that enabled surgeons to do the prostatectomy through small incisions in the skin without directly touching the patient; instead, the robot does the work under the guidance of the surgeon who sits at a table several feet from the operating table. This operation usually is completed in two to four hours, although much longer operations have been reported. Most men go home after one night's stay in the hospital.

The advantages of a RALP are similar to the perineal and laparoscopic methods; it also has less blood loss, rarely requires a blood transfusion, has a slightly shorter time in the hospital, and has a more rapid recovery than the retropubic operation. Also, it does provide the surgeon with a larger view of the surgical area than the retropubic and perineal methods, which some doctors believe makes the operation easier to do. Another advantage of this method over the perineal approach is the ability to remove the lymph nodes. The disadvantages of this method are that the surgeon cannot feel the lymph nodes or the pelvic nerves and it has a steeper learning curve than the laparoscopic method. Some experts believe that several hundred RALPs are needed as experience before good results are obtained by a surgeon. That means you should definitely ask how many your doctor has done so that you are not part of his or her "learning curve."

Which Surgical Method Is Best?

If you read the advertisements on billboards or websites, you would think that the robot-assisted method is the only way to go. In fact, it is now the most common method used to remove the prostate. However, is it the best method? The answer remains unknown. No good study has ever proven that this method does a better job at controlling the cancer, or causes less urinary leakage or fewer problems with erections. For that reason, they are all equally good choices for removing your prostate. The most important message here is *choose your surgeon rather than the surgical method that will be used!*

How to Choose a Surgeon

Some studies have shown that surgeons who do more than 20 or 40 radical prostatectomies per year have fewer side effects and get better results than less-experienced surgeons. The problem is that most urologists in the United States do not do that many. A survey in 2005 found that 80% of urologists perform no more than 10 of them per year.

So, how do you choose a surgeon? Should it be the urologist who found your cancer, another doctor in the community, or do you need to go to someone who specializes in performing this operation? Don't expect urologists to volunteer how many they have done or offer to refer you to someone else who might have more experience. *If you want to have the best chance for a good result, have your surgery done by a very experienced surgeon.* Many cities have "specialists" who focus almost entirely on doing this operation and caring for men with prostate cancer. The only way to find out your doctor's experience is to ask, "How many of these operations do you do each year? How many have you done in your career? How often do the different complications occur in those patients?" Don't be afraid to do this because you have every right to know the answers. It is not your concern if the doctor's ego gets hurt. You are the one who will have to live with the results and that depends greatly on the surgeon's experience. Although doing less than 20 per year does not mean a surgeon always will get worse results, it is more likely compared with someone doing more of them annually. The following questions were listed in chapter 6 and are repeated for emphasis. The answers can help you decide who should do your operation. You are encouraged to write them on a piece of paper and take them with you when you have a consultation regarding your treatment, or take this book with you.

- What percentage of your patients with erections before surgery is able to have intercourse without any aids 12 to 18 months after surgery?

- How many of them use aids such as a medication or a pump?

- What percentage of your patients has the same urinary control one year after surgery as they did before the operation?

- What percentage of your patients develop other complications?

If you decide to ask any of these questions, you also should ask how your doctor got this information: Was it estimated, or was a written survey used that has been shown to provide more accurate results? Asking patients during a follow-up visit, "How are you doing?" or "Are you having any problems?" *underestimates the true complication rate.* The problem is that very few doctors use written surveys, which means most do not know their true results. The best advice to give you is to choose a surgeon who uses a written survey, assuming you can find one nearby. If none is available in your community, at least choose a surgeon who has done many of these operations.

When asked about side effects, some doctors quote results reported in medical journals. Keep in mind that the best surgeons in the country write these papers, so if your doctor is not one of them, his or her results probably are not as good.

Some surgeons may try to make you feel more comfortable by giving you the names of previously treated men whom you can call to ask about their own experience. The problem is that talking to someone with a "good" result really will not allow you to evaluate that doctor. In many ways it is the same as the references you put on your own résumé. Would you ever name someone who would not give you a good report? No, of course not! If you do decide to talk to other patients treated by your doctor, you may find it helpful to ask them these questions.

- How long did you stay in the hospital?

- How long was the catheter left in your bladder?

- Was your pain well controlled after surgery?

- How was the nursing staff?

- What complications did you develop?

- How was the bedside manner of the physician?

- Was the doctor compassionate about your discomfort and feelings?

- Have you regained your urine control and sexual function, and how long did it take after surgery?

- Did the doctor do a good job of explaining everything to you?

If you do decide to have a specialist perform your surgery, the next question is, how do you find a good one? It may be necessary to call different doctors in your area to ask how many of these operations are done each year and how they assess their results. The best place to start is at a university hospital or a major medical institution. If none is nearby, consider going to another city. Although traveling out of town may be inconvenient, you will be living a long time so it is worth a trip to get the best result possible. After you recover from your operation, a local doctor can do the follow-up care so you will not need constant traveling.

Some men look at "Best Doctor Lists" published in books and magazines to find their surgeon. You should know that these are more like popularity contests rather than a true measure of excellence. They are not based on any surgical results. Some doctors on those lists may not be very good surgeons while others left off the list might be excellent.

What Happens before the Operation

Regardless of how the prostate will be removed, you first must have a preoperative evaluation that is done about one or two weeks before the surgery date. A complete physical examination and a heart test called an *electrocardiogram*, or *EKG*, will be performed. Blood will be taken to measure your blood count, called a *CBC*, as well as the amount of *sodium, potassium, chloride, carbon dioxide, blood urea nitrogen,* and *glucose* in the bloodstream. Additional tests may be ordered depending on your medical history. The goal of these tests is to make sure nothing is wrong that might increase your risk from having the operation.

For at least one week before surgery, you should not take over-the-counter medications that can increase your risk of bleeding. That includes any drug belonging to a group called *nonsteroidal anti-inflammatory drugs*, or *NSAIDS* such as aspirin, Motrin, ibuprofen, naprosyn, Aleve, and Celebrex. Vitamin E also should be avoided for the same reason. If one of these is taken by mistake within seven days of surgery, you should notify you doctor right away. Also, you should not eat or drink anything after midnight of the evening before surgery.

What to Expect on the Day of Surgery

You will be told to arrive at the hospital or surgical center a few hours before the scheduled time of the operation. Once there, you will change into a surgical gown and then be placed on a cart. Some surgeons doing a retropubic prostatectomy will ask that a blood sample be sent to the blood bank to crossmatch blood in case it is needed. An intravenous line is inserted into your arm to administer fluids and medications. You may receive a drug to relax you before being taken into the operating room.

The retropubic operation is performed under *general* or *spinal anesthesia*. General anesthesia means you are put to sleep and usually a tube is placed down your windpipe through your mouth. A ventilator will control your breathing and deliver a gas that keeps you asleep. Spinal anesthesia means you are awake but you will be unable to feel any pain in the lower half of your body. You still will breathe on your own. The spinal is done by injecting a local anesthetic under the skin in your lower back and then inserting a small needle into the fluid surrounding your spinal cord. An anesthetic drug is then injected into the needle. During the surgery, the anesthesiologist can give you other medication to make you feel sleepy so that you don't have to listen to the sounds in the operating room. The perineal, laparoscopic, and robot-assisted laparoscopic operations usually are done under general anesthesia. After the anesthetic takes effect, the skin is washed and covered with an antiseptic solution; sterile drapes are placed over the surgical site, and then the operation can begin.

What Happens during the Surgery

The retropubic prostatectomy begins with the surgeon making a cut in the skin from just below the navel down to the pubic bone. The length of the incision varies depending on a man's height but is usually about 8 to 10 centimeters long. No muscles are cut; they are simply spread apart to allow the surgeon to reach the prostate. The tissues holding the prostate in place are divided and then the surgeon feels behind the prostate to determine whether the cancer is growing outside the gland. If the cancer appears to be localized inside the prostate, then the pelvic nerves are preserved. However, if the surgeon feels a lump, hardness, or any other abnormality near the nerves, the safest approach is to remove one or both of them along with the prostate. Of course, this is a very subjective evaluation because there is no completely accurate way to tell whether cancer has grown near a pelvic nerve without removing it. If the doctor is uncertain, the safest approach for getting rid of the entire cancer is to remove the nerve.

Doctors sometimes take a different approach when they are unsure about saving the nerves. Initially the nerves are left in place while the prostate is removed and a *frozen section* is requested with the patient remaining under anesthesia. This means the pathologist will immediately examine the prostate under a microscope to see whether cancer has grown outside the gland near the location of each nerve. If that has happened, then one or both nerves can be removed before the operation is completed.

Because of the potential blood loss, many doctors ask their patients to donate one or two pints of blood a few weeks before surgery. It is given back during or shortly after the operation. In recent years this has been done less often because the blood obtained from the blood bank is much safer now and the amount of blood loss infrequently requires a transfusion. The following table shows the current odds of getting a side effect from a transfusion.

Table 9.1

Complications of Blood Transfusion	Frequency
Allergic reaction	1 out of every 333 pints
Hepatitis B	1 out of every 205,000 pints
Human immunodeficiency virus (HIV)	1 out of every 2,135,000 pints
Fever	1 out of every 100 pints

If you are going to have a retropubic prostatectomy, ask how often your doctor gives a transfusion and then decide whether you want to donate your blood, accept blood from the blood bank, or choose a different surgeon if he or she transfuses too many patients. Donating your own blood is not necessarily a good thing to do because it will lower your blood count going into the operation. Combining a low blood count before starting the operation with the amount of blood lost during surgery can raise the chances of your need for a transfusion. A side effect such as a fever or other allergic reaction can happen even from receiving your own blood.

The reason for requiring general anesthesia when a perineal prostatectomy is performed is because the patient must be placed in the lithotomy position with his legs raised off the table while he lies on his back. This operation begins by making a curved cut in the skin underneath the scrotum in front of the rectum, called the perineum. The length of this cut is about 6 to 8 centimeters. The surgeon separates the prostate from the rectum and can feel the backside of the gland to determine whether the nerves should be preserved. The tissues holding the prostate in place are divided so that the gland can be removed.

The laparoscopic prostatectomy begins by passing a small needle through the skin near the belly button and into the abdominal cavity. Carbon dioxide is passed through the needle, which separates the abdominal wall from the internal organs. This creates a space to do the surgery. Four skin openings are made in the lower abdomen, each one about 5 to 10 millimeters in length. A surgical instrument is inserted through three of the sites and a telescopic lens is passed through the fourth site. A camera is connected to the lens, which shows the surgical area on a TV screen located in the operating room. The surgeon performs the operation by looking at the TV screen rather than at the patient. After the prostate has been separated from the surrounding tissues, a 4 to 6 centimeter incision is made above the pubic bone to remove it from the body.

The robot-assisted prostatectomy begins in the same way as the laparoscopic prostatectomy with placement of the needle, inflating the abdomen with carbon dioxide, and then inserting the surgical instruments and a telescopic lens through the skin. Next, robotic arms with special cables are attached to each of them. The cables connect to a console at a separate table positioned several feet from the operating table. The surgeon sits at this table and looks through two eyepieces that give a three-dimensional view of the inside of the belly. Controls on the console and on the floor are used to move the instruments inside the patient. Every movement by the surgeon causes an identical movement of the robotic arms connected to the patient. After the prostate has been separated from the surrounding tissues, it is removed through a 4-centimeter cut made on the skin.

Completing the Operation

After the prostate has been removed, the remainder of the operation is the same for all four methods. Since the prostate was attached to the bladder and the urethra, these two structures must be reconnected to each other by placing several stitches. A rubber tube called a *Foley catheter* is inserted through the penis and passed into the bladder to drain urine while healing occurs. It is left in place for 3 to 14 days depending on the surgeon's preference. The catheter is held in place by a small water-filled balloon located at the end sitting in the bladder. The other end is connected to a bag that collects the urine. Patients are taught how to empty the urine from the bag, which is easy to do. They are sent home with two bags. A large one is used mostly at night to avoid overfilling. It lies on the floor or attaches to the lower part of the bed. Patients are told to keep the bag lower than the bladder, otherwise the urine will not drain properly and an infection may occur. The smaller bag is used during the day because it straps to the leg and is hidden under a man's pants allowing him to walk around without people noticing it. It is emptied directly into the toilet through a valve located at the lower end of the bag.

Toward the end of the operation, another rubber tube, called a *surgical drain*, is placed near the connection between the bladder and urethra. Many doctors performing a laparoscopic or robot-assisted prostatectomy have stopped inserting a surgical drain but it is still used for the retropubic and perineal methods. When it is used, the drain comes out of the body through another small opening in the skin that is made near the surgical incision. The drain helps avoid an infection by removing any fluids that collect in the pelvic area. It is held in place by a suture connecting it to the skin where it remains for one or two days.

What Happens after the Operation

When the operation is over, the patient is transferred to the recovery room and remains there until the anesthetic has worn off. Pain medication and intravenous fluids are given as needed. Patients are transferred to a hospital bed when stable. Usually, they can begin drinking fluids and possibly eating later in the day or the following morning. Patients are encouraged to cough and take deep breaths to avoid getting pneumonia. They are sent home when they are eating and walking, have a normal temperature, pills control their pain, and there is no evidence of an infection. Before being discharged, the drain is removed by cutting the suture and slowly sliding it out through the opening in the skin. This causes very little discomfort. The drain site then is covered with a bandage, which can be changed at home if needed.

What Happens after Leaving the Hospital

Doctors usually advise waiting one or two days before showering. After 5 to 10 days patients must return to have the wound checked and possibly the Foley catheter removed. The sutures used to close the skin incisions after the perineal, laparoscopic, and robotic operations are placed under the skin so there is no need to remove them. They will dissolve within 10 days. The staples used to close the incision made during the retropubic operation will be removed and covered with Steri-strips™. Some doctors perform an x-ray examination called a cystogram before taking out the catheter to make sure the connection between the bladder and urethra has healed. A dye is placed into the bladder through the catheter just before the x-ray is done. If a leak is seen, the catheter is left in place for one or two more weeks. The Foley is removed after first taking out the fluid from inside the catheter balloon. This is done using a syringe that connects to a valve on the catheter. The Foley then is slowly withdrawn, which takes less than two minutes and usually causes only a minor discomfort.

In most cases, urine leaks from the penis after the catheter is removed. Bringing a pair of Depends or some other absorbing material to wear underneath your clothes can avoid embarrassing leakage until you get home. Wearing dark colored pants also is recommended because they hide any leakage that might occur.

The amount of urine leakage and how long it will last vary between patients. You can help yourself by doing *Kegel exercises*. The way to learn how to do them is to start to urinate while in the shower and then tighten the pelvic muscles until the urine flow stops. Good studies have shown that starting these exercises either *four weeks before the operation* or just after the catheter has been removed can shorten the time of leakage. It also can result in better urinary control one year after the operation. The following schedule was used in one study that showed these exercises were helpful.

• Alternate 10 contractions of the pelvic muscles lasting 5 seconds with 10 seconds of muscular relaxation.

• Perform the exercises sitting, standing, squatting, and going up and down stairs.

• Perform three sets of exercises daily for six months.

Most doctors probably are not aware of the results of these studies, so the best course of action is to begin these exercises on your own a few weeks before surgery. You should be patient about regaining your urinary control. Some men regain complete control very quickly, but up to one year may be required before urine control returns to near normal. Unfortunately, leakage does not stop in all patients. Treatment options for urinary incontinence are explained in chapter 18.

Another important part of your recovery is doing something to help your sexual function. Opinions vary on what to do. Most doctors have no specific advice while others suggest taking Viagra, Levitra, or Cialis on a regular basis or using a *vacuum pump* device. The options available for improving your sexual function also are discussed in chapter 18.

Follow-Up Care

Most men begin to feel reasonably well within two weeks of surgery but this is quite variable. Vigorous exercise or heavy lifting or straining should be avoided for two weeks following a perineal operation, four weeks after the robot-assisted or laparo-scopic operation, and about six weeks after the retropubic operation. Most doctors have their patients return for an evaluation about every three months during the first year and every three to six months in the second year. At each visit, a prostate-specific antigen (PSA) and digital rectal examination (DRE) will be performed. Any decision about additional treatment will be made based on your pathology report from surgery and the PSA level. Even if you get a good result, you should continue to have regular PSA tests because the cancer can reappear many years later.

What Are the Potential Complications of Radical Prostatectomy?

The lack of randomized studies presents a challenge for comparing the odds of getting side effects or complications for the different treatments. Uncontrolled studies can, however, give you some idea of how they compare. You should be aware that the true results depend on many factors including a man's age and health, the specifics about his cancer, and most importantly, the experience of the doctor doing the operation.

Short-Term Complications

Short-term complications are defined as those occurring within the first 30 days after surgery. The most common ones and their frequency for each operation are shown in the next table and explained below.

Table 9.2 Short-Term Complications after Radical Prostatectomy

Complication	Retropubic	Perineal	Laparoscopic	Robotic
Blood transfusions	21%	7.25%–11%	2.2%	0%–2%
Deep venous thrombosis/ pulmonary embolus	0.1%–2%	Not available	0.6%	0%–0.5%
Rectal injury	0.5%–0.6%	1.4%–11%	0.4%–2.2%	0.7%–4.1%
Lymphocele	3%–14%	15%	2%–5%	0%
Urethral stricture	2%–9%	3%	2.2%–5%	0.6%
Death	0.1%–0.5%	0.5%	0.1%	0.1%

- **Deep Venous Thrombosis/Pulmonary Embolus:** A blood clot that forms in a leg vein causing pain, fever, and swelling. It is treated in the hospital with *anticoagulants* to "thin the blood." Sometimes the blood clot moves to the lungs, forming a *pulmonary embolus*, which can be life-threatening. It also is treated with blood thinners but surgery might be needed in rare cases to remove the clot.

- **Rectal Injury:** An opening into the rectum may occur because it is separated from the prostate by only a few millimeters. The injury is fixed by placing sutures into the rectum. Sometimes, however, the risk of infection is too high. In those cases, the intestine must be brought to the skin creating a *colostomy*. A bag is worn over the opening to drain the bowel contents. About six weeks later, another operation is done to close the colostomy, restoring normal bowel function. Sometimes an injury to the rectum is repaired at surgery but it does not heal properly. About 7 to 10 days later, bowel contents are seen coming through the skin or in the urine, called a *recto-cutaneous* or *rectourethral fistula*. Placing a catheter in the bladder may allow the latter type to heal without other therapy. Often, however, another operation is needed to repair the opening in the bowel and do a colostomy until the repaired area heals. The colostomy can be closed at another operation six weeks later.

- **Lymphocele:** When lymph nodes are removed, sometimes lymph fluid leaks into the surrounding tissues and forms a fluid collection called a *lymphocele*. It usually causes pain and fever. The proper treatment is to drain the fluid. In most cases, an x-ray can be used to guide a needle through the skin and into the fluid collection to help drain it. Sometimes a lymphocele becomes infected and then it also must be treated with antibiotics.

- **Urethral Stricture:** At the end of the operation, the bladder is connected to the urethra, which sometimes leads to scarring. Another name for this is a *bladder neck contracture*. Treatment consists of dilating it with an instrument or cutting it with a laser passed through a cystoscope that is inserted into the urethra through the penis after medicine is given to minimize discomfort.

- **Heart Attack, Congestive Heart Failure, and Death:** All of these also can occur with any operation. A heart attack and congestive heart failure require hospitalization and in some cases surgery or placement of a stent into blood vessels supplying the heart.

Several other injuries can also occur including an infection at the skin, damage to an internal organ such as the bladder, a ureter or an artery, and vein. All of these can be repaired immediately provided the surgeon is aware one of these has occurred. On rare occasions, these injuries are not found until sometime after surgery and then another operation is needed to correct the problem. Respiratory complications may result secondary to the anesthesia.

Long-Term Complications

The long-term complications are anything occurring beyond the first 30 days of surgery. Comparing long-term complications following the different surgical methods is difficult to do because no randomized studies are available and each uncontrolled report contains patients with very varied characteristics. The range of the common complications reported from many studies is shown in the following table with an explanation included afterward. Remember, the chances you might get one or more of these side effects depend mostly on the skill of your surgeon. Men are encouraged to ask their surgeon about their specific results.

Table 9.3 Late Complications of Radical Prostatectomy

Complications	Odds They May Occur
Leaking urine (urinary incontinence)	3%–30%
Difficulty having erections (impotence)	20%–90%
Urethral stricture	5%–14%
Inguinal hernia	7%–21%
Penile shortening	15%–80%
Pain during ejaculation	10%–15%
Dry orgasm	100%

Urinary Incontinence: This means urine leaks out from the penis. It can vary from a few drops with heavy exertion to leaking urine every minute of the day. Urinary incontinence probably is the most embarrassing side effect of radical prostatectomy. It happens to almost every man immediately after surgery. Some improve very quickly while others take up to a year to fully regain control. A small percentage never get back to normal and require either medication, the use of pads inside their underwear, or even surgery to correct the problem.

Impotence (Erectile Dysfunction): This is defined as being unable to have an erection good enough for sexual intercourse. Even when a nerve-sparing prostatectomy is done properly, some men become impotent for reasons doctors cannot explain. It occurs immediately after surgery in almost all men but can get better over time. In some cases erections return within a few weeks but it can take up to two years. Some men never regain spontaneous sexual function.

Urethral Stricture: This is a scar that forms in the tube carrying urine from the bladder out through the tip of the penis. It results in slowing of the urinary stream and in some cases men are unable to urinate. Once treated, a urethral stricture may recur, requiring repeated treatments.

Inguinal Hernia: This is an extension of a portion of the intestine down the inguinal canal toward the scrotum. It feels like a bulge in the groin area. The development of an inguinal hernia has not been widely recognized as a side effect of a radical prostatectomy, but recently, several good studies have shown that it does occur. Doctors think that some men have an undiscovered hernia that is made worse by the operation rather than being caused by it. If you are planning to have this treatment you should ask your doctor to examine you while standing and straining. This is called a *Valsalva maneuver*. If a hernia is found, it can be fixed during the prostatectomy; otherwise, another operation will be needed. A hernia is not a side effect of the perineal prostatectomy method.

Penile Shortening: This side effect rarely is discussed with patients prior to surgery. It is determined by measuring the length of the stretched penis before surgery and again after the operation. The loss is greatest at the time the catheter is removed from the penis and it can improve gradually. The average loss is one centimeter. It may completely resolve within four years. The incidence may be less in men having both pelvic nerves preserved.

Painful Orgasm: This is another side effect seldom discussed by surgeons. It usually lasts for about one minute during sexual activity. Some men report it is so severe that it interferes with normal sexual function.

Dry Orgasm: During the operation, the tubes carrying seminal fluid to the penis are cut, preventing any fluid from coming out following an orgasm. This will be permanent and there is no treatment for it. Some men report this decreases their pleasure during sexual activity.

By now you might be overwhelmed as you read about all these side effects and the odds they might occur. Because so many factors affect the results, the best thing you can do is be ready to ask your doctor how often each of them occurs in his or her practice. That way you can decide whether the odds are acceptable or whether you want to go find a doctor with more expertise.

What Are the Chances the Cancer Will Return?

After the prostate has been removed, the predominant source of PSA is gone so the value usually drops to less than 0.05 ng/ml. In most cases it becomes undetectable. Since this takes about four weeks, measuring it before this time could give a falsely high number. Does a low PSA level mean you are cured? Not necessarily. A few cancer cells might still be in your body but they don't produce enough PSA to be detected by the test. Where would they be located? Some could have grown into the area surrounding the prostate, some may have spread to other parts of the body, or some could be in multiple locations. As the cells multiply, the PSA eventually will rise, but it could take 15 years or more. That is why you should continue to have the test.

Because you can't be sure whether you have been cured, you might begin to wonder about your odds of getting a recurrence. Fortunately, tools now are available that can give you this information. One is called *Kattan nomogram*, which is based on several characteristics about your tumor as shown in the table.

Table 9.4 Information Used for the Kattan Nomogram

1. The PSA level before surgery

2. The tumor stage before surgery

3. The primary and secondary Gleason grade on the radical prostatectomy

4. The extent of cancer found at surgery

5. The presence or absence of cancer in the seminal vesicles and lymph nodes

This calculator is freely available at the Memorial Sloan Kettering Hospital website (www.mskcc.org). Once you log on to the site, enter "prostate" as the type of cancer. Then click on "prostate cancer prediction tool" and select "prediction tool after radical prostatectomy." You can get your personal results if you enter the information found on your pathology report, which you can get from your doctor. The information you will need includes:

Primary and Secondary Gleason Grades: As explained in chapter 3, every prostate cancer is given two numbers, each from 1 to 5. It is based on how the cells appear when viewed under a microscope. The first number is called the *primary Gleason grade*. It is the number given to the most common type of cancer cells seen in the tissue. The second number is the *secondary Gleason* grade. It is the number given to the second most common type of cancer cells. Most operative reports provide these numbers. For example, a report may say, "Gleason score 3+3=6" or "4+3=7." If the report only gives the total Gleason score without the primary and secondary numbers, then you can contact the pathology department and ask for the individual numbers. If the Gleason score is reported as 4, 6, or 8, you can assume that the primary and secondary Gleason grades are very likely the same. It is very rare for a man to have two Gleason grades that are two numbers apart such as 1+3, 2+4, or 3+5.

Clinical Stage: As also explained in chapter 3, the clinical stage is partly based on what the doctor feels during a digital rectal examination. The pathological stage is what is found on the biopsy report. If you do not know it, ask your doctor to provide it to you. The possibilities include T1a, T1b, T1c, T2a, T2b, T2c, T3a, T3b, T4a, and T4b (see chapter 3).

Tumor Margin: After the prostate is removed, the pathologist will coat the outside of the prostate with ink before processing the tissue. A positive margin means cancer cells are touching the ink.

Capsular Penetration: The capsule is a very thin layer of tissue that surrounds the prostate. Capsular penetration means cancer cells are growing outside the capsule.

Seminal Vesicle Invasion: The seminal vesicles are two small glands attached to the prostate. Seminal vesicle invasion means cancer cells have grown in one or both of the seminal vesicles.

Lymph Node Invasion: The pathology report will state whether lymph nodes were removed during surgery and whether any of them contain cancer. If the lymph nodes were not removed then enter N0 into the computer if you are using the prostate cancer prediction tool.

The Kattan nomogram was developed using results from thousands of patients. It has been rechecked on many other patients and appears to be very reliable. You should realize what it does and does not do. It *does* tell you what happened to a group of men with similar types of tumors as yours. It *does not* tell exactly what will happen to you.

Two cases below show the information provided by this tool. The first patient is 55 years old, his Gleason score is 3+3=6, the tumor stage is T1c, the tumor margins are negative, the capsule is not penetrated, and the seminal vesicles and lymph nodes do not show cancer. The second patient has a more aggressive cancer. He is 62 years old, his Gleason score is 4+4=8, the tumor stage is T2b, the tumor margin is positive, and cancer has invaded into the seminal vesicles and the lymph nodes.

Although the two men only have a slightly different chance of dying from prostate cancer in the next 15 years, the second man has a much greater chance that his PSA will go up. Knowing that the recurrence rate is high, this patient might be willing to have radiation therapy to the prostate bed to reduce his risk of recurrence. The first patient does not need to consider additional therapy at this time.

The information from the Kattan nomogram can help you with your care. If you have a very low risk of developing a rise in your PSA, monitoring can be done less often, perhaps every one or two years. If the PSA does go up, you may not feel the need to have it treated right away because it has a low chance of harming you. If you have a higher risk of recurrence, you would continue to be tested more often and may want to have additional treatment.

A less helpful tool for predicting the likelihood of developing a significant increase in the PSA is a test called the *ultrasensitive PSA*. It can detect smaller amounts of PSA in a blood sample than the standard test and if the level is very low, the chance of your PSA going up also is very low. For example, when the ultrasensitive PSA level is below 0.01 ng/ml, the odds of it rising in the next three years are only 4%, but it is almost 90% when the ultrasensitive PSA is at least 0.04 ng/ml.

Table 9.5 Examples Using the Kattan Nomogram

Patient Characteristic	Patient 1 (age 55)	Patient 2 (age 62)
Age at surgery (years)	55	62
PSA before surgery (ng/ml)	6	11
Primary Gleason grade	3	4
Secondary Gleason grade	3	4
Clinical stage	T1c	T2b
Tumor margins positive	No	Yes
Extracapsular extension	No	No
Cancer in seminal vesicles	No	Yes
Cancer in lymph nodes	No	Yes
Chances for Recurrence	**Patient 1**	**Patient 2**
Chance of PSA rising above 0.4 ng/ml in 5 years	3%	55%
Chance of PSA rising above 0.4 ng/ml in 10 years	5%	74%
Chance of dying from prostate cancer in 10 years	1%	1%
Chance of dying from prostate cancer in 15 years	1%	3%

This tool is not as useful as the Kattan nomogram for several reasons. First, more time is needed after surgery for the PSA to drop to its lowest level. You can have a standard PSA test done four to six weeks after surgery, but one study found the ultrasensitive PSA took 8 to 10 months before it dropped below 0.01 ng/ml. The only way to be sure that an ultrasensitive PSA level has "bottomed-out" is by performing additional PSA tests several weeks or months later to see whether it remains stable. This may cause you considerable anxiety while waiting for that to occur.

A second and more important problem with the ultrasensitive test is that doctors do not definitely know what to do with the information. If your result is higher than 0.01 ng/ml, should you get treated immediately or wait until the PSA is rising? Treating all men with this ultrasensitive PSA result would mean many of them would get a treatment they would never need. For example, treating 100 men with an ultrasensitive PSA of 0.02 ng/ml means that at least 85 are getting unnecessary treatment. Based on these concerns, the standard PSA is sufficient for follow-up testing until studies report results with a longer follow-up using the ultrasensitive test.

What to Do If the Risk for Recurrence Is High

If you are uncomfortable with the estimated risk of getting a recurrence of your cancer, what should you do? Should you have radiation therapy to the area where the prostate was located, ADT, or both? Only one good study has been done to answer this question. It assigned men to get radiation within 18 weeks of the prostatectomy or be observed until the disease recurred. All of them had cancer growing outside their prostate. With more than half the men followed longer than 12.5 years, the key results were:

- Metastatic disease occurred in 54% of the men in the control compared to only 46% in the group getting immediate radiation. These results mean that radiation therapy must be given to about twelve men to prevent one from getting metastatic disease over the next 12.5 years.

- One-half of the men treated with radiation lived slightly more than 15 years compared with slightly more than 13 years in the control group. This means about nine men must be treated to prevent one from dying over the next 12.5 years.

- Five years after surgery, ADT was started in 10% of the radiation group compared with 21% in the control group.

- Complications were more common in men receiving radiation including:
  Bowel irritation (proctitis) or rectal bleeding (3% vs. 0%)
  Urethral strictures (18% vs. 10%)
  Urinary incontinence (7% vs. 3%)

- Two years after radiation, both groups had similar bowel and sexual function, but urinary frequency was more common in the group getting radiation.

This study shows a small but definite benefit from immediate radiation. The trade-off is that many men get a treatment that does not help them and they end up with slightly worse urinary function. You will have to decide whether the benefits are worth the risks. If your cancer is outside the prostate and you want to do everything possible to survive, then have the radiation early rather than waiting for the PSA to rise. It is even possible that getting radiation today will give better results than that shown in the study. The reason is a higher dose now can be given compared with the amount given in the past without causing more side effects.

What to Do If the Prostate-Specific Antigen (PSA) Is Detectable after Surgery

In a small percentage of men, the standard PSA does not drop to the desired level after surgery. The reasons could be:

- **Someone else's blood sample was tested.** Though rare, mistakes can occur and most doctors will confirm the result with a second test.

- **Some prostate tissue was left behind.** Although the goal is always to remove the entire prostate, sometimes the surgeon makes a technical error and leaves some prostate tissue in the body, which will make PSA whether it contains normal cells or cancer cells. The only way to find out whether cancer is still present is by following the PSA over time or eventually doing a biopsy. No other test can accurately explain the reason for an abnormal PSA.

- **Cancer cells already had spread outside the prostate before the operation.** The pathology report might be useful since most pathologists coat the outer surface of the prostate with colored ink before it is processed. When the specimen is viewed under a microscope, the pathologist may see cancer cells touching the ink. This could mean cancer is still in that area.

- **Cancer has spread to some other area of the body.** These cancer cells continue producing PSA after the prostate is gone, which prevents the PSA from dropping to an undetectable level. If the PSA continues to rise, either a bone scan or ProstaScint® scan eventually may show where the cancer is located.

How do you decide what to do if this happens to you? The first thing to know is that you are in no immediate danger, but it does mean that your PSA is likely to keep going up. Should you have radiation therapy, ADT, or both? In the study discussed earlier in this chapter, about one-third of the men had a PSA above 0.2 ng/ml following surgery. Getting radiation within three months also improved their survival. This means radiation also helps men with a measurable PSA after surgery. Good studies have not yet been done to find out if adding ADT to the radiation will make things even better. Even so, it is an option that may cause side effects that may reduce your quality of life.

Another option is to *not get radiation right away* but instead wait to see whether and when your PSA eventually goes up. It may allow you to avoid getting an unnecessary treatment. At this time, doctors do not know whether starting the radiation later will be as helpful as getting it very soon after surgery. Also, studies are not available that tell what happens by adding ADT. The key thing to remember is radiation offers some benefits but it does have trade-offs. More information about managing a rising PSA after radical prostatectomy is provided in chapter 19.

The Bottom Line on Radical Prostatectomy

Each treatment you read about in this book has reasons to choose it and reasons to avoid it. Surgery is the right choice if you want the most aggressive treatment for your cancer provided you are willing to accept the possible side effects. More information is available about the results with this treatment than any other option. That means the long-term results with other treatments are more uncertain. You must realize, however, that no good study has proven that surgery definitely is better than any of the other options. In chapter 17, information will be provided that compares this treatment with some of the other options and ways to think about them so that you can determine which one is right for you. Knowing the right questions to ask is the best thing you can do to help you make a decision.

Removing the Lymph Nodes: If, When, and How?

If you decide to have a radical prostatectomy, a question that must be addressed before surgery is what to do about the pelvic lymph nodes: Should they be removed or left in place? You need to be aware that doctors have very different ideas about what to do. The following three approaches are being used:

1. Remove the lymph nodes in all patients.

2. Leave them alone if they feel normal and the estimated risk of cancer having spread into them is less than 15%, but take them out if the risk is higher.

3. If the risk is higher than 15%, they should be removed and sent for frozen sections before deciding whether to take out the prostate. If cancer is found in the lymph nodes, the operation should be discontinued and other treatments should be offered after the patient recovers.

Understanding the pros and cons of each approach will enable you to share the decision with your doctor about what to do. First, you need to know several facts about the lymph nodes and treatment results when prostate cancer cells invade them:

- The term for cancer in the lymph nodes is *lymph node metastases*.

- If cancer has not spread into the lymph nodes, meaning they are normal, there is no benefit to the patient from taking them out. The surgeon, however, benefits by collecting a higher fee.

- No test can tell if cancer is in the lymph nodes. The only way to know for sure is to remove them and examine them under the microscope. Doctors remove them by doing an operation called a *pelvic lymphadenectomy* or *pelvic lymph node dissection* (PLND).

- Lymph nodes are named according to a nearby blood vessel. Those closest to the prostate are called the *external iliac and obturator* nodes, followed by the *hypogastric, internal iliac, and presacral nodes,* and then the *common iliac and aortic nodes.* In the past, surgeons routinely performed a *limited pelvic lymphadenectomy,* which removes only the external iliac and obturator nodes. They thought that if the lymph nodes closest to the prostate were negative, then the others further away also would be negative. Recently, this thinking has changed, however, because studies have found that prostate cancer sometimes skips the close lymph nodes and invades others further away. That means doing only the limited operation will miss some men who have lymph node metastases. To be more certain whether cancer has spread, an *extended pelvic lymphadenectomy* is needed. The disadvantages of this procedure are that it takes longer to perform, requires more time for the pathologist to do the frozen sections, and has a slightly higher complication rate.

- No good studies have proven that patients will benefit from a radical prostatectomy when cancer has spread to the lymph nodes. That is why some doctors remove the lymph nodes and wait for the pathologist to do frozen sections on the tissue to see whether cancer is present. This takes about 15 to 30 minutes to complete. If they are negative, meaning cancer is not present, then the prostatectomy is completed. If they are *positive*, meaning cancer is in the lymph nodes, the prostate is not removed, the wound is closed, and a different treatment is done after the person recovers from surgery. The reason for this approach is to spare a patient from the side effects of the prostatectomy when it doesn't definitely improve survival.

- The chance that cancer has spread into the lymph nodes can be estimated based on the prostate-specific antigen (PSA) test, the Gleason score, and the clinical stage, as was explained in chapter 3. This information can be used to decide whether the lymph nodes can be left alone or should be removed.

The Pros and Cons of Removing the Lymph Nodes

You may find it helpful to understand why doctors have these different opinions about managing the lymph nodes.

Approach #1: Those who routinely remove the lymph nodes in all patients, even those with a low risk of lymph node metastases without doing frozen sections, argue:

- It is easy to do and takes very little time.

- Even if it doesn't improve survival, the chances that a limited lymph node dissection will cause complications are low.

- If cancer is found in the lymph nodes you can get androgen deprivation therapy (ADT), which will increase your chances for survival.

- Doing a frozen section and waiting for the results before completing the prostatectomy should be avoided because it keeps you under anesthesia for a longer time.

Approach #2: Doctors who leave the lymph nodes in place in men at low risk for metastases, but remove them in men at high risk for lymph node metastases and immediately take out the prostate without doing frozen section, argue:

- Although no studies prove you will live longer by taking out the prostate when cancer has spread to the lymph nodes, there is a possibility. Even if the odds of benefitting are very small, you could be the one who is helped by it, so why not go for it?

- Removing the prostate helps avoid urinary problems in the future.

Approach #3: Doctors who leave the lymph nodes in place when the risk of lymph node metastases is low but do frozen sections when the chances of spreading are high and wait for the results before deciding whether to remove the prostate, argue:

- Removing negative lymph nodes offers no benefit, so why do it when it may increase your risk of complications?

- There is no proven benefit from taking out the prostate when cancer is in the lymph nodes. So, why should you be subjected to an operation that could reduce your quality of life without improving your chances for survival?

- The standard way of surgically removing lymph nodes misses many that are positive. To be more accurate, an extended lymph node operation is needed, which has a higher risk of complications. For this reason, it should be done only in men with a high (greater than 15%) risk for lymph node metastases and omitted when the risk of metastases is lower.

Should You Have Your Lymph Nodes Removed?

Now that you understand the reasons why doctors vary in their approaches, your next question probably is, what should I do? Of the three options available, the most prudent approach is number three: leave the lymph nodes alone when the risk of metastases is very low and do an extended lymphadenectomy with frozen sections when the risk is high. If the lymph nodes show cancer, then leave the prostate in place, and if they are negative, finish the prostatectomy. This provides the best balance between the potential for benefit and the potential for harm. Fortunately, more than 80% of all new cases diagnosed today have only a 0% to 1% chance of cancer in the lymph nodes. If these are your odds, removing the lymph nodes makes no *sense*. Your chance of having an unnecessary operation would be 99%. The only good reason to remove the lymph nodes is if they feel suspicious when the doctor examines them during surgery.

Despite the arguments made for this approach, you may want to be as aggressive as possible and may be willing to accept the risks. In that case, tell your doctor you want the lymph nodes and the prostate removed and do not want frozen sections performed.

What Are the Complications of a Pelvic Lymph Node Dissection?

Although the complication rate of removing the lymph nodes is much lower today than it was 20 years ago, some that occur are very serious. Of course, the frequency of side effects will vary depending on the surgeon. The results from one good study of a limited dissection are shown in the next table.

Table 10.1

Complications of PLND	Frequency
Bowel injury	1%
Injury to obturator nerve	1%–2%
Deep venous thrombosis	5%–6%
Lymphocele	9%–11%
Pulmonary embolism	1%–2%

Some of these complications could be due to taking out the prostate along with the lymph nodes rather than just from removing the lymph nodes themselves. Very little recent information is available about the frequency of side effects in men having a PLND without the prostatectomy. Injuries to the bowel and obturator nerve can be serious if not treated properly. They must be recognized during surgery and repaired immediately. The other three complications can be serious and life-threatening.

What Should Be Done If Cancer Is in the Lymph Nodes?

Doctors continue to disagree about the best treatment for men with cancer in the lymph nodes. The options depend on whether it is found during the frozen sections or several days after the prostate has been removed when the tissue has been examined. If metastases are found on the frozen sections, the treatment options include:

- Leave the prostate in place and give immediate ADT, or delay it until the PSA rises.

- Take out the prostate and give ADT immediately, or delay until the PSA rises.

- Leave the prostate in place and give radiation combined with immediate or delayed ADT.

Since no well-done studies have been completed, all three options are reasonable. If you want to be conservative and avoid the risk of impotence, incontinence, and other complications of surgery, then leave the prostate in place and delay the ADT. If you want to be aggressive, then take out the prostate and start ADT right away.

If lymph node metastases are discovered several days after the prostate has been removed, then your choices are immediate or delayed ADT. Radiation at that time has not been properly tested so its value remains uncertain. Only one randomized study has been done in this group of patients. Men were given either immediate ADT or it was delayed until the cancer had spread into the bones. With half the men followed for almost 11 years, those getting immediate ADT were almost twice as likely to be alive as those getting delayed treatment. This study has been criticized for enrolling fewer men than initially intended, which could have biased the results. Even so, it was well done and does provide useful information that can help guide your decision.

The Bottom Line on Removing the Lymph Nodes

You should be part of the decision about your lymph nodes. If you want to do everything possible that might improve your survival, then have the lymph nodes and the prostate removed. Do not bother having frozen sections done. However, the operation should include an extended, rather than a limited, pelvic lymphadenectomy.

If you prefer to have a more balanced approach that avoids unnecessary risk, then be more selective. Do not have the lymph nodes removed unless your odds of lymph node metastases are at least 15% as estimated from the Partin tables. If they are removed, then it should be done by an extended PLND with frozen sections. Your prostate should be removed only if the lymph nodes are negative. Here again, the best advice is to discuss the options with your surgeon and ask the necessary questions.

External Beam Radiation

When doctors talk about radiation therapy for prostate cancer, they may use different terms including *external beam radiation*, *XRT*, and *EBRT*. They all mean that the source of the radiation is located outside a patient's body. In the next chapter you will read about ways to deliver radiation with the source placed inside a person's body. Fortunately, for those men considering external radiation, this treatment has gone through many changes over the past 20 years, resulting in more ways of doing it with fewer complications. The challenge is trying to decide which approach is a good option for treating your localized prostate cancer.

What Is Radiation and How Does It Work?

Before discussing details of the different types of external radiation that are available, you should know some basics about what it is and how it works. Radiation is a type of energy. It can occur naturally such as the radiation from the sun or it can be man-made such as the energy from your microwave oven. The level or intensity of the energy determines how it affects our body. For example, a microwave produces a low level of energy, making it very safe. In contrast, the sun produces a very high level of energy, making it potentially more dangerous.

All living cells contain DNA, which controls their ability to divide. Cancer cells harm us because they continue to divide without limitation. The different types of radiation used to treat prostate cancer deliver energy that is so strong it can either damage the DNA in cancer cells, causing them to die or make them unable to divide.

What Are the Benefits and Risks of External Radiation for Prostate Cancer?

The advantage of external radiation is that it may cure your disease without having an operation. The potential disadvantages include the side effects that may occur and the greater difficulty of doing surgery if the cancer is not eliminated. Also, some studies suggest that radiation slightly increases the risk of developing bladder or rectal cancer more than 10 years after the treatment. Doctors are uncertain how this risk will be affected by changes that have occurred in the equipment delivering the radiation and the amount of radiation patients are now receiving. The most common side effects of radiation are shown in the following table.

Table 11.1

Side Effects of External Radiation
Impotence
Incontinence
Bowel dysfunction (diarrhea, bloody stool, urgency to have a bowel movement)
Sexual dysfunction
Hematuria
Anejaculation

Bowel changes may begin within a few weeks of starting treatment and gradually go away in several months, although a small percentage of men continue to have problems permanently. Impotence, incontinence, and hematuria may not fully develop until one or two years later. Another side effect rarely reported is *anejaculation*, meaning no fluid comes out of the penis following an orgasm. One recent study of men using written surveys found that by three years, 69% had this problem and at five years it occurred in 89%. The exact frequency of these side effects depends on many factors including the experience of the radiation therapist, a patient's age and health, the amount of radiation delivered, and the equipment used. Making conclusions is nearly impossible when studies include men who differ in so many ways. Rather than quote you percentages that may be inaccurate, your best course of action is to ask your doctor for the results seen in his or her patients. Remember to ask how those results were gathered. Written surveys completed by patients are much more accurate than answering a nurse's or doctor's questions during an office visit.

How Are Side Effects Rated?

Radiation therapists have created a scoring system for the short-term and long-term bowel and bladder side effects that occur following this treatment. It ranges from 0–5. For both short- and long-term effects, grade 0 means no side effect has occurred and grade 5 means a patient has died as a result of this complication. The definitions of the other grades are shown in the next four tables. The same grades apply to external radiation, as well as to temporary and permanent brachytherapy.

Table 11.2 Short-Term Bowel Side Effects following Radiation Therapy

Grade 1	Grade 2	Grade 3	Grade 4
Increased frequency or change in quality of bowel habits not requiring medication Rectal discomfort not requiring analgesics	Diarrhea requiring medication Mucous discharge not needing pads Rectal or abdominal pain requiring drugs	Diarrhea requiring IV fluids Severe mucous or blood discharge needing pads Abdominal distention	Acute bowel obstruction Hole in bowel wall Bleeding requiring transfusion Abdominal pain or cramping requiring tube placement or colostomy

Table 11.3 Long-Term Bowel Side Effects following Radiation Therapy

Grade 1	Grade 2	Grade 3	Grade 4
Mild diarrhea Mild cramping Five bowel movements a day Slight rectal discharge Rectal bleeding	Moderate diarrhea More than five daily bowel movements Daily rectal mucus Intermittent bleeding	Obstruction or bleeding requiring surgery	Dead bowel tissue Opening in bowel wall Bowel contents leak into body

Table 11.4 Short-Term Bladder/Urinary Side Effects following Radiation Therapy

Grade 1	Grade 2	Grade 3	Grade 4
Frequent urination	Frequent urination	Frequency, urgency, and urinating at night at least hourly	Blood in urine requiring transfusion
Urinating twice per night	Urinating at night less often than hourly		Acute bladder obstruction not secondary to clot passage
Urgency to urinate not requiring medication	Burning, urgency, or bladder spasms requiring medication	Burning, pelvic pain, or bladder spasm requiring narcotics	
		Blood in urine without clots	Bladder ulceration or dead bladder tissue

Table 11.5 Long-Term Bladder Side and Urinary Side Effects following Radiation Therapy

Grade 1	Grade 2	Grade 3	Grade 4
Minor areas of bladder irritation	Moderate urinary frequency	Severe urinary frequency and burning	Necrosis/ contracted bladder (capacity <100 cc)
Microscopic bleeding in urine	Redness throughout bladder lining	Severe generalized redness in bladder	
	Intermittent visible blood in urine	Frequent bloody urine	Severe bleeding
		Reduction in bladder capacity (<150 cc)	

Options for External Radiation

Several options are available now for treating men with external radiation. The list includes:

- External beam radiation therapy (EBRT)

- Three-dimensional conformal radiation (3D-CRT)

- Intensity-modulated radiation therapy (IMRT)

- Image-guided radiation therapy (IGRT) or stereotactic guided radiation therapy (SGRT)

- Proton beam radiation therapy (PBR)

External Beam Radiation Therapy

Of all the radiation options, EBRT has been used for the longest time. Before treatment can begin, a CT scan is done so the radiation therapist can create a treatment plan. The size and shape of your prostate will determine where the radiation will be given and how much will be used. Radiation is measured in units called *rads* or *gray*. Rad stands for radiation absorbed dose and gray is a metric term that is being used more often when discussing prostate cancer. It is abbreviated as Gy. The total amount of radiation used for prostate cancer usually is between 6600 and 7000 rads or 66 and 70 Gy.

Before you begin your treatments, ink markings are placed on your body to help direct the beams to the right location for each treatment. Traditional external beam is delivered by a *linear accelerator or LINAC*. The treatment is aimed a few millimeters beyond the outer capsule of the prostate to help ensure that any cancer cells growing beyond the prostate are also killed by the treatment. Some doctors also direct radiation to the pelvic lymph nodes.

Treatment is given once a day, five days a week, until all the radiation has been delivered. This takes about seven to nine weeks depending on the total dose chosen by your doctor. Each day, you will lie on a table and then an x-ray will be taken to make sure you are in the proper position. After you have been properly positioned, the treatment only takes a few minutes and then you can go home. You will not feel anything during these treatments. All of your daily activities can be resumed immediately after leaving the treatment center.

However, after many years of doing EBRT, doctors rarely do it this way now because studies have shown that the doses used were often inadequate for killing all the cancer cells.

Three-Dimensional Conformal Radiation

Improvements in the LINAC equipment have made it possible to focus radiation beams more directly on the prostate and less on the surrounding tissues. This has enabled patients to receive higher doses of radiation without causing more complications. In fact, the complication rates have declined. 3D-CRT is done using computers, which plan the treatment from different angles to the body according to the shape of the prostate. The dose used with this approach ranges from about 68 Gy to 81 Gy. Before beginning, a body mold of the pelvis is made and each day the patient fits into the mold to keep him close to the same position during treatment. Here too, the radiation is delivered very quickly, and after leaving the radiation site, patients can resume all activities right away.

Intensity-Modulated Radiation Therapy

The next improvement was a modification of 3D-CRT. The radiation is broken up into a large number of narrow beams rather than a single, wide beam. The intensity of each beam is adjustable, allowing greater control of the dose given to the prostate and the surrounding organs. A computer determines the amount of radiation delivered from each beam. The net result is that more radiation reaches the cancer without greatly increasing the amount to the bladder or rectum. A CT scan is performed to plan the treatment and a body mold is made to keep the patient in the same position each day while being treated.

Image-Guided Radiation Therapy or Stereotactic Guided Radiation Therapy

With standard IMRT, the treatment is planned based on a single CT scan done before the treatment begins. One of the challenges of delivering radiation is that each day the prostate may be in a slightly different position due to the bladder filling with urine or the rectum filling with air and stool. This can result in undertreating the cancer or overtreating the surrounding tissues. A solution for this problem is to constantly monitor the position of the prostate using a CT scan that is built into the radiation machine. Before each treatment, the scan will identify the proper area to treat. This is IGRT.

Another way to locate the prostate for each treatment is to use *fiducial markers* that will enable the radiation machine to identify the correct area to radiate. They are placed into the prostate through the rectum using ultrasound guidance. Some of them emit a signal that can be detected by the radiation equipment, which aids in properly targeting the radiation. These sensors send off signals 10 times per second that deliver information about the location of the prostate. It functions like a Global Positioning System that you may use in your car to guide you to a destination. Some call it a "GPS for the body." The *CyberKnife®️ system* of SGRT uses this approach. One week after the markers are placed in the prostate, the radiation will begin. None of the methods using these markers have shown superiority, so for now any of them can be used. Long-term results are not yet available to know how this method compares with IMRT.

One potential advantage of IGRT or SGRT is that doctors can give even higher doses of radiation without significantly increasing the odds of experiencing side effects. Total doses over 80 Gy are being used. Another advantage is the ability to increase the daily dose of radiation. The term for this is *hypofractionation*. The treatment is completed in four to five weeks and even in as short as one week.

Placing the markers will cause some side effects in some men such as urinary frequency, blood in the urine, rectal bleeding, and burning during urination. Over 90% of them go away within two weeks. Burning during urination, frequency, and urinary obstruction are the most common symptoms lasting more than two weeks.

Proton Beam Radiation

This type of radiation comes from a proton *accelerator* instead of from a LINAC. The difference is that radiation from a linear accelerator delivers its energy as it passes through the tissues. That means normal tissue is getting some of the energy. Protons only deliver their energy when they reach the target. The result is that PBR may deliver less radiation outside the prostate. Considerable publicity promoting this treatment is occurring around the United States. This is partly because the machines are expensive to build, costing from $100 million to $200 million. The marketing message is that in theory, the treatment can focus less radiation on normal tissues, potentially causing fewer symptoms. In reality, however, no study has yet shown either better results or fewer side effects compared with other forms of external radiation.

Actually, two recent nonrandomized studies have found more side effects with PBR compared with conventional radiation. Other problems are that no study has reported long-term survival with this treatment and it is much more expensive than IMRT. The bottom line is that until good studies show better results or until long-term survival has been reported, PBR offers no clear advantage for patients. Another disadvantage is that the number of centers offering this therapy is limited at present, which means that most patients must travel out of town and reside there for several weeks until the treatment is completed.

Which Type of Radiation Is Best?

With so many options, you now want to know, "Which radiation method is best?" The answer is not available right now because no good studies have compared them. Since prostate cancer often grows slowly, these treatments cannot be reliably compared unless the patients have been followed for many years. Valid conclusions cannot be made based on short-term results and that is all that is available for IGRT (SGRT), PBR, and even IMRT. However, though such results are not yet available, you still can get some guidance on what to do.

First, if you decide that radiation is the right treatment for you, make sure that newer equipment is being used. The older LINAC machines are no longer adequate. After reading about the differences between 3D-CRT and IMRT, you might want to know, "Is IMRT better?" Uncontrolled studies suggest a slightly lower percentage of bowel side effects with IMRT but no difference in urinary side effects. Without good evidence that IMRT is definitely better, either approach is reasonable, although most radiation therapists are likely to prefer IMRT. If both are available in your area and you have a choice, IMRT may give you a better result.

What about IGRT (SGRT) and PBR? They all have theoretical advantages over 3D-CRT and IMRT, but not one comparison has been done and no long-term survival results have been reported. If you like the idea of these newer options, you should know that no one can tell how they will compare to IMRT with longer follow-up. That means they have more uncertainty. PBR has the longest track record of these newer options. It has been used to treat thousands of patients in California over the last 15 years. Despite this experience, only one study has been published and it did not report survival results nor did it assess side effects using written surveys. Also, recent studies have found that PBR had a higher complication rate than IMRT. Although it is more costly, most insurance companies are covering it. If you decide this is for you, be aware that only about 11 centers currently offer this treatment and about 7 more are nearing completion in the United States, so most men will need to travel to have it done.

If you prefer to get your treatment completed quickly, IGRT (SGRT) is for you; however, the long-term results will not be known for many years. Also, it is not known whether the much higher daily dose of radiation will lead to higher complications in the future.

Your choice of radiation methods should depend in part on your goals and motivation. If you are willing to try something new without knowing exactly how well it might work, then any of these options can be selected. If you want a more established treatment, then 3D-CRT or IMRT would be a better choice right now.

What Is the Optimal Dose of Radiation?

Regardless of the type of radiation you choose, information has been accumulating about how much radiation one should get. One well-done study assigned men with localized prostate cancer to receive 70.2 Gy or 79.2 Gy. With more than one-half of them followed for about nine years, the survival rates were about the same. One difference is that fewer men with a low-risk cancer had a rise in their PSA if they got the higher dose.

Another good study compared men's quality of life three years after getting 68 Gy or 78 Gy and found no difference. Does that mean you are better off getting a higher dose of radiation? At this time, the answer is not clear. The PSA is not a reliable way to predict long-term survival results. Still, most doctors are recommending a higher dose because it can be done very safely. For now, a higher dose of radiation may do a better job of getting rid of your cancer. Doctors still don't know whether it will cause more long-term side effects or help you live longer. If you decide to have radiation, be sure to ask the doctor how much they plan to give you in addition to what equipment they use. If your goal is to avoid any problems from prostate cancer, then a higher dose may be best without making your quality of life much worse. Most doctors now use over 76 Gy or higher to treat localized prostate cancer.

The Role of Androgen Deprivation Therapy (ADT) in Men Treated with External Radiation

Despite improvement in radiation methods, not all men are cured of their disease, particularly those with intermediate- or high-risk disease. As discussed previously, intermediate cancers have a PSA between 10 and 20 ng/ml, a Gleason score of 7, and a clinical stage of T2b. High-risk cancers have a PSA over 20 ng/ml, a Gleason score of 8–10, or a clinical stage of T2c or T3. Doctors have questioned whether combining androgen deprivation therapy (ADT) with external radiation could improve survival. ADT is described in detail in chapter 14. It involves lowering the male sex hormone, testosterone, because normally it helps prostate cancer cells grow. Studies have shown that reducing testosterone kills prostate cancer and improves symptoms caused by the disease. Years ago, studies suggested that lowering testosterone might make radiation more effective.

Several randomized studies have been done so far. In one study, patients with localized prostate cancer received either radiation alone or radiation plus two months of ADT before and two months during radiation. The ADT used was called *combined androgen blockade*, which is described in detail in chapter 28. Patients received two drugs; one is called an *LHRH agonist* (chapter 27) and the other is called an *antiandrogen*. LHRH stands for luteinizing hormone releasing hormone. This drug stops the testicles from producing testosterone. The LHRH drugs used were either *leuprolide* or *goserelin*. They are injected either into a muscle or under the skin. The *antiandrogen*, which stops testosterone from stimulating cancer cells is a pill taken either one or three times a day. The drugs used are called *flutamide or bicalutamide*.

The study found that the estimated survival at 10 years was significantly higher in the group getting both radiation and ADT. It was 62% for those getting combination therapy compared with only 57% for those getting radiation alone. The chance of dying from prostate cancer was 4% in men getting both treatments compared with 8% in men only getting radiation. Although the ADT improved survival, the odds of benefitting were small. It helped only about 1 out of every 20 men live longer and about 1 out of every 25 men avoid dying from prostate cancer in 10 years. The combination therapy also resulted in a lower chance of having cancer on a prostate biopsy done two years after treatment; it occurred in 20% of the men having both treatments compared with 39% in those having only radiation.

When the results were looked at according to risk groups, ADT helped men with intermediate-risk disease; the estimated survival increased from 54% without ADT to 61% with ADT. This means about 1 out of every 14 men in this group is benefitting. Adding ADT provided no benefit for men with low-risk disease. Caution is needed regarding this last result because the study was not intended to look at low-risk disease. That means the conclusion that ADT wasn't helpful might not be correct and only another study can make that determination. The most common side effects caused by the ADT were worsening of sexual function at one year in 58%, minor liver toxicity in 20% (caused by the flutamide), urinary side effects in 6% to 8%, and severe bowel problems in 1% to 3%.

Although this was a well-done study, the radiation dose was lower than recommended by many doctors today; patients only received a total dose of 66.6 Gy. Some doctors question whether the ADT really would be helpful or necessary when men are given 74 to 76 Gy. Until another study is done, this question cannot be answered.

The second randomized study began in 1995 and enrolled mostly men with intermediate-risk disease and some with high-risk disease. ADT again consisted of combined androgen blockade or CAB. Men received flutamide three times per day by mouth and either leuprolide or goserelin for six months. The total dose of radiation was 70 Gy.

The estimated survival at eight years was 61% in men getting radiation alone compared with 74% for men getting both treatments. That means one out of every seven men getting hormone therapy benefitted by living longer. Also, men getting radiation alone were four times more likely to die from prostate cancer. The benefit was limited to men who were generally in good health, but not those with other illnesses.

The odds of developing urinary or bowel side effects were similar in the two groups. The main difference was in the odds of developing breast enlargement, which occurred in 18% of the men on combined androgen blockade compared with 3% of the control group. This is a known side effect of flutamide.

Other studies have been done in men with high-risk disease. Although many of these patients are thought to have localized tumors, in reality a high percentage of them are growing outside the prostate. These tumors definitely are more difficult to treat.

In the best study done so far, survival was 18% higher in men receiving ADT that started when radiation began. Only about 10% of them had high-risk localized cancer and the remainder had cancer extending outside the prostate. Another study would be needed to find out whether men with only high-risk localized disease would benefit from this same treatment.

Another well-done study was done in men with tumors growing outside the prostate or localized tumors with a Gleason score of 8, 9, or 10. All the patients received two months of combined ADT (flutamide plus goserelin) before and two months during radiation. They were then randomized to receive no additional treatment or another 24 months of goserelin. Overall survival was 32% for the men getting short-term ADT compared with 45% in those getting long-term therapy. Men had a much better survival if they received radiation and a total of 28 months of ADT compared with only 4 months. The ADT consisted of the LHRH agonist by itself or it was combined with one month of an antiandrogen. Again, although well designed, the study was not intended to look at men with high Gleason scores. For that reason, the conclusion is not completely reliable and another study would be needed to make sure there is a benefit.

As expected, the addition of ADT increased the rate of side effects including hot flashes, a decreased sex drive, and decreased sexual function. These side effects decrease but do not always completely disappear after the ADT is stopped.

Other randomized studies have been done, but they are not discussed here because their end point was not survival and this could lead to incorrect conclusions about the value of a particular therapy.

The Bottom Line on Combining ADT with External Radiation

Now that you have read about all these different studies, you probably want to know what to do. As mentioned earlier, some doctors argue the only reason ADT was helpful in these studies is because the dose of radiation was too low. For that reason, they believe you should not receive ADT if you are going to receive more than 70 Gy of radiation. Others will say that while higher doses of radiation may lessen the need for ADT, for now it may be better to do combination therapy if your goal is to maximize your chances for survival. Remember, there are side effects from the ADT, but they are uncommon and will disappear in most patients some time after the treatment is stopped. At this time, the best advice is the following:

1. If you have low-risk prostate cancer, there is no good evidence that combining ADT with the radiation will significantly improve your survival.

2. For intermediate-risk disease, ADT for six months does improve survival but the odds of benefitting are not very high. The treatment is appropriate if you feel that maximizing survival is your primary goal.

3. For high-risk disease, ADT beginning two months before the radiation and continuing for a total of 28 months, or starting at the beginning of radiation and continuing for 36 months, appear to improve survival significantly.

Some doctors use a combination of external radiation and brachytherapy (seed implantation, discussed in the next chapter) to treat localized prostate cancer, and some also add hormone therapy. Little information is available to assess how often side effects occur or whether the brachytherapy offers any added benefit. Therefore, it cannot be recommended as a good treatment option at this time, but you should be aware that some doctors heavily promote it.

Follow-Up Care after External Radiation

After radiation is complete, patients are seen at regular intervals to assess and treat any side effects that may have occurred. Doctors vary in the frequency of follow-up visits they recommend after treatment. A reasonable approach is to measure the PSA every three months for one or two years and then every 6 to 12 months if the test remains stable. Beyond five years, it can be done once a year unless it is rising. Most doctors also do a digital rectal examination to determine whether the cancer is growing although that is probably unnecessary because the PSA is far more reliable. It should gradually decline and then remain stable.

One difference between surgery and radiation is that the PSA declines more slowly after radiation. It may not reach its lowest level, called the nadir, for up to two years after treatment has been completed. Following surgery, the nadir occurs within four weeks. Some men feel very anxious when the PSA does not drop right away. Knowing that the decline normally takes time should make you feel a little more comfortable. Some patients ask whether a slowly dropping PSA predicts a worse result. Currently, there is no good evidence that the rate of decline in the PSA has any impact on the cancer coming back.

In some cases, the PSA may begin to rise again, which may mean that the cancer has not been eliminated. A bone scan and CT scan will be done to determine whether the cancer is in the bones or other parts of the body, but usually not before the PSA reaches at least 10 ng/ml. More information about managing a rising PSA will be discussed in chapter 19.

Researchers are working on ways to predict what will happen after radiation, as they have with their predictions after surgery. Several problems may complicate this task. Most importantly, higher doses of radiation and newer methods of delivering it could affect the way this cancer behaves after the treatment has been completed.

Some predictions are possible using the nadir PSA. One retrospective study separated men into two groups: those with a PSA over 1.5 ng/ml and those with a PSA less than or equal to that value two years after completing radiation. The results are shown in the following table.

Table 11.6 Chance of Developing Metastatic Disease following External Beam Radiation

PSA Result 2 Years after Radiation	Metastases at 5 Years	Metastases at 10 Years
0–1.5 ng/ml	2.4%	7.9%
Over 1.5 ng/ml	10%	17.9%

Men with a PSA below 1.5 ng/ml at two years were much less likely to have cancer appear in other parts of their body at 5 and 10 years after radiation. Although the study was not ideal, it does show that even if the PSA is greater than 1.5 ng/ml, the vast majority of men will not have metastatic disease at 10 years.

The Bottom Line on External Radiation

Radiation offers men a way to get rid of their cancer without having an operation. It may be a better choice than surgery for older or less healthy men. Also, this treatment does appear to have a lower risk of developing urinary incontinence or impotence but a higher risk of bowel problems. For men with a very long life expectancy of greater than 15 years, surgery may be a better option because 15-year results with the latest radiation methods are not yet available. For men with low-risk prostate cancer, no studies have proven that external radiation offers a better survival than active surveillance, radical prostatectomy, or seed implantation. A small percentage of men with intermediate- or high-risk disease will benefit from combining ADT with the radiation. However, it is not known whether this combination is as good as, or better or worse than, radical prostatectomy. Most, but not all of the side effects of the ADT will go away after it is discontinued. IMRT appears to cause fewer side effects than older technology while allowing higher doses of radiation to be used. IGRT and PBR offer similar short-term results compared with IMRT, but without knowing the long-term outcomes, they have more uncertainty about what to expect. At this time, there is no evidence to support the claims that proton beam therapy will give better results or cause fewer side effects than IMRT. Chapter 17 will provide additional help in deciding which treatment is for you.

Brachytherapy

Another way to deliver radiation to the prostate is called brachy-therapy or *seed implantation*. In Latin, the word "brachy" means short distance, which is appropriate for a treatment in which the radioactive material is placed inside the body very close to the cancer. It works like external radiation by damaging cancer cells so they die or can no longer divide and multiply.

This treatment can be done two ways. One option is to leave the source of radiation in the body, which is called *permanent brachytherapy*. The other option is to place it in the prostate for a short time and then remove it, which is called *temporary brachytherapy*. The radioactive materials used for permanent brachytherapy are *iodine-125 (I-125)*, *palladium-103 (Pd-103)*, and *cesium-131 (Cs-131)* while temporary brachytherapy is done using *iridium-192 (Ir-192)*.

The radioactivity in the seeds used for permanent brachytherapy does not last forever; it gradually disappears. The time required for it to disappear varies for each source of radiation. The *half-life* is the number of days it takes for 50% of the radiation to go away. For I-125 it is 60 days, Pd-103 is next at 17 days, and it is only 9.7 days for Cs-131. This translates into I-125 losing about 97% of its radiation in 300 days compared with 85 days for Pd-103 and 49 days for Cs-131.

Another way that these materials differ is the intensity or strength of radiation they deliver to the body. This is measured by the *dose rate*. A low dose rate, or LDR, means the material gives off small amounts of radiation each day. A high dose rate or HDR means a large amount is given off. I-125, Pd-103, and Cs-131 have low dose rates, which is the reason they can be put in the body permanently. Ir-192 has a much higher dose rate so it can only be put in the body for a short time. Otherwise it will cause too much damage to the prostate and surrounding tissues.

Permanent Brachytherapy

The radioactive material used for permanent brachytherapy is contained inside tiny "seeds" or tubes made of titanium. They look like birdseeds, each one measuring a few millimeters in length. That is why the treatment is often called *seed implantation*. The radiation is able to penetrate outward through the titanium tubes.

Prostate brachytherapy began in the 1970s but it was not very successful because the seeds were placed by hand during an open operation. The development of transrectal ultrasound in the 1980s significantly improved the technique because the seeds could be placed more accurately and without the need for an open operation.

What Are the Advantages and Disadvantages of Permanent Brachytherapy?

The main advantage of permanent brachytherapy is a higher dose of radiation can be given to the prostate compared with external radiation. The total dose is about 145 Gy for I-125, 125 Gy for Pd-103, 115 Gy for Cs-131, and only 81 to 91 Gy for Intensity Modulated Radiation Therapy (IMRT). Other advantages are that the treatment is completed quickly, it causes few side effects during the first few months after treatment, and it allows the patient to resume all activities in just a few days. One disadvantage is the prostate is more difficult to remove if the cancer is not eliminated. The other disadvantages are the potential short-term and long-term side effects as listed in the next table.

Table 12.1

Side Effects of Permanent Brachytherapy
Urinary retention
Urinary incontinence
Urinary frequency
Blood in urine
Erectile dysfunction
Bowel dysfunction
Urethral stricture
Seed migration to the lung or bladder
Anejaculation

The most common short-term side effects are urinary frequency, urgency, difficulty emptying the bladder, and blood in the stool. How often they occur depends on many factors including:

- The experience of the doctor implanting the seeds.

- The patient's age and health.

- The radiation material used for the implant.

- The total amount of radiation delivered to the prostate.

The side effects usually occur within the first few weeks after the implant and gradually improve. Blood in the stool rarely needs any treatment. The chances of having urinary problems after treatment also will depend on a man's urinary function before treatment. The *International Prostate Symptom Score* (IPSS), is a survey

Table 12.2 IPSS Questionnaire

	Not at All (0)	Less Than 1 in 5 (1)	Less Than Half the Time (2)	About Half the Time (3)	More Than Half the Time (4)	Almost Always (5)
Over the past month, how often have you had a sensation of not emptying your bladder completely after you finished urinating?						
Over the past month, how often have you had to urinate again less than 2 hours after urinating?						
Over the past month, how often have you found you stopped and started again several times when you urinate?						
Over the past month, how often have you found it difficult to postpone urination?						

	Not at All	Once	Twice	Three Times	Four Times	Five or More Times
Over the past month, how often have you had a weak urinary stream?						
Over the past month, how often have you had to push or strain to begin urination?						
Over the past month, how many times did you most typically get up to urinate from the time you went to bed at night until you got up in the morning?						
Total Score						

143

used to measure urinary symptoms. It has seven questions, each with five possible answers so the total score can range from 7 to 35. You can answer the survey and find out your score before considering this treatment. A higher IPSS score means you are having more urinary symptoms.

These symptoms usually occur because brachytherapy causes inflammation in the urethra and prostate for several weeks. Occasionally this leads to a complete blockage called *urinary retention*. Passing a rubber tube called *urethral catheter* into the penis can relieve the obstruction. The tube is connected to a bag that collects the urine, which the patient empties when it is full. The inflammation usually goes away within a few weeks and the catheter can be removed. In some cases, anti-inflammatory drugs or steroids are prescribed.

Brachytherapy can have long-term effects on bladder, bowel, and sexual function. They may develop soon after treatment and persist or occasionally they develop one to two years later. If bloody stool persists, a biopsy of the rectal wall should be avoided because it can result in a *fistula*, an opening in the rectum that allows bowel contents to leak out. In some cases, fistulas do not heal and a surgery is required.

The frequency of side effects is most accurately determined using written surveys completed by patients, but most doctors do not use them. If you are considering this treatment, make sure to ask about the results obtained by your doctor and whether surveys were used. Some results are presented in chapter 16.

What Are the Results with Permanent Brachytherapy?

As stated several times before, no good study has compared the long-term effectiveness of the different treatments for prostate cancer. Only short-term information is available about brachytherapy using Cs-131 because it was not approved until 2004. One short-term randomized study did compare radical prostatectomy to brachytherapy using I-125 seeds. All the patients had low-risk disease, and at five years only 9% of the surgery group and 8% of the seed group had a rising PSA. No information is available about survival and so no conclusions are possible. One problem with this study is that it included men who would do very well without any therapy, which makes it hard to know whether either the surgery or brachytherapy was helping these patients.

The rest of the published studies on permanent brachytherapy are from uncontrolled trials. A comprehensive review attempted to compare permanent brachytherapy, external radiation, and temporary brachytherapy and concluded that temporary implants were best. However, there are so many variations in the study populations, methods used, durations of follow-up, and definitions of treatment failure that these conclusions may be incorrect.

Only two studies have reported the estimated 10-year overall survival rate following I-125 implants. In one of them, it was 65% in a group of 152 men with a range of Gleason scores, PSA levels, and clinical stages. About 15% of the men in this study had cancer detected in a follow-up biopsy. This study has several problems. First, few of the cancers were detected by a screening PSA because the study was done in 1987–1988, before the test was widely used. Also, the study combined the results for men with low-, intermediate-, and high-risk patients rather than showing them separately. These problems make the results less helpful for counseling men who are diagnosed today.

The second study was much larger, enrolling about 1100 men with low-risk disease and almost 800 men with intermediate-risk disease between 1988 and 2001. The estimated overall 10-year survival rate of the entire group was 44%. There can be many reasons for the worse results in this study compared with the first one. Here again, without separating the patients into low-, intermediate-, and high-risk groups, conclusions about brachytherapy are difficult to make.

Many other uncontrolled studies have reported the effect of seed implantation on preventing a rise in the serum PSA. However, this is not nearly as helpful as looking at survival results because:

- PSA is not a reliable way to assess the true impact of a therapy; what happens to the PSA does not reliably predict what will happen with survival.

- Many men also were given androgen deprivation therapy (ADT) or external radiation, which can make the PSA results look better.

- Different definitions of PSA failure are used in many of the studies, which makes it hard to compare results.

- Most studies *estimate* the results using statistical methods, which can give misleading information.

The bottom line is that no reliable conclusion can be made about the long-term survival after brachytherapy. It could be as good as, or better or worse than, other treatments. For now, this treatment is considered as reasonable an option as radical prostatectomy and external radiation, particularly for men with low-risk disease.

Who Is a Good Candidate for Permanent Brachytherapy?

Although brachytherapy by itself is a reasonable option for men with localized prostate cancer, it is not for everyone. The most important requirements are that a man is healthy enough to be able to have general anesthesia with a life expectancy of at least 10 years. Brachytherapy might not be an ideal choice if someone has a life expectancy greater than 15 years and his goal is to minimize the chance of being harmed by prostate cancer. The reason is that little is known about the percentage of men surviving for that long, which means the treatment has more uncertainty than radical prostatectomy.

This treatment is best for men with low-risk and possibly for inter-mediate-risk prostate cancer. Some doctors question whether combining ADT with brachytherapy will improve survival in men with intermediate-risk tumors similar to the finding for external beam radiation plus ADT. So far, no well-done studies have tested this idea and mixed results were found in nonrandomized studies. That means for now, the value of this combination treatment remains uncertain.

What about the high-risk group? Here too, no proper studies have been done. One retrospective study suggested that brachy-therapy alone was as good as external beam radiation, but no valid conclusions could be made because of the study design. Many doctors will combine external radiation with brachytherapy and possibly add ADT because these men have a much greater risk for recurrence with one therapy alone. Studies are underway to test these approaches. For now, however, the value of brachytherapy alone in high-risk disease is less certain.

Who should not get brachytherapy? One group is men with a very large prostate. Some doctors set an upper limit of only 40 cubic centimeters (cc) while others will treat a prostate up to 60 cc. The reason is that the pubic bone may prevent proper positioning of some of the needles into the prostate gland. If your prostate is above these limits, you still may be a candidate by getting ADT for several months, which can shrink the size of the gland by about 30% over three to six months. Details about this therapy are provided in chapter 14.

Another exclusion is men who have many urinary symptoms such as a slow stream, getting up at night to urinate, or urinary fre-quency. As described earlier, these symptoms can be determined using the IPSS questionnaire. Many doctors will not do brachyther-apy if the score is higher than 15. Again, you still may be able to have this treatment if your symptoms improve after taking a drug called an *alpha-blocker* or *5-alpha reductase inhibitor*. Brachytherapy also is less appropriate for anyone who has had surgical removal of part of the prostate to improve urinary symptoms. The reason is that the risk of urinary side effects following brachytherapy is increased.

How Is Brachytherapy Performed?

Before the procedure can be done, the prostate size must be carefully determined by doing a *volume study*. This occurs about two weeks before the operation with the same ultrasound equipment used for the prostate biopsy. First, a catheter is placed into the bladder through the penis so the urethra can be identified on the ultrasound. It is removed after the study is finished. Measuring the prostate volume does not require an anesthetic and is completed in about 15 minutes. The information from this study is entered into a computer, which determines the best location to place the seeds and how many will be needed.

Some doctors use a different approach to determine the number of seeds needed. Instead of preplanning the treatment, it is done by a computer while the patient is under anesthesia for the implant. This approach is used because the size and shape of the prostate may change slightly between the time a volume study was done and the day of the implant. More seeds must be ordered for this real-time approach and some of them may be wasted if they are not used. No study has determined which approach is best, so either is reasonable. During the visit for the volume study, an anesthesiologist or nurse will evaluate you to make sure you are suitable for general anesthesia. Also, an electrocardiogram and blood tests will be performed.

Beginning one week before the implant, you will be told to stop taking any drugs that can increase your risk of bleeding. The most common ones are nonsteroidal anti-inflammatory drugs or NSAIDs. They include Motrin, ibuprofen, naprosyn, Aleve, and Celebrex. Vitamin E also should be avoided. If one of these is taken by mistake within seven days of the procedure, you should notify your doctor right away. No eating or drinking should be done after midnight on the day before the procedure.

The decision about whether to use I-125, Pd-103, or Cs-131 will be made by the doctor performing the procedure. Since no studies have proven that a particular one gives better results, they are all reasonable options. Cs-131 has a theoretical benefit of delivering more intense radiation, which could more effectively kill the cancer cells, but few doctors are using it. One difference among the three seeds is their effect on urinary function. A randomized study measured the IPSS in men assigned to receive I-125 or Pd-103. The score was higher in the Pd-103 group at one month but lower at six months. Uncontrolled studies suggest that CS-131 results in even higher IPSS scores within the first few weeks after the implant, but they decline sooner than with Pd-103. Does that mean Cs-131 is a better choice? The answer is not really. It simply shows that either you get the most severe side effects for a shorter time with Cs-131, less severe but for a slightly longer time with Pd-103, or the least severe side effects for the longest time with I-125. In the United States, iodine seeds are used more often for low-risk tumors because they have the longest track record. Many doctors favor the I-125 for low-risk cancers and Pd-103 for intermediate- or high-risk cancers. You can discuss the three options with your doctor and ask which one they think is best for you and for what reason.

What to Expect on the Day of the Implant

On the day of your implant, you will take an enema and arrive at the treatment center about 60 to 90 minutes before the procedure. After you change into a hospital gown, a needle will be placed in your arm to administer intravenous fluids. When it is time for the procedure, you will be taken into a treatment room, transferred onto a table, and put to sleep by the anesthesiologist. The staff will position you with your legs elevated, cleanse the rectal area, and cover it with surgical drapes.

The procedure begins by placing an ultrasound probe into the rectum. A specially designed needle guide is attached to the probe and pushed against the perineal skin above the rectum. This guide has many labeled, small openings positioned close to one another. It is secured in place with a clamp connected to the operating table. The radioactive seeds are either preloaded into the needles before the procedure begins or they are filled in the operating room at the time of the procedure. Each needle containing the right number of seeds for the selected location is inserted into a specific opening on the needle guide. The seeds are left in the prostate as the needle is withdrawn. About 50 to 120 seeds will be placed during the procedure, which usually is completed in 60 to 90 minutes.

The ultrasound probe is then removed and a telescopic instrument called a *cystoscope* is inserted into the penis and passed into the bladder to look for any bleeding or to remove any seeds that did not stay in place in the prostate. A catheter is inserted into the bladder and then you will be transferred to the recovery room. The catheter will be removed when you're fully awake. You can go home when you are able to eat, drink, and urinate. If you can't urinate, the catheter will be inserted again and remain there for one or two weeks. Most men are able to urinate after this time but some need to be treated with medication for several weeks. In rare cases, surgery is needed to enable the person to urinate.

What Happens When You Are Home

Daily activities can be resumed within one or two days after the procedure. You will be instructed to urinate into a strainer to look for any seeds coming out of the prostate. Doctors recommend avoiding or limiting very close contact with children or pregnant women until the risk of radiation exposure is very low. They can be in a room with you if they are more than six feet away. Close contact is safe after approximately 300 days after an implant using iodine seeds, 85 days after palladium seeds, and 49 days with cesium seeds. Some men will see blood in the urine, called *hematuria*. No treatment is needed unless the bleeding is very heavy. Call your doctor right away if you see blood clots or have severe burning when you urinate. Within the first few weeks after the implant, some men get acute pain or burning during urination from severe inflammation. In a small percentage of cases, steroids are needed to reduce these symptoms.

One month after the procedure, a CAT scan is performed to determine the exact location of each seed. This information is used to calculate the amount of radiation that is being delivered to your prostate.

A DRE and PSA test are done starting at three months and then again at three- to six-month intervals to monitor the cancer. After five years, an annual test is enough, provided the PSA is not rising.

Temporary Brachytherapy (HDR)

Brachytherapy can also be done using temporary radioactive implants. This is called *high dose rate* or *HDR brachytherapy* because the radioactive material gives off more radiation each day than the permanent seed implants.

What Are the Advantages and Disadvantages of HDR Brachytherapy?

HDR has advantages and disadvantages compared with permanent brachytherapy and external radiation as listed in the following tables.

Table 12.3 Advantages of Temporary Brachytherapy

Potentially more precise delivery of radiation to the prostate
No radioactive seeds left in the body
Treatment completed in several days
No risk of radiation to other people

Table 12.4 Disadvantages of Temporary Brachytherapy

Requires anesthesia and two nights in the hospital
More inconvenient than permanent brachytherapy
Limited number of centers offering procedure
Long-term results not available using HDR by itself

The primary advantage of this treatment is the potential ability to more effectively tailor the radiation to the shape of the prostate. In theory, this might cause fewer side effects, but it has not yet been proven in well-done studies. Another advantage is no radiation is left in your body. HDR brachytherapy is more inconvenient for a patient than a permanent implant because it requires two nights in the hospital, each about one-week apart, two anesthetics, and four to six treatment sessions. The patient must remain still while the implant is in place, which can make some men very uncomfortable.

The biggest problem is that long-term survival results have not been reported for HDR. More information is available using HDR brachytherapy combined with external radiation for men with intermediate- or high-risk cancers, but no well-done studies have been done and long-term survival has not been reported. One report combined results from several studies and found a significantly better overall survival at eight years for HDR compared with external beam radiation alone or combined with permanent seed implants. Whether this finding is valid or not is unclear because the study was not randomized. It is also unclear how often the external radiation was given using the latest equipment, what dose was given and whether ADT was used. The bottom line is that HDR has potential advantages but not enough is known to determine whether it is better, worse, or the same as other options for treating this disease.

Who Is a Good Candidate for HDR Brachytherapy?

Not enough information is available to be sure who is a good candidate for HDR brachytherapy. For men with low-risk disease, it probably is a reasonable option but certainly requires a more involved procedure than the permanent implants. The only clear advantage of HDR is that patients are able to have close contact with a child or pregnant woman immediately after it's done rather than having to wait. The absence of 10- and 15-year survival results makes it difficult to recommend as the sole treatment for intermediate or high-risk disease. As long as a patient understands this limitation, it can be considered. Whether combining it with external radiation will give better results than external radiation plus ADT for men with intermediate- or high-risk disease remains an unanswered question. Also, more information is definitely needed to know how this treatment compares with surgery, external radiation, or seed implantation.

What Happens before You Undergo HDR Brachytherapy

Approximately one week before the procedure, the patient will be examined and an electrocardiogram and blood tests will be obtained to make sure that anesthesia is safe to use. Any drugs that may cause bleeding should be stopped at that time.

How Is HDR Brachytherapy Performed?

On the day of the procedure, the patient arrives at the hospital, changes into a hospital gown, and is given fluids intravenously. After transferring the patient to the operating room, general or spinal anesthesia is administered and both legs are placed in stirrups. The area around the rectum is washed and coated with an antiseptic. A Foley catheter is placed through the penis and into the bladder and an ultrasound probe is placed in the rectum. About 20 thin plastic tubes are pushed through the perineal skin and into the prostate, guided by the ultrasound. They are held in place with a flexible needle guide sewn to the skin. The anesthesia is stopped after the legs have been lowered onto the table. Patients then are transferred to radiology where a CAT scan is performed to plan the amount of radiation needed.

The next stop is the radiation treatment room where the patient is positioned on the table and connected to a computer-controlled machine. It pushes the radioactive Ir-192 wires through the catheters and into the prostate. They remain in position for a limited time and then are moved to a new location until the whole prostate has been treated. The setup and positioning may take more than an hour but the actual treatment is completed in about 20 minutes. Patients have little discomfort during the procedure. They are transferred to a hospital room where they must remain in bed with the catheters in place. Unlike permanent seed implantation, no radiation is left in the body after HDR brachytherapy is completed.

The following day, the treatment is repeated one or two times and then the catheters in the skin and bladder are removed and the patient is sent home. Normal activities can resume in a day or two. The entire process is repeated within a few weeks, although some centers now are completing the entire procedure in a single hospital visit.

What Happens after HDR Brachytherapy?

Since no radiation remains in the body after the patient goes home, there is no need to avoid contact with children or pregnant women. All activities can be resumed immediately. A PSA will be measured starting about three months after the implant and then again every three to six months usually for five years. It gradually declines but can take six months before leveling off. Additional tests may then be done annually if the PSA value remains stable. A digital rectal examination is also done at each visit.

The Bottom Line on Brachytherapy

Current methods of performing permanent brachytherapy have been in use for more than 15 years. Like surgery and external radiation, it is a reasonable alternative for treating localized prostate cancer despite an absence of any direct comparisons with other therapies. It also causes changes in bowel, bladder, and sexual functions, which may be permanent and can alter your quality of life. The most appropriate candidates are those with low-risk or intermediate-risk disease. It may be less suitable in men with a life expectancy of 15 years or longer because the long-term effect is not known. Permanent brachytherapy by itself may not be a good choice for high-risk tumors. Although temporary brachytherapy has some potential advantages, not enough information is available about how well it works when used alone or in combination with external radiation.

Cryotherapy or "Freezing the Prostate"

What Is Cryotherapy?

Cryo means cold or freezing, so cryotherapy is a treatment in which very cold temperatures are delivered to the prostate. Other terms often used for this treatment are *cryosurgery* and *cryoablation*. How does it work? When cancer cells are cooled to very low temperatures and then rewarmed, several things happen that eventually lead to the death of those cells. Cryotherapy for prostate cancer began in the 1960s without great success. However, the methods have greatly improved over the last 15 years, making it safer and more effective.

What Are the Advantages and Disadvantages of Cryotherapy?

Cryotherapy often is described as a "minimally invasive" treatment with several potential advantages. First, it may cure your prostate tumor provided all the cancer cells are inside the prostate and they are cooled to the proper temperature. Second, the treatment can be completed in few hours as compared with external radiation, which takes six to eight weeks. Next, it is an easier treatment to go through with less blood loss and a shorter recovery time than radical prostatectomy. It avoids having radiation in the body like permanent brachytherapy. Unlike surgery or any type of radiation, cryotherapy may be repeated if the cancer is not completely eliminated.

One of the disadvantages is that the technology keeps changing, so long-term survival rates using the latest methods are not known. Originally, liquid nitrogen was used to freeze the prostate. Currently, argon gas does the cooling, which appears to cause fewer complications. Although cryosurgery initially was promoted as having fewer side effects than other treatments, this has not been the case. Short-term side effects include urinary retention requiring a urinary catheter, and penile and scrotal swelling lasting one to two weeks. Some men complain of numbness in the penis lasting one to two months. The next table shows the range of doctor-reported complications from several uncontrolled studies.

Table 13.1 Complications of Cryotherapy

Complication	Percentage of Patients
Erectile dysfunction (at one year)	41%–88%
Urinary incontinence	2%–15%
Rectal fistula	0.4%–2.4%
Urethral sloughing	0%–15%
Urinary obstruction	3%–23%
Perineal pain	0.4%–12%

Since none of them are based on written questionnaires, the true complication rates are likely to be higher.

Other long-term complications include urinary incontinence, fistula formation, and urinary obstruction resulting from dying prostate tissue. All except the last one were explained in previous chapters. Prostate tissue that has been destroyed by the cryotherapy can cause an obstruction. It is treated by a minor operation that requires cutting away the tissue blocking the urethra using an instrument inserted into the urethra through the penis.

What Are the Results with Cryotherapy?

There are several difficulties in telling you what to expect if you choose this treatment including:

- No randomized studies have been performed comparing cryosurgery to other treatments.

- The only uncontrolled study reporting long-term survival is based on only 51 men with localized disease treated from 1973 to 1977 using outdated technology. Cancer recurred in 78% of them, with 47% dying from prostate cancer.

Without information about survival, doctors report the following results:

- How often the prostate-specific antigen (PSA) goes up.

- The percentage of men needing more treatment.

- How often the cancer spreads to other parts of the body.

One problem with comparing studies that used PSA results as the measure of success is that the definition of failure was not uniform. They used one of the following:

- A PSA greater than 0.4 ng/ml

- A PSA greater than 0.5 ng/ml

- A PSA greater than 1.0 ng/ml

- Three consecutive increases in PSA

- An increase of 2 ng/ml above the lowest, or nadir, PSA.

Some of these definitions will make the results look better than others and none of them is an accurate predictor of long-term survival. How well does cryotherapy prevent the PSA from going up? One uncontrolled study used statistical methods to *estimate* the results because many of the men had not been followed for 10 years. They divided the patients into those with low-, intermediate-, or high-risk cancer. The definition of treatment failure was a rise in PSA of 2 ng/ml above the nadir level.

Table 13.2 Ten-Year PSA Results following Cryotherapy

Patients Without Rise of 2 ng/ml above Nadir	Low-Risk Cancers	Intermediate-Risk Cancers	High-Risk Cancers
Estimated result	81%	74%	46%
Range	64%–90%	62%–83%	32%–58%

These results again show why comparing different treatments is so difficult. When results are *estimated*, the true result could fall anywhere within the reported range. For example, in the low-risk group, the estimated odds of the PSA not rising by 2 ng/ml above the nadir is 81%, but the real value could be as low as 64% or as high as 90%. There is no way to know the exact result. Now, suppose that these results are compared with a different treatment that has similar estimated results. Are these treatments equally effective? An accurate answer is not possible. The treatments could have the same effect or they could differ by as much as 25% (90%–64%). This is important to understand because most doctors who recommend a treatment based on studies that estimated PSA failures do not explain this limitation. Another problem is that many studies do not even report the range of results. The end result is that you may receive misleading information about how well a treatment works. The truth is that no one can say that two treatments are equally effective without comparing them in a randomized study.

Who Is a Good Candidate for Cryotherapy?

The best candidates for cryotherapy are men with low-risk disease who are not suitable for radical prostatectomy because of previous pelvic surgery. Radiation also is not a good option because of previous pelvic radiation to treat a different disease, inflammatory bowel disease, or rectal disorders. Men should be healthy enough to undergo general or spinal anesthesia and have at least a 10-year life expectancy. This treatment is not appropriate for individuals who are concerned about their sexual function, have a large prostate gland, or have had previous prostate surgery to improve urinary symptoms. Men with a larger prostate gland may be able to have cryotherapy if the size is reduced after three to six months of androgen deprivation therapy (ADT).

How Is Cryotherapy Performed?

About one week before getting your treatment, you will be sent for a preoperative assessment by someone from the anesthesia department. Several blood tests will be ordered and an electrocardiogram will be performed to make sure it is safe to undergo anesthesia. Any blood-thinning medications such as non-steroidal anti-inflammatory drugs (NSAIDs), aspirin, Coumadin, or vitamin E should be stopped at least one week before the procedure. On the night prior to the cryosurgery, an enema should be taken and you should not eat or drink anything after midnight.

What to Expect on the Day of Cryotherapy

Patients arrive at the treatment center a few hours before the procedure. They change into a surgical gown, an intravenous line will be started, and nurses will give relaxing medication. Next, the patient is transferred to the operating room and either given general or spinal anesthesia. He is positioned on the table in the dorsal lithotomy position with legs elevated off the table that are held in place with stirrups. The perianal area is washed and coated with an antiseptic and then covered with sterile drapes.

An ultrasound probe like the one used for your prostate biopsy is placed into the rectum. A special rubber tube called a *urethral warming catheter* is inserted through the penis into the bladder. It allows water to be circulated through the urethra to keep it from getting too cold, which lowers the chance of injury. Temperature-sensing needles are placed through the skin near the rectum and into the prostate and surrounding tissues. They measure the temperature during the treatment to make sure it gets cold enough inside the prostate without overcooling the surrounding tissues. Six to eight special "freezing" needles then are placed through the skin in front of the rectum. A computer determines the best location for these needles based on the size and shape of the gland. They are guided into those locations using the ultrasound.

After all the needles are in position, *argon gas* is passed through the cooling needles to freeze the prostate. This creates an "ice ball" which can be viewed on the ultrasound. The goal is to cool the prostate to a temperature of minus 40 degrees Centigrade for several minutes and then allow the prostate to rewarm, which causes the cells to rupture. The procedure is repeated, which is thought to increase the chance of killing all the cells. Afterward, the needles and warming tube are removed and a tube called a *Foley catheter* is placed into the bladder through the penis to drain the urine. It may be left in place for a few days because swelling often occurs, making urination difficult. The procedure usually is completed in two to three hours, the anesthesia is discontinued, and then the patient is returned to the recovery room. After the anesthetic has worn off and the patient can drink and urinate, he is sent home. The catheter usually causes only minor discomfort. The patient returns in a few days to have the catheter removed.

What to Expect after Going Home

You will be advised to limit activity for several days and place ice packs in your perineal area to reduce swelling and discomfort. Some doctors will prescribe antibiotics for several days to reduce the chance of getting an infection. Do not be alarmed if you see blood at the tip of the penis or in the urine as these often occur. Both should stop within several days. If you get a fever or chills, contact your doctor right away. Long-term complications such as urinary leakage or sexual problems usually do not occur for many months.

How You Are Monitored after Cryotherapy

No guidelines have been established for follow-up care. A reasonable approach is to perform a PSA and digital rectal examination approximately every three months for one or two years and then every 6 to 12 months unless the PSA is changing. After five years, an annual test is sufficient. Some doctors recommend doing another prostate biopsy within one to two years because the PSA level may not accurately predict whether cancer has been eliminated. If cancer cells are still present, the treatment may be repeated.

No further therapy is needed provided the PSA remains stable and a follow-up biopsy does not show any cancer. However, if the PSA begins to rise or if the biopsy shows cancer, additional treatment may be needed. A bone scan and CT scan or an MRI will be ordered if the PSA rises above 5 or 10 ng/ml. Management of a rising PSA is discussed in chapter 19.

What Is Focal Cryotherapy?

Most of the prostate cancers now being detected are very small. For that reason, doctors have questioned whether cryotherapy could be done only to the areas of the prostate containing the cancer cells rather than to the entire prostate. A potential advantage of this approach is it might cause less damage to the pelvic nerves, thereby preserving a man's sexual function. Treating only a portion of the prostate is called focal cryotherapy. Some doctors are calling it a "male lumpectomy." The treatment either is directed to any area of the prostate where cancer was detected or it is limited to one entire side of the prostate.

The Advantages and Disadvantages of Focal Cryotherapy

The main advantage of focal treatment is the possibility of reducing the side effects that result from treating the entire gland. Also, if cancer is not completely eliminated, treatment may be repeated.

The main disadvantage is that prostate cancer is a *multifocal* disease, located in more than one area of the prostate. Biopsies are not 100% accurate in identifying all the areas containing cancer. Therefore, treating only one-half of the gland may fail to cure many men of their disease. This concern is supported by several studies. One of them was done on men undergoing radical prostatectomy who were thought to have disease on only one side of the prostate. After the prostate was taken out, 71% of the men were found to have cancer on the other side of the gland. Although the treatment may be repeated, by the time the remaining cancer is discovered some cancer cells already may have spread to other parts of the body. That would mean the patient has missed out on a chance to be cured by not having the entire cancer treated from the beginning.

What Are the Results of Focal Cryotherapy?

Focal cryotherapy is relatively new, so long-term survival results will not be available for many years. Also, the studies done so far have included only small numbers of patients. One study included 70 men whose first biopsy showed a small amount of cancer on one side of the prostate. Treatment was done to that side only. Follow-up biopsies were done on 48 men at 6 and 12 months after the procedure and then annually. Although only one man had cancer seen on the side treated with cryotherapy, 12 more were positive on the opposite side. This means the first biopsy failed to find all the cancer. Sexual function was preserved in 86% but this was not based on written surveys. Hopefully, larger series with longer follow-up will become available in the next several years.

Who Is a Candidate for Focal Cryotherapy?

Obviously, focal cryotherapy can be done only if the cancer is found in very few locations on one side of the gland. The challenge is to make sure a patient meets this requirement. Studies have shown that taking 10 or 12 samples of prostate tissue during a biopsy often underestimates the amount and location of all the cancer. Therefore, relying on just one set of biopsies is not enough to tell where all your cancer is located. Patients who may be candidates for focal therapy usually undergo mapping biopsies during which more samples are taken. Ideal candidates have low-risk disease limited to one side of the gland. The treatment is performed similar to whole gland treatment.

How Men Are Followed after Focal Cryotherapy

Since focal cryotherapy is so new, the best way to follow men has not been established. Using PSA will be difficult for two reasons. First, the PSA will not drop nearly as low as when the entire gland is treated because normal prostate cells are still alive and they make PSA. No level can guarantee all the cancer cells have been killed nor can a stable PSA. The best option may be to repeat the mapping biopsies, but more studies are needed.

The Bottom Line on Cryotherapy

Cryotherapy is an option to consider for your localized cancer provided you understand what is known and not known, especially if you have low-risk disease and want to avoid a major operation or radiation therapy. However, if your goal is to have the best chance of getting rid of your cancer, this treatment is not the right one for you. The reason is that doctors do not yet know the survival results at 10 years or beyond using the latest methods, so the treatment has more uncertainty. Cryotherapy also would not be the right choice if you place a high priority on preserving your sexual function. Focal therapy is too new to know how it will compare with other therapies and should be considered experimental. It may be reasonable to do as part of a clinical study or if you are a good candidate for active surveillance but want to do "something" rather than just watch it.

Androgen Deprivation Therapy (ADT)

Testosterone is a male hormone called an *androgen* that is normally responsible for hair growth, muscle development, sperm production, and sexual function. In 1946, Dr. Charles Huggins discovered that testosterone causes prostate cancer cells to grow. He also found that reducing the amount of this hormone in the body improved symptoms of men with widespread prostate cancer. This treatment became known as *hormone therapy*. Other names include *androgen deprivation therapy (ADT)*, *androgen ablation*, and *castration*. As for this book, androgen deprivation therapy or ADT is the preferred term for this therapy. Although initially used to treat advanced disease, over the past 20 years ADT has also been used to treat men with localized prostate cancer.

How Is ADT Done?

When ADT was first discovered, men had only two options. One was to remove the testicles by a minor operation called a *bilateral orchiectomy*, because that organ produces most of the body's testosterone. This is called *surgical castration*. A second option was to give men female hormone pills called *diethylstilbestrol* or *DES*, which stopped the body from making testosterone. Since then, other drugs were discovered that had a similar effect. They are called *LHRH agonists* and *LHRH antagonists*. The chemical names are *leuprolide*, *goserelin*, *triptorelin*, *leuprolide acetate*, and *degarelix* and the commercial names are *Lupron and Eligard, Zoladex, Trelstar, Viadur,* and Firmagon. Using a drug for ADT is also called *medical castration*. They all have the advantages of enabling men to avoid an operation and the psychological stigma of losing their testicles. The drugs are given by an injection into a muscle or under the skin every one, three, or six months, or by an implant under the skin every 12 months. The side effects of these drugs are the same as removing the testicles, which are described later in this chapter.

Another group of drugs that affect the male hormones are called *antiandrogens*. They work by blocking testosterone from stimulating prostate cancer cells. Three drugs are available, each given by mouth. The chemical names are *bicalutamide, flutamide, and nilutamide* and the commercial names are *Casodex, Eulexin, and Nilandron*. The FDA approved these drugs for men with advanced disease, in combination with the LHRH agonists but not as a stand-alone treatment. So far, no good studies of antiandrogens have been done in men with localized disease, and conflicting results were found in men with more extensive disease. Even so, some doctors do use these drugs "off-label" to treat localized disease because of their lower rate of side effects. Men are less likely to have problems with erections and libido is preserved more often. Also, these drugs cause less weight gain and are less likely to affect cholesterol, triglycerides, or glucose. More information about them is contained in chapter 28.

What Are the Results with ADT?

A thorough review of medical journals yields few good studies of ADT for men with localized disease. One large study done between 1990 and 1999 randomized men to receive either immediate or delayed ADT. The delayed group was treated when disease progression occurred, but almost 50% of the men in this group had not yet received any treatment because their disease remained stable. With one-half of the men followed for seven years, overall survival was higher in the group receiving immediate therapy; it was 47.8% for immediate therapy versus 42.4% for delayed treatment. However, the percentage of men dying from prostate cancer was similar in the two groups (19.1% with immediate ADT and 20.1% in the delayed group). Also, the time until symptoms developed or the disease progressed was similar. The conclusion from this study is that immediate ADT slightly increased overall survival but it had no impact on the chance of dying from prostate cancer.

A different conclusion was made following an analysis of nearly 20,000 men who had immediate or delayed ADT for localized disease. It found a slightly higher risk of men dying from prostate cancer in 10 years with immediate therapy (19.9%) compared with delayed treatment (17.4%) but no difference in overall survival. This study was not randomized so the results are less reliable than the previous one discussed.

Since neither study offers any comparison to other treatments such as surgery or radiation, what should be the right take-home message about ADT? Some doctors might make the following argument:

- Delayed ADT is really the same as watchful waiting because those men eventually get ADT when the disease progresses. For that reason, the randomized study of immediate ADT versus delayed ADT is really a comparison of immediate ADT versus watchful waiting and it showed no difference in overall survival.

- Since the randomized study of radical prostatectomy versus watchful waiting also showed no difference in overall survival, then it is reasonable to conclude that there is no difference in overall survival between radical prostatectomy and immediate ADT.

Although logical, this argument may not be correct and only a randomized study can prove whether or not it is true. Until that occurs, the bottom line is that immediate ADT is a reasonable option for localized disease, but men might do nearly as well by delaying ADT until the disease progresses. Only those with high risk disease may be better off with early rather than delayed ADT.

What Are the Side Effects of ADT and How Are They Treated?

Both surgical and medical castrations cause side effects, which can have a negative impact on men's quality of life and sometimes may cause serious problems. Most of the information is obtained from retrospective studies making the true incidence of side effects less unclear. The most common ones and the reported frequencies are shown in the following table and explained below together with a brief discussion of how they are treated.

Table 14.1 Side Effects of ADT

Side Effect	Frequency and Extent
Hot flashes	21%–73%
Decreased sex drive	40%–60%
Problems with sexual function	50%
Decreased muscle mass (average loss)	1%–4%
Weight gain (average increase in 75% of patients)	3%
Osteoporosis (thinning of the bones; per year)	2%–3%
Bone fractures	6%–9%
Increased lipid levels:	
Cholesterol	8%
Triglycerides	27%
Low-density lipoproteins	9%

(continued)

Table 14.1 Side Effects of ADT (continued)

Side Effect	Frequency and Extent
Decreased cognitive function (thinking, calculating, memory)	Progresses over time
Anemia (decreased blood count)	90% of men have 10% drop 13% of men have 25% drop
Fatigue	2%–18%
Breast enlargement (gynecomastia)	10%–25%

Hot Flashes: These are similar to the hot flashes women have when they go through menopause, but doctors are not sure why they occur in men. It feels like a sudden sense of warmth in the face and upper body that may last a few seconds or minutes. Although they often occur several times a day, hot flashes usually are mild but occasionally they are very bothersome. Over time, they tend to become less severe. The FDA has not yet approved any drugs to treat this problem in men, but studies show that some used for other illnesses can be helpful. They are:

- Megestrol acetate (Megace) 20 mg two times a day

- Gabapentin (Neurontin) 900 mg a day

- Medroxyprogesterone (Provera) acetate 10 mg two times a day

- Venlafaxine (Effexor) 75 mg once a day

Decreased Sex Drive (Decreased Libido) and Impotence: Men's sex drive is controlled by testosterone. As it declines, so does a man's libido. The only way it can be treated is by allowing the testosterone level to rise, but that could make the cancer get worse.

The following drugs are available for men with decreased erections but they have no effect on libido. They work by increasing blood flow into the penis. Other treatments are described in chapter 18.

- Sildenafil (Viagra) 50 mg per day

- Tadalafil (Cialis) 10 or 20 mg taken every 36 hours

- Vardenafil (Levitra) 10 mg per day

- Avanafil (Stendra) 100–200 mg per day

Decreased Muscle Mass and Weight Gain: Testosterone plays a role in regulating normal metabolism. When the level goes down, metabolism slows down, weight gain may occur, muscle mass decreases, and fat content increases. No well-done studies have been done to show how best to treat these problems. One option is to eat differently. Men may benefit from meeting with a dietitian to plan out a well-balanced meal with the right amount of calories for a person's body size. Also, doing weight-bearing exercises several times a week can help burn calories while protecting the bones. These include walking, weight lifting, jogging, climbing stairs, aerobics, and dancing. If regular exercise has not been part of a person's daily life, he should consult with a fitness expert to develop a safe and effective program.

Osteoporosis and Fractures: Many aging men develop thinning of the bones called *osteoporosis*. This process happens faster when the testosterone level is lowered and can lead to an increased risk of fractures. Experts recommend that all men on ADT take *calcium carbonate* (500–1000 mg daily) and a daily multivitamin containing 400 IU of vitamin D. Decreased smoking and regular weight-bearing exercises also can help.

Bone health should be checked with a *DEXA scan (dual-energy x-ray absorptiometry)* when treatment begins and then repeated annually. Many doctors do not order this test so you will have to make sure to discuss it and request one. Every man should ask for a copy of his DEXA scan results to keep on file. They usually contain three numbers or scores: the bone mineral density (BMD), the T score, and the Z score. A normal BMD is from +1 to −1. The higher the number the better is a person's bone health. When the number is between −1 and −2.5 a person has *osteopenia* and anything lower than −2.5 means a person has osteoporosis. The other two values compare a patient's score to either a woman in her 30s (T score) or a person of similar age (Z score). The scoring is the same as the BMD.

Using this score, men can get some idea of their risk for fractures by using a fracture risk assessment tool called FRAX, which can be obtained for free on the Internet by typing "FRAX calculator" in your web browser. It will ask for some personal information and then calculate the probability of developing a pelvic fracture in the next 10 years. Patients with a FRAX value over three warrant a careful follow-up. Anyone with osteoporosis can be treated with one of the following FDA-approved medications for osteoporosis.

- Denosumab (Prolia, 60 mg given subcutaneously [under the skin] every six months for 6 doses). In a large randomized study, this drug reduced the risk of fractures from 3.9% to 1.5% over 3 years. That means it helps 15 men out of every 1000 that receive it. It is FDA approved for improving BMD and reducing fractures.

- Pamidronate disodium (Aredia, 60 mg given intravenously for two hours every 12 weeks) starting when hormone therapy begins can decrease bone loss during ADT. It is not known whether this drug will reduce the number of fractures.

- Alendronate (Fosamax, 70 mg orally once per week) was found to increase BMD in men with osteoporosis but it has not been studied in men on ADT. Also, its effect in preventing fractures is unknown.

- Risedronate (Actonel, 35 mg by mouth once per week or 150 mg once per month) is another approved oral bisphosphonate for men with osteoporosis, but not for preventing it in men on ADT.

- Ibandronate (Boniva, 150 mg orally once per month) improved BMD in men with osteoporosis.

- Zoledronic acid (Reclast, 5 mg given intravenously over 15 minutes once every 12 months) reduces bone loss and improves BMD in men with osteoporosis. Its effect on fractures at this dose is unknown and it does not have a specific approval for men on ADT without osteoporosis.

- Toremifene (Fareston, 80 mg orally each day) is one of a group of drugs called *selective estrogen receptor modulators or SERMs*, that have estrogen-like activity. In a recent randomized study, it was compared with a placebo in men on ADT. At the end of two years, fractures occurred in 4.9% of men on placebo compared with 2.5% of men on toremifene. This means it helped one out of every forty men taking it. The FDA has approved this drug for women but not yet for men on ADT.

No studies have been done comparing the different drugs for osteoporosis in men on ADT so the optimal treatment is not known. All of the ones described are reasonable options. Although they are all appropriate to treat osteoporosis, only denosumab and toremifene reduced fractures in men on ADT, and so far only denosumab is approved for that indication. More studies are likely to provide helpful information in the near future.

Some severe side effects can occur with these drugs. The bisphosphonates can irritate the stomach. They should be taken in the morning with a full glass of water on an empty stomach, before eating a meal. Food intake should be delayed for at least 30 minutes after taking the drug. Patients should sit or stand but not lie down for at least a half-hour to avoid heartburn. These drugs should not be taken late in the day. The bisphosphonates and denosumab can cause a drop in calcium in the blood and jaw problems called *osteonecrosis of the jaw* or ONJ. Patients having dental surgery should inform their dentist when they are taking these drugs. The bisphosphonates also can affect kidney function and require periodic testing. Men also should take calcium supplements while on one of these drugs. Another side effect of toremifene is deep vein thrombosis or pulmonary embolus, which occurred in 2.6% of the patients compared with 1.1% of the controls.

Metabolic Syndrome: This occurs when an individual has at least three of the following findings. It is associated with a significantly higher risk of developing heart disease.

- Elevated levels of cholesterol

- Elevated triglycerides

- Waist size greater than 40 inches

- Low levels of good cholesterol (HDL)

- High level of fasting glucose

An ongoing debate is whether ADT increases the risk for heart attacks in men without heart disease. This controversy is addressed later in this chapter.

Decreased Cognitive Function: Some good studies have found that, over time, castration results in decreased memory and a decreased ability to perform certain mental tasks such as doing calculations. These do not generally interfere with normal day-to-day activities. At this time, no studies have shown what should be done to treat this problem.

Anemia and Fatigue: All adults make a protein in their kidneys called *erythropoietin*, which helps make red blood cells. ADT lowers the production of this protein, resulting in a drop in the blood count within one or two months of starting treatment. A low blood count is called *anemia*, which can cause decreased energy, increased fatigue, and weakness. In men with heart disease, anemia can result in shortness of breath, chest pain, and even a heart attack.

Anemia usually is not treated unless symptoms occur, which happens in about 10% to 15% of men on hormone therapy. One option is to give a blood transfusion, but the blood count will drop again one to two months later. Iron supplements are not helpful for this problem.

A controversial option recommended by some doctors is to use a laboratory-made drug belonging to a group called *erythropoietin stimulating agents (ESAs)*. They work by helping the body to make more red blood cells. Well-done studies have shown they are able to reduce the need for blood transfusions in cancer patients treated with chemotherapy. A few good studies done outside the United States showed that giving an ESA to anemic prostate cancer patients on ADT reduced their need for a blood transfusion and improved their quality of life. However, ESAs are not approved in the United States for patients on this therapy, and they may be harmful. Well-done studies in breast and lung cancer patients have shown that ESAs can shorten survival, increase disease recurrence, and increase the risk of getting blood clots. Without further testing, your best advice at this time is *not to get an ESA* if you get anemic from ADT. Given the increased safety of donated blood, blood transfusions are a better approach if you have symptoms from a low blood count. The use of an ESA is appropriate if anemia develops while being treated with chemotherapy.

Weakness and Decreased Energy: Many men notice decreased energy, less ability to be active, and generalized weakness several months after starting ADT. Well-done studies show that men who participate in a resistance exercise program had less interference from fatigue, a higher quality of life, and higher levels of upper body and lower body muscular fitness than men not doing exercise. The program consisted of nine upper and lower strength-training exercises performed three times a week under the supervision of a fitness expert. Few doctors in the United States advise men to do any formal exercise program so you may have to seek out your own fitness trainer to set up a program for you.

Breast Enlargement (Gynecomastia): All men have both testosterone and estrogen in their body. Normally, the ratio of estrogen to testosterone is low but this changes during ADT, resulting in breast enlargement. Fortunately, only a small percentage of men are very bothered by it. In rare cases, plastic surgery is needed to reduce breast size. One to three radiation treatments directed at the breasts before starting treatment can reduce the chance of it occurring. Some drugs also are helpful; tamoxifen (Nolvadex) is a hormonal drug used to treat breast cancer and it can reverse the gynecomastia. The FDA has not approved it for use in men. Even so, before considering surgery, taking tamoxifen off-label might be an option to discuss if you are severely bothered.

Does ADT Increase the Risk of Heart Attacks?

Several poorly designed studies suggest the risk of dying from heart disease is increased in men on ADT. However, none of the randomized studies on the effect of ADT found an increased risk of dying from heart disease. A recent study combined eight randomized studies of ADT and found that regardless of the duration of treatment, deaths from cardiovascular disease were not increased. Nevertheless, the concern was important enough for the American Heart Association to issue the following advisory statements in 2010.

- There may be a relation between hormone therapy and cardiovascular risk.

- There is no clear indication to refer men for evaluation before starting hormone therapy.

- Men should be referred to their primary care doctor for periodic follow-up examinations.

Until new information is available, men should know that ADT can cause many side effects, but an increased risk of dying from heart disease does not appear to be one of them. As a precaution, the safest thing to do is check with your family doctor or heart specialist when starting this treatment. Dietary changes, exercise, and careful monitoring of glucose, cholesterol, and triglycerides should be part of a good treatment plan.

Who Is a Candidate for ADT?

Clearly, without a randomized study doctors can't be sure how the survival rate with ADT compares to the other treatments. Until then, ADT is most appropriate for a man with a life expectancy of less than 10 years who is not concerned about curing his cancer. It is a good option for someone who is satisfied to slow disease progression because he has other health concerns that are more likely to affect his survival. This treatment is not appropriate for someone who wants to do everything possible to avoid dying or suffering from prostate cancer. It also may not be a good choice for a man with low-risk disease (Gleason score less than 7, clinical stage less than T2b, and prostate-specific antigen (PSA) less than 10 ng/ml) because he is much more likely to die of something other than prostate cancer. For that reason, he may not want to suffer the side effects resulting from this therapy. ADT may be reasonable to consider for someone who has intermediate- or high-risk localized disease but does not want surgery or radiation. Be aware that it will result in a lower survival compared with getting ADT plus external radiation.

Suppose someone has severe heart disease; can he still consider having this treatment? The answer is a qualified *yes*, pending a consultation with the cardiologist.

What Is Intermittent Androgen Deprivation Therapy (IADT)?

More than 15 years ago, laboratory studies suggested that giving hormone therapy intermittently might be as good as or better than using it continually. This approach is called *intermittent hormone therapy* or *intermittent androgen deprivation therapy* (IADT). It is done by giving men one of the drugs that lower testosterone for several months and then stopping it after the PSA reaches a certain level. It is restarted either when the PSA rises to a certain number or after a set number of months. This process is repeated until the PSA no longer decreases when the treatment is restarted.

The benefits of IADT are that it lowers testosterone and the PSA similar to continuous therapy while minimizing the side effects. The reason side effects improve is that when ADT is stopped, the body usually regains its ability to make testosterone. As this hormone rises, some of the side effects go away until the treatment is restarted and then the side effects reappear. The net result is some men on IADT will have a better quality of life compared with those on continuous therapy.

No study of intermittent therapy has been done on men with localized disease but two have been done on other groups of patients. In one of them, men with a rising PSA after radiation therapy were given either continuous or intermittent therapy. No significant difference in survival was seen after half of the men had been followed for seven years. Men on IADT did have better physical function, with less fatigue, urinary problems, and hot flashes. They also had a better libido and better erectile function. A second study done on men with metastatic prostate cancer found that intermittent therapy gave a worse survival rate than continuous therapy. For now, intermittent androgen deprivation for a man with localized prostate cancer is an option, but there is uncertainty about its long-term effect. It does offer an improved quality of life, but it is less likely to maximize a man's survival. Also, doctors have not yet determined the best way to do this treatment. They do not know how long a man should be on therapy before stopping it or how long they should be off therapy before restarting it.

The Bottom Line on ADT in Localized Disease

In the absence of good studies, hormone therapy can be considered as an option, but it is unlikely to help men maximize their survival. Also, it does cause side effects that can significantly affect a man's quality of life. As with every treatment, the potential benefits comes with risks and each person will have to decide whether those risks are acceptable.

High-Intensity Focused Ultrasound (HIFU)

15

High-intensity focused ultrasound (HIFU) is a treatment that uses the energy from ultrasound waves to produce very high temperatures in the prostate of about 100 degrees Celsius or 212 degrees Fahrenheit. This is the same ultrasound used during a prostate biopsy with a different probe inserted into the rectum that delivers the energy. Laboratory studies have shown that HIFU can destroy cells in several organs, including the prostate gland. It has been tested as a method of treatment for different diseases for more than 50 years. In the last 10 years, the instruments have improved, making it safer and potentially more effective.

What Are the Advantages and Disadvantages of HIFU?

There are several reasons for HIFU being used as a treatment for localized prostate cancer. One is that some men with low-risk disease have trouble accepting active surveillance. They cannot live with the idea of leaving their cancer untreated even for a short time. They also are unwilling to accept the possibility of getting the complications that occur with radical prostatectomy, radiation, or seed implantation. They would rather have something done that can kill cancer cells if it is easy to do, even if its long-term benefit is unproven.

A second reason for its use is that HIFU is "minimally invasive," which means there are no cuts on the body. This enables men to recover quickly and avoid some of the side effects of radical prostatectomy such as blood loss, shortening of the penis, pain during an orgasm, or the development of a hernia. Another benefit is that permanent urinary leakage may be less common with HIFU than with surgery. Lastly, patients do not need to be routinely hospitalized following HIFU in contrast to all men needing at least one or two nights in the hospital after their prostate is removed.

HIFU also has potential advantages over radiation therapy. Men do not have to avoid close contact with children or pregnant women as they do with seed implantation. The treatment is completed in a few hours compared with six to eight weeks with external radiation. Lastly, HIFU can be repeated if some cancer cells survive, which is not possible after any form of radiation. Of course, the same is true for cryotherapy.

Although HIFU is minimally invasive, it still does have definite risks and disadvantages. Most importantly, the FDA has not yet approved it for use in the United States because its benefits still are unproven. That may change soon as the companies making the equipment have submitted an application for approval to the FDA. Also, long-term survival rates have not been reported. That also may change soon because older studies continue to report on patient outcomes. Until then, anyone wanting this treatment must have it done outside of this country. Some U.S. doctors are performing HIFU by taking their patients to treatment centers in Canada, Mexico, the Bahamas, or the Dominican Republic. Without FDA approval, Medicare and other insurance companies are unlikely to pay for it so you will have to pay for it yourself. The current fee ranges from $10,000 to $25,000 per treatment. If the cancer is not cured and the procedure is repeated, then you will need to pay an additional fee.

Another disadvantage is that side effects may occur. Despite its use for many years around the world, the true frequency of getting side effects has not been determined through use of written surveys. Without them, a valid comparison between HIFU and other treatments cannot easily be done. Although it has been marketed as having a low chance of impotence, that does not appear to be the case. The following table shows the approximate complication rates for men treated with either of the two HIFU machines in use today (Ablatherm and Sonablate 500).

Table 15.1 HIFU Complications

	Ablatherm	Sonablate
Retrograde ejaculation	NR	NR
Bladder neck/urethral stricture/stenosis	2%–17%	4%–30%
Urinary tract infection	2%–58%	4%–24%
Urinary incontinence	2%–34%	1%–2%
Urinary retention	3%–14%	1%–13%
Impotence	NR	20%–39%
Rectal burn	0%–15%	NR
Rectourethral fistula	0%–3%	NR

NR: not reported.

An explanation of these complications is provided below.

Retrograde ejaculation: The absence of fluid coming out through the tip of the penis after an orgasm. Instead, it goes into the bladder and comes out when a man urinates. Many men say that retrograde ejaculation decreases their pleasure during sexual activity. There is no good treatment and usually it will be permanent.

Bladder neck/urethral stricture/stenosis: A a scar that forms in the urinary tract. A rubber tube called a dilator or a metal instrument, called a *sound* is passed into the penis and through the scar to stretch it. Another option is a minor operation called a *visual internal urethrotomy (VIU)* in which a telescope is passed into the urethra and an attached knife or a laser can cut the scar. Some patients require these treatments more than once.

Urinary tract infection: Although an antibiotic is given before the HIFU is done, some men still get an infection, which usually responds to more antibiotics.

Urinary incontinence: Some men leak urine following HIFU, which gradually goes away in most cases. A small number are left with severe and permanent leakage, which may require surgery.

Urinary retention: Following HIFU, patients usually have a catheter left inside their bladder for one to two weeks because of difficulty urinating. The catheter is placed either through the penis or through the skin over the lower abdomen. After the catheter is removed, some men will still have difficulty urinating, which requires another catheter. Approximately 10% to 20% of patients will need additional treatment. To avoid this problem, some doctors are now doing a *transurethral resection of the prostate*, or *TURP*, just prior to the HIFU during the same anesthetic. It will remove prostate tissue that may block the urine.

Impotence: The inability to have an erection, which may be permanent or may improve over time. The treatment options are discussed in chapter 18.

Rectal burn: Sometimes the surface of the rectum is overheated during the procedure, causing a burn, which usually resolves without therapy.

Rectourethral fistula: Since the rectum is very close to the back of the prostate, intense heat can cause damage to the rectal wall leading to a small opening called a *fistula*. It may close on its own without any treatment, but in some cases it may require an operation.

What Are the Results with HIFU?

Although HIFU has been done for many years, no well-done studies have reported long-term survival. One recent retrospective study did report their results for 538 consecutive cases treated over 14 years with an average follow-up of eight years. The estimated results for low-, intermediate-, and high-risk tumors at 10 years are shown in the table.

Table 15.2 Ten-Year HIFU Results Using Ablatherm Device

Result	Low Risk	Intermediate Risk	High Risk
Biochemical disease-free survival (bDFS)	71%	63%	32%
No metastatic disease	99.6%	94.3%	84.6%
Died from prostate cancer	0%	3.3%	11%

The definition of *biochemical disease-free survival* used in this study was a PSA not increasing by 2 ng/ml over the lowest level achieved following treatment. Other studies use different definitions, which makes it hard to compare the results.

These results raise concern over the effectiveness of HIFU because almost 30% of low-risk and almost two-thirds of men with intermediate-risk disease developed recurrent disease. The side effects are also a concern because only 25% of men who were potent before treatment retained their erections.

Another way to evaluate this therapy is to look at the percentage of men with a positive biopsy some time after the treatment has been completed. Some published studies show cancer in 8% to 30% of the biopsies. The reasons for the wide range are that the proportion not having a biopsy and the number of cores removed varied widely in the studies reporting this result. Also, some studies counted HIFU successful in a patient if the first biopsy showed cancer but another biopsy was negative after the patient was re-treated. This also overestimates the success of this treatment.

Another controversy about evaluating HIFU is the definition of success based on the lowest PSA occurring after treatment. Studies show that an undetectable level is reached in only 50% to 70% of patients. Cancer recurred in 30% of men whose lowest PSA reached after treatment was between 0.2 and 1.0 ng/ml.

Who Is a Good Candidate for HIFU?

Until HIFU receives FDA approval and has long-term survival results, it must be considered a more uncertain way to treat prostate cancer. It would not be a good treatment for men who want to minimize being harmed by prostate cancer, those with high-risk disease, or those who have a prostate volume greater than 40 grams, unless the gland size can be reduced with medication. However, for men who understand its limitations, have a low-risk prostate cancer, and want to avoid surgery or radiation, it may be an option to consider.

How Is HIFU Performed?

On the night before and the morning of the HIFU treatment, an enema is given to clean the bowels. HIFU is performed under a general or spinal anesthetic to prevent you from moving during the procedure. After you are properly positioned on the treatment table, the anesthetic is administered and the HIFU probe is inserted into the rectum. It is similar to the ultrasound probe used to perform your biopsy, except it can focus the sound waves to a single point. Pictures then are taken and a computer determines the best location to focus the ultrasound. The procedure begins by sending a pulse of energy through the probe, generating intense heat that destroys several grams of prostate tissue. After one area is treated, the probe is focused on a different area until the entire prostate has been treated. The procedure is completed in approximately two to four hours depending on the size of the gland. Some doctors are also doing an operation called a transurethral resection of the prostate to remove tissue that may cause urinary blockage after a patient has been treated.

At the end of the procedure, a catheter is inserted into the bladder either through the abdomen or the penis. It remains in place for one to two weeks and then is removed. Before going home, patients are taught how to place a catheter into the penis in case they have difficulty urinating. Men can leave the hospital after recovering from the anesthetic.

The two machines currently in use are the *Sonoblate 500* and the *Ablatherm*. The Sonoblate 500 does have a theoretical advantage over the Ablatherm instrument; the doctor can see the prostate with the ultrasound and perform the treatment at the same time. The Ablatherm device requires that the ultrasound be performed first. The pictures taken are fed into a computer that plans the treatment. The actual treatment cannot be visualized while it is occurring. This might permit better control with the Sonoblate 500 device, but no study has compared the two. Until then, treatment with either machine is reasonable.

How Are Patients Monitored after HIFU?

Since HIFU is still evolving, no one has determined the optimal timing of follow-up visits. In many of the published reports from other countries, PSA tests are done about every three months for two years. Most patients reach their nadir PSA (lowest level) within six months, which is below 0.5 ng/ml in the majority of patients. Many surgeons also recommend performing a biopsy about three months after the procedure. HIFU either can be repeated or surgery or radiation can be offered if the biopsy does show cancer. Men continue to be monitored by a PSA and digital examination if the biopsy is negative.

The Bottom Line on HIFU

When you weigh all your options for treating localized disease, be aware that the current information is inadequate to determine whether HIFU is as effective for localized prostate cancer as surgery or radiation in terms of long-term survival or quality of life. Therefore, you should be cautious when (1) reading testimonials from men who have had this treatment, (2) consulting with doctors who perform it, or (3) visiting websites that promote it. They all have biases favoring HIFU and are not presenting all the information accurately. Many of the men followed for less than 10 years may appear to be doing well after HIFU not because the treatment was effective but rather because their cancer was not dangerous. Without longer follow-ups and better studies, you will not know what to expect from HIFU. Studies are underway in the United States, but until they are completed I feel it's important to repeat the following statement that most accurately summarizes the current status of HIFU:

> *The current information is inadequate to determine if HIFU is an effective treatment for localized prostate cancer with long-term survival and quality of life comparable to surgery or radiation.*

Hopefully, more information will become available in the next few years.

The Effects of Treatment on Men's Quality of Life

Making a decision about treating your prostate cancer would be so much easier if none of the treatments affected your quality of life, but unfortunately that is not the case. They may cause changes in urinary, sexual, and possibly bowel functions, and have other effects as well. Because no one can exactly predict what will happen to you, the best that can be done is to tell you what happened to other men following their treatment.

The most accurate way to determine the effects of a therapy is by having men complete a written or telephone survey containing questions that have been tested for their reliability. Not enough doctors use these surveys, which makes it hard to know the true results occurring with most treatments. Instead, side effects are simply estimated, which is far less accurate. Fortunately, a growing number of studies have used these surveys and the results from some of them are contained in the tables included in this chapter.

What Are the Results from Quality-of-Life Surveys?

In the first study, surveys were sent about four years after 380 men were enrolled in the randomized Scandinavian study comparing watchful waiting and radical prostatectomy that was discussed in detail in chapter 7. The results are shown below in tables. The last column shows the difference between the two treatments; a plus (+) sign means it was more common after radical prostatectomy and a minus (–) means it was more common with watchful waiting.

Table 16.1a Sexual Function of Men following Watchful Waiting or Radical Prostatectomy

Outcome	Watchful Waiting	Radical Prostatectomy	Difference
Erection seldom or never sufficient for intercourse	45%	80%	+35%
Spontaneous erections seldom or never sufficient for intercourse	61%	90%	+29%
Moderate or severe distress from erectile dysfunction	43%	58%	+15%
Intercourse less than once per month	59%	80%	+21%
Moderate or great distress from decreased intercourse	43%	59%	+16%

Table 16.1b Urinary Function of Men following Watchful Waiting or Radical Prostatectomy

Urinary Outcome	Watchful Waiting	Radical Prostatectomy	Difference
Weak urinary stream on more than one in five occasions	44%	28%	−16%
Leak urine at least once per week	21%	49%	+28%
Some urinary leakage	35%	62%	+27%

(continued)

Table 16.1b Urinary Function of Men following Watchful Waiting or Radical Prostatectomy (continued)

Urinary Outcome	Watchful Waiting	Radical Prostatectomy	Difference
Moderate or severe distress from urinary leakage	9%	29%	+20%
Use some aid for urinary leakage	10%	43%	+33%
Moderate or severe stress from all urinary symptoms	18%	27%	+9%

As you can see, urinary and sexual functions were worse for the men having surgery except for the strength of their urinary stream. That was worse with watchful waiting, which is explained by the prostate increasing in size. One of the important results of this study is that it shows that the quality of life for men on conservative therapy does decline over time, but it clearly is worse for men getting surgery.

There are some limitations to this study. First, no baseline surveys were done, which prevents determining how men were changed by their treatment. Second, it was done in Sweden and Finland, enrolling patients from 1989 to 1999. It is unclear how men treated in the United States would respond if treated now. Also, the results are not 100% accurate because some men did not complete their assigned treatment and were treated differently. Lastly, not everyone who received a survey completed it. Despite these limitations, however, the results begin to provide you with some idea about how men are affected by these two treatments.

In a second study, phone surveys were done before and up to two years after 1200 men were treated with external radiation, permanent brachytherapy, or radical prostatectomy. The patients were enrolled between 2003 and 2006. Table 16.2 shows the change in the percentage of men having each complaint before

Table 16.2 Quality of Life Two Years after Radical Prostatectomy, External Radiation, or Brachytherapy

Quality of Life	Difference from Baseline to Two Years		
	Radical Prostatectomy (%)	External Radiation (%)	Permanent Brachytherapy (%)
Weak urinary stream	−8%	−3%	+4%
Urinary frequency	−7%	−2%	+9%
Leaking urine more than once/day	+10%	+1%	+5%
Using pads in underwear	+7%	+4%	+6%
Urine leakage a moderate/big problem	+6%	No change	+8%
Urgency to have bowel movement	+1%	+13%	+5%
Frequent bowel movements	None	+8%	+4%
Blood in stool	None	+4%	+2%
Bothered by bowel function	None	+8%	+6%
Poor erections	+44%	+23%	+21%
Difficulty with orgasms	+30%	+18%	+21%
Erections not firm	+47%	+18%	+22%
Poor sexual function	+41%	+24%	+18%
Sexual function a moderate or big problem	+31%	+19%	+18%

treatment compared with two years after treatment. A plus sign (+) means more men had that complaint following their treatment and a negative sign (–) means fewer men had it.

You can interpret this table as follows. The first complaint is *weak urinary stream*. It occurred in 8% fewer men after surgery, in 3% fewer men after external radiation, but in 4% more men after permanent brachytherapy. As you can see, at two years, more men had problems with sexual function after surgery but fewer problems with bowel function compared with either form of radiation. Urinary frequency was most common in men having seed implantation. This study also found that African American men had less satisfaction following their treatment than other races. Another feature of this study was assessing responses from the spouses and partners of patients. Not surprisingly, their distress level due to side effects was similar to their partner's.

The potential weaknesses of this study are that the patients were not randomly selected for their treatment. As a result, the groups differed in several ways including the average age of the patients, their tumor stage and grade, and overall health status. Also, although the men having surgery were younger and healthier, many of them did not have nerve-sparing surgery. This could partly explain why more of them had poor sexual function compared with that reported in many recent studies from the United States. As for the radiation group, there are two possible reasons for the worsening sexual function. First, some of the men received hormone therapy. Secondly, the average age of this group was higher, and older men have a more rapid decline in sexual function than younger men due to natural aging. Another problem with the study is that only 60% of the patients completed both surveys. This could bias the results if those men not responding would have answered the questions differently. Even so, this study adds to your information about the frequency of side effects after treatment.

In another study, interviews based on standardized surveys were conducted on more than 1600 men under age 70 who were treated in Australia between 2000 and 2002 by community-based doctors.

Table 16.3 Difference in Percentage of Patients with Problem before Compared with Three Years after Treatment

Symptoms	Active Surveillance	Hormone Therapy	RP Nerve-Sparing	RP Non-Nerve-Sparing	XRT	XRT + Hormones	LDR Seeds	HDR
Urinary incontinence	−3%	−2%	+9%	+14%	+3%	+1%	+5%	+7%
Moderate/ severe bowel problems	−7%	−4%	No change	−3%	+4%	+4%	No change	+7%
Impotence	+27%	+21%	+52%	+59%	+38%	+43%	+17%	+52%

Treatments: RP = radical prostatectomy, XRT = external radiation, LDR = permanent seed implantation, HDR = temporary brachytherapy.
Urinary incontinence defined as leakage that required one or more pads per day.
Bowel problems defined as moderate or big problem with bowel habits.
Impotence defined as being unable to obtain an erection sufficient for sexual intercourse.

The table on the facing page shows the difference in the percentage of men having one of these problems before and three years after treatment. Similar to the previous table, a plus (+) sign means the problem was more common at three years and a minus (−) sign means it was less common.

This table shows that the smallest change in sexual function occurred with permanent seed implants and the biggest increase in the percentage of men with impotence or incontinence occurred following radical prostatectomy. Men undergoing nerve-sparing surgery did not do that much better than men not having a nerve-sparing operation. This could be due in part to the experience level of the surgeons. You might wonder why 27% of the men on active surveillance had worse sexual function at three years. Since this management often is done to help preserve sexual function, the expectation is it should have been much better. However, many of the men stopped active surveillance and switched to definite therapy, most often surgery. Since the results were still counted in the active surveillance group, it made the outcomes for that group look worse.

Here again, several factors may have affected the results. The men were not randomized to each treatment so the groups did not consist of men with the same age, tumor stage, or health status. A second problem is all men were treated outside the United States. Also, not all men completed the three-year survey and those not responding might have had different results. Lastly, better results might have occurred if "prostate cancer experts" had done each treatment.

The next three tables (16.4a, 16.4b, and 16.4c) provide information from the U.S. Prostate Cancer Outcomes Study, or PCOS, comparing radical prostatectomy and external radiation. The report is based on almost 1200 men in the age range of 55 to 74, who were treated between 1994 and 1995 in one of six regions in the United States. Each patient was sent a survey to complete at two and five years. Since the studies discussed earlier reported their results at two and three years after treatment, only the five-year results from this study are shown in the following tables. The last column shows the difference between the two groups in the percentage of men having each side effect. Here again, a plus (+) sign means it was more common after radical prostatectomy and a minus (−) sign means it was less common.

Table 16.4a Urinary Function Five Years after Radical Prostatectomy or External Radiation

Urinary Function	Percentage of Men Affected by Each Treatment		
	Radical Prostatectomy	External Radiation	Difference
No urinary control or frequent leakage	14%	5%	+9%
Leak urine more than once per day	15%	4%	+11%
Wear urinary pads	29%	4%	+25%
Bothered by urinary leakage	14%	3%	+11%

Table 16.4b Sexual Function Five Years after Radical Prostatectomy or External Radiation

Sexual Function	Percentage of Men Affected by Each Treatment		
	Radical Prostatectomy	External Radiation	Difference
Erection insufficient for intercourse	77%	73%	+4%
Bothered by sexual dysfunction	47%	42%	+5%
No sexual activity	49%	51%	−2%

Table 16.4c Bowel Function Five Years after Radical Prostatectomy or External Radiation

	Percentage of Men Affected by Each Treatment		
Bowel Function	Radical Prostatectomy	External Radiation	Difference
Bowel urgency	18%	33%	−15%
Wetness in rectal area	14%	21%	−7%
Diarrhea	23%	29%	−6%

This study also found men had worse urinary and sexual function five years after radical prostatectomy and worse bowel function after radiation. Here too, potential biases and other factors may have affected the results. Again, the study was not randomized so the groups differed in age and health status. Another potential bias is that many men did not complete the five-year survey. Also, improvements in radiation and surgery methods over the last 20 years would likely result in better outcomes today. Lastly, different results may be expected today if experts in prostate cancer therapies do the treatments. Despite these problems, this is one more piece of information to consider when choosing your treatment.

As you have just read, each of these studies has shortcomings but they were selected because of the number of men included and the methods used. Smaller studies or those not using validated surveys are much less likely to be accurate and that is all that is available for other treatments. Perhaps one day, truly reliable information will become available, but until then, this is what you will have to use as you weigh your options.

The Bottom Line on Quality of Life following Treatment of Localized Disease

What do all these numbers mean? Despite the limitations of each study cited, these results should help "paint a better picture" for you of what has happened to other men following their treatment for localized prostate cancer over the last 20 years. As you can see, there is some consistency to the results. With radical prostatectomy, men have the greatest problem with sexual function and urinary control immediately after surgery and then gradually they improve. Those individuals treated with some form of radiation have little change in urinary control or sexual function immediately after treatment, but then they may get worse with time. The main problem is leaking urine, and in all the studies it becomes worse after surgery. By five years, the differences between surgery and radiation get smaller but they still persist. In contrast, men treated with radiation have persistent problems with bowel function consisting of urgency and frequency of their bowel movements. As time goes on, this problem still persists. More studies using validated surveys are needed in men having other forms of treatment, which will provide a better picture of what happens. As stated before, the results probably would be better today than reported in these studies and the exact changes will still depend on each man's age, health, tumor type, and the experience of his doctor.

The goal in this chapter has been to provide you with much more information than simply what *can* happen after each treatment. By having some idea of *how often* each problem has occurred in other patients and combining it with the odds each treatment will get rid of your cancer, you are now more equipped to decide how to proceed. Remember, each treatment offers a package of good and bad effects, and only you can decide if the trade-off is acceptable. The next chapter will help you make the decision about which treatment is right for you.

How to Decide Which Treatment Is Right for You

At this point, you have read about nearly every treatment for managing localized prostate cancer and yet you may be no closer to knowing what to do. You understand the pros and cons of each option and find that each one has things you like and dislike. As you have heard before, each treatment has its combination of good and bad results. Hopefully, you have a better understanding of those packages. Now it's "crunch" time as you try to answer the question, "Which treatment is right for me?" Although it may feel like a purely emotional decision, you can still be objective. It begins by reviewing what you have read. The following table shows the strengths, weaknesses, and optimal patients for every available option.

Table 17.1 Summary of Treatment Options

Treatment Options	Strengths	Weaknesses	Optimal Patients
Watchful waiting	Avoid side effects of local treatment	Could result in shortened survival or developing metastatic disease. May miss an opportunity for cure. Psychologically stressful	Low-risk and intermediate-risk tumors. Life expectancy less than 10 years. Quality of life is highest priority
Active surveillance	More than 50% of patients may avoid treatment for at least 10 years. Less risk than watchful waiting	Limited information about 10-year survival results. No long-term results for patients getting delayed treatment. Psychologically stressful	Low-risk and some intermediate-risk tumors. Life expectancy less than 10 years. Quality of life is high priority
Radical prostatectomy	Has the most information available about long-term survival. May cure localized cancer. Causes more sexual dysfunction and urinary problems than other options. Most aggressive way to get rid of cancer	Has immediate effect on sexual and urinary function that often improves with time Sexual function often does not return to baseline level	Low-, intermediate- and high-risk tumors. Life expectancy greater than 15 years. Want immediate results. Survival matters more than quality of life

External radiation using 3D-CRT or IMRT	Higher doses now safer and more effective	10–15 yr survival not available with higher doses. Poor choice if bowel dysfunction present. Delayed effect on bowel, urinary, and sexual function. Fewer bladder and sexual function side effects than surgery. More bowel side effects than surgery	Low-, intermediate-, and high-risk tumors benefit from hormone therapy. Life expectancy greater than 10 years. Want to avoid surgery. Survival matters more than quality of life. Minimal bowel problems
Brachytherapy	Quick and convenient. Sexual function maintained initially. Resume normal activities more quickly than with surgery	Side effects increase over two years. Poor choice if urinary problems are present. Must avoid close contact with pregnant women and children for several months	Low- and intermediate-risk cancers. Life expectancy greater than 10 years. Want to resume normal activities quickly. Gland size less than 40–50 g

(continued)

Table 17.1 Summary of Treatment Options (continued)

Treatment Options	Strengths	Weaknesses	Optimal Patients
Proton beam radiation	Theoretical advantages over 3D-CRT or IMRT, but recent studies show opposite results	No 10-year survival results. No proven advantage over external radiation. Limited studies have not shown better quality of life. More expensive than external radiation Few treatment centers in U.S.	Low-, and intermediate-risk tumors. Willing to accept new treatment without knowing effectiveness
IGRT (Calypso tracking) or SGRT (CyberKnife system)	Theoretical advantages over 3D-CRT or IMRT. Treatment completed in a shorter time	Poor studies assessing survival or quality of life. 10-year results not available Treatment centers limited No studies proving it delivers better results	Low-risk tumors Unclear if ADT improves results for intermediate- or high-risk tumors. Willing to accept new treatment without knowing effectiveness
Cryotherapy	May destroy cancer without surgery. Treatment can be repeated	High risk of erectile dysfunction 10-year survival results not reported Impact on quality of life not assessed well.	Low-risk tumors Life expectancy greater than 10 years. Want immediate results.

			Sexual function not important. Not bothered by limited follow-up. Gland size must be less than 60 gm
High-intensity focused ultrasound	May destroy cancer without surgery or radiation. Treatment can be repeated	10-year survival not reported. Impact on quality of life not assessed well. Not FDA approved in U.S.	Low-risk tumors. Life expectancy 10 years or less. Willing to accept new treatment without knowing long-term effectiveness. Want to avoid surgery and radiation
Androgen deprivation therapy	Avoids surgery and radiation. Delays disease progression. Uncertain impact on survival	Many side effects cause decrease in quality of life. Impact on survival unknown. Does not kill all cancer cells	Low-, intermediate-risk tumors. Life expectancy less than 10 years. Getting rid of tumor not primary concern

3D-CRT = Three-dimensional conformal radiotherapy; IMRT = Intensity-modulated radiation therapy; SGRT = Stereotactic guided radiation therapy, FDA = Food and Drug Administration; ADT = Androgen deprivation therapy; IGRT = Image Guided Radiation Therapy.

Factors to Consider as You Make Your Choice

The most important point to remember as you make your decision is that the right treatment for you is not necessarily the right treatment for other men. Of course, it should partly depend on your age, health, and tumor properties. But equally important is the need to factor in your personal goals and fears and your personality type. As a first step, you should try to answer the following questions:

- What is most important to you, to maximize your survival or your quality of life?

- What kind of person are you? Are you a risk taker or do you prefer to minimize uncertainty?

- Do you like immediate results or are you willing to be patient?

- Are you a worrier who will think about your cancer day and night, or can you let it go and go about your normal daily activities without much anxiety?

Recognizing characteristics about yourself is an important part of this decision because some treatments may "fit" your personality better than others. For example, suppose you have a low-risk cancer (PSA under 10 ng/ml, Gleason score less than 7 and stage T1c or T2a). Given the most recent study results (see chapter 7), you may feel that the odds of benefitting from treatment are not high enough to justify taking the risk of getting side effects. Instead, maximizing your quality of life is your highest priority. In this case, watchful waiting or active surveillance is the right choice for you. Your quality of life may get worse in the future, as you age or if you eventually need treatment for your cancer, but at least nothing will change right now or for many years after your diagnosis. Focal cryotherapy may be worth considering if you do not want to leave the cancer untreated. Even though doctors do not know if it will effectively treat the cancer, it is a better way to preserve your quality of life than the other options. It also offers a psychological benefit, by enabling you to believe that you are doing something to treat your cancer.

What if you cannot accept the possibility of missing out on a chance to be cured even if you have a low-risk tumor? Or perhaps you may not be comfortable rolling the dice, hoping the cancer never harms you. The possibility of a decrease in your quality of life is a small price to pay to have "peace of mind." In this case, the treatments that would not be good for you include watchful waiting, active surveillance, high-intensity focused ultrasound (HIFU), cryotherapy, proton beam therapy, temporary brachytherapy, and stereotactic guided radiation. None of them have been in use long enough to know how well they will control prostate cancer at 10 or 15 years. The bottom line on these options is that too little is known for any of them to be a good choice for someone who wants the best chance of getting rid of his cancer. This does not mean they are definitely inferior treatments. However, until more information becomes available, they would not be the best fit for someone with these concerns.

Probably the best fit here is a radical prostatectomy provided the person has a low- or intermediate-risk cancer. It will provide some helpful details about the risk for recurrence that can't be obtained with any other treatment and the cancer will be "out of your body."

If no studies have proven that surgery is better than radiation or brachytherapy, you may be wondering why some doctors consider it to be the most aggressive treatment. Think of the answer this way: if all the cancer cells are located inside the prostate and the entire gland is removed, then the cancer is gone and you will be cured. The reason radiation and seed implantation are considered to be less aggressive is because these treatments *may not kill all the cells all of the time.* Even if they are combined with hormone therapy, some cancer cells may survive. Over time, they may grow and spread and eventually may cause harm. The bottom line is that surgery immediately gets rid of all the cancer *when it is located inside the prostate,* but the different types of radiation may not do so in all cases. Furthermore, one to two years may be needed to find out if all the cancer has been killed following radiation. Some day randomized studies comparing these treatments may become available. Until then, all that can be said is that these three treatments are reasonable alternatives for low- and intermediate-risk disease, with surgery fitting better for men who want to be very aggressive.

Of course, radical prostatectomy does not cure everyone because sometimes cancer cells already have left the prostate and they are unaffected by the surgery. Over time, they continue to grow. Patients with high-risk tumors often fit into this group. The best option for these men is radical prostatectomy or radiation combined with ADT. Combining IMRT either with temporary or permanent seed implantation plus ADT is a more aggressive option than radiation plus ADT. So far, however, no studies have shown that the results are better. It definitely will result in the greatest chance of getting side effects. At this time, the role of permanent seed implantation, SGRT, cryotherapy, HIFU, or ADT in these men is very unclear. If you choose one of them, be aware that you are taking more risk because very little is known about their ability to control these more aggressive cancers. Although you still are able to have surgery if any of these methods fail to eliminate the cancer, the odds of getting complications would be higher than if you had surgery first.

Suppose you have a low- or intermediate-risk cancer and want to be cured, but you are afraid of surgery and you do not need immediate results. In this case, 3D-CRT, x-ray therapy, IMRT, or permanent brachytherapy would be the best fit. Brachytherapy is the most convenient option because it only takes a few hours to complete without your needing to stay in the hospital. Temporary brachytherapy is more inconvenient, requiring one or two nights in the hospital confined to bed. The benefit is that you go home without any radiation in your body. The main problem with temporary brachytherapy is long-term survival results are still unknown.

Lastly, perhaps you are an "adventurer," someone who likes taking chances. Clear proof that the treatment works is not that important. You feel comfortable gambling on new treatments because they sound exciting and you are willing to accept the consequences. In that case, proton beam radiation, temporary brachytherapy, SGRT, cryosurgery, or HIFU may appeal to you. The bottom line is that your personality should be an important part of choosing your therapy.

Health issues should also be considered. If you have a low-risk tumor and have other health problems that are likely to shorten your life span to 10 years or less, active surveillance makes the most sense. If you have a high-risk cancer, then treatment might be helpful even if your life expectancy is only five years, with any option worth considering. Perhaps you already are unable to have an erection and various options for improving erections have not helped. If you choose surgery, a nerve-sparing radical prostatectomy makes little sense because your sexual function is already impaired. You should just have both nerves removed along with the prostate to reduce the chance of leaving cancer behind. Perhaps you already have difficulty urinating or go frequently. In that case, brachytherapy will worsen these symptoms more than the other options and surgery will make it better. Lastly, if bowel problems already exist, external radiation will have a more negative effect on your quality of life and probably should be avoided. The bottom line is that you should combine your knowledge about each option with your goals, fears, and personality when deciding what to do.

The Role of Your Partner

If you are married or have a life partner, he or she should be part of this decision too, because what happens to you also will affect your spouse or partner. It should be no surprise that your partner may have different goals than you do. Many men, particularly those under 60, place the highest priority on sexual function when survival is the highest priority for their partner. What are you supposed to do if you are strongly considering watchful waiting or active surveillance but they want your prostate removed tomorrow? There is no easy solution and certainly no "right" answer. The best advice is to gather the facts and talk about them with your partner. Then you can make a decision together. There even may be a role for a counselor to help you discuss any differences you may have. Bringing your spouse or partner to the doctor to ask questions and hear about each treatment will be good for both of you.

Your Family Doctor's Role in Selecting Your Treatment

As you work through this decision process, two obvious places to turn for help are your family doctor and your urologist or radiation therapist. By now, you have already been informed about your options and probably have heard a "recommendation" from the specialist. Nothing is wrong with a doctor offering an opinion, but it should be made clear to you that it is just an opinion and there may be a bias. The newer therapies are likely to be recommended by those doctors who are performing them and not by other doctors. Remember, of the 14 options available, only watchful waiting and radical prostatectomy have been compared in a randomized study. For that reason, no one can really say which treatment has the best chance of curing your cancer.

Increasingly, doctors are becoming more balanced when discussing the options, choosing to explain the pros and cons of each option and letting their patients decide rather than telling them what to do. Although that may be unsettling to you, it's the most honest way to help you. Right now, doctors do not have all the answers. Do you really want them to decide for you when they really don't know what's best? Also, since you will have to live with the side effects—not your doctor—you should be part of this decision.

Some patients put the question to the doctor directly by asking, "What would you do if you were me?" Unfortunately, the answer is not really very helpful, again because of possible biases. Years ago, an interesting survey was done in which urologists, oncologists, and radiation therapists were asked, "What treatment would you recommend for a 60-year-old, healthy member of your family who has localized prostate cancer?" Not surprisingly, nearly all the surgeons answered surgery, nearly all the radiation therapists answered radiation, and the oncologists were split. It is not very different from asking a Cadillac salesperson "What car should I buy, a Cadillac or a Volvo?" That person would have trouble staying in business if he or she recommended the Volvo! Similarly, the radiation therapist would have a problem by routinely recommending surgery.

What about getting a second opinion? That might be reasonable provided you tell your doctor you want only an unbiased assessment of your situation and not someone else to treat you. Otherwise the advice given also might be biased. What about asking your family doctor for a second opinion since he or she has no particular interest in which treatment you choose? That might seem to be helpful, but only if the family doctor has all the facts you have read in this book, which is highly unlikely. Otherwise, your family doctor, too, will have biases. What your family doctor can do, however, is provide you with information about your current health and life expectancy, which is important to know when making your decision. The bottom line is that after reading this book, you have the best information available to enable you to make a decision.

Talking to Other Patients

Getting information from other men who have been treated for prostate cancer can sometimes be helpful and sometimes can be the opposite. They can tell you about their experience, what problems they had, and how they made their choice, which is valuable information. However, you should be careful because their response may depend on how well they are doing, which can be misleading. If you talk to someone who had an excellent response to his treatment, he is highly likely to recommend it. If he had a bad result, then the opposite is likely to happen. Asking someone,

"Would you do the same thing again?" also is not very helpful because the question is meaningless; they can't undo their treatment. Also, men do not like to admit they made a mistake. If you want to talk with a number of men having different treatments, the prostate cancer support groups are an excellent place to go. You can either ask your doctor if there is a group nearby or search the Internet for prostate cancer-support groups. Some type of group is present in most cities.

The Bottom Line on Choosing Your Treatment

No doubt, you have been going through a difficult emotional experience for several weeks or months starting with your PSA test. First you had anxiety worrying about the result. Then you had to go through a biopsy and worry if it would show cancer. Finally, you have probably spent considerable time learning about your options while you struggle with the choice of which option to choose. You should now have all the information you need and you do not have to make your decision quickly. Your cancer did not develop yesterday and is highly unlikely to get worse if you take a few weeks to decide how you want to be treated. Make sure you have all your questions answered and then review the ones raised at the beginning of this chapter. That should enable you to decide which treatment is right for you.

How to Improve Your Quality of Life

After your treatment has been completed, the priority can shift to maximizing your quality of life. The most important message in this chapter is that several treatments are available to help you, and you should make sure all of them are discussed. If your doctor does not bring them all up, then be sure to ask questions so you can get the information you need. The most common problems occurring following treatment affect your sexual, urinary, and bowel functions, but other things can also occur. There are two parts of treatment to help maintain your quality of life. One is to do things that will reduce the chance of having problems following your treatment. The other is to treat any side effects as soon as they occur.

Changes in Sexual Function after Prostate Cancer Treatments

Men's sexual function may be affected in several ways following treatment for prostate cancer. The ability to have erections good enough for sexual intercourse may be reduced. Some men notice a decrease in the length of the penis, which may limit their ability to satisfy their partner. Lastly, men also can have psychological reasons for poor sexual function such as depression. This can lead to a decreased desire to have sexual relations.

One difference between some of the cancer treatments is at what point a man will develop problems with his sexual function. Those who are treated with radiation or seed implantation usually keep their erections initially, but this ability may get worse with time. In contrast, men undergoing nerve-sparing radical prostatectomy, cryotherapy, or high-intensity focused ultrasound usually have erection problems immediately after treatment. They may get better with time, but it might take up to two years before knowing how well they will function. Treatment is aimed at maintaining adequate blood flow into the penis to prevent scarring until normal functions return.

Options for Penile Rehabilitation and Treating Sexual Dysfunction

Studies have been done to determine whether any treatment can increase the chance that a man will regain his pretreatment sexual function. The term for this is *penile rehabilitation*.

The options tested include *phospho-diesterase-5 inhibitors* (PDE-5 inhibitors), *penile injections*, and a *vacuum erection device* (VED).

- **PDE-5 Inhibitors:** Normally, an enzyme in the body breaks down a chemical that helps a man maintain an erection. PDE-5 inhibitors block that enzyme, which increases blood flow to the penis, thus helping to improve erections. This is the easiest treatment available and usually is the first one offered to patients. The PDE-5 inhibitors that have been approved by the FDA include *sildenafil (Viagra)*, *tadalafil (Cialis)*, *vardenafil (Levitra)*, and *avanafil (Stendra)*. None of these have been compared in a randomized study so it is unclear which one would be best. However, the effects of tadalafil can last for up to 36 hours. Some doctors let patients make the decision after trying samples of each of them. If you try one and it does not work, then ask your doctor about trying the others.

- **Penile injections:** Drugs are available that can cause an erection within 5 to 10 minutes when injected into the side of the penis through a very small needle. They work by opening or dilating blood vessels to allow more blood into the penis. One of them is called *alprostadil* (*Caverject, Edex*). It is self-administered about 10 to 15 minutes before sexual activity. The main side effect with both methods is pain in the penis or a bruise from the injection. A rare side effect is an erection that does not go away called *priapism*, which requires immediate medical attention. Some men get better results injecting a mixture of three drugs called trimix instead of the alprostadil.

- **Vacuum erection device:** This is a hollow plastic cylinder that fits over the penis and is pushed firmly against the skin. Air is pumped out of the chamber by a battery-operated motor located at the end of the device. This creates a vacuum, which draws blood into the penis resulting in an erection. A special band is slipped onto the penis to maintain the erection. When the band is removed, the blood flows out of the penis and the erection goes away. Several companies make these devices, which can be seen by searching the Internet. None has been shown to be superior, so any of the options are acceptable.

Two other treatments are available to help a man resume sexual intercourse.

- **MUSE (Medicated Urethral System for Erection)** is a small suppository containing alprostadil that is placed inside the urethra at the tip of the penis. It works similar to the penile injection by increasing blood flow into the penis. It often produces an erection within 10 minutes that can last several hours. The main side effect is pain in the penis.

- **Artificial penile implant** is a device that is placed inside the penis during a two-hour operation. Some implants are inflated at the time of sexual activity by activating a small pump placed into the scrotum. Others are semirigid and work without any adjustments. The main side effect is infection, which sometimes requires that the device be removed.

After reading about these options, your first reaction may be that taking a pill is okay but the others are not. The idea of putting a needle into the side of your penis, placing something inside the tip, or using a pump or penile implant sounds unappealing. You are not the first person to have those reactions, but the truth is that most men and their partners find every one of them acceptable and satisfying. You are encouraged to consider all of them and even try them as a possible solution. At least you have several choices that can enable you to resume sexual intimacy with your partner.

Results of Penile Rehabilitation Studies

Doctors have tried to find ways to help men improve more quickly after their therapy. One randomized study compared vardenafil (Levitra) to a placebo in 300 men under age 65 who were recovering from a nerve-sparing radical prostatectomy. One group took 20 mg of the drug "on demand," meaning when the man was interested in sexual activity. The other group only took a placebo. The reason that the drug only was used on demand is because a previous study had found that "on demand" worked better than routinely taking the drug several times a week. This study found that men had a significant benefit from the vardenafil; about 22% to 26% more men on the drug had successful intercourse or adequate erections compared with only 3% to 4% of those on placebo. Also, a higher percentage of men taking the active drug achieved normal erections by the end of the study. The most common side effect was headache, occurring in 20% of the men.

A small, randomized study in 30 men recovering from radical prostatectomy compared taking alprostadil injections three times per week for 12 weeks against no treatmentat. Sixty-seven percent of the men getting the drug were able to have erections compared with only 20% in the control group. One problem was that many men did not continue the program long term due to discomfort from the injections.

Two small studies compared the use of a VED pump starting one month after radical prostatectomy to those men who waited five or six months before using the device. The early intervention group used the device daily without a constriction band for five months. Men using the VED shortly after surgery had better sexual function and the stretched length of the penis was significantly longer compared with the men not using the device.

Little information is available on penile rehabilitation following other treatments for prostate cancer. One small, randomized study found that men with reduced erections after external radiation that received 50 mg or 100 mg of sildenafil had better sexual function compared with those men on placebo. Without proper studies, however, doctors cannot say whether any of the treatments are worth doing for men having one of the other nonsurgical treatments for their prostate cancer. Certainly, all the options can be tried to see whether they will help.

Another complaint of some men after prostate cancer therapy is a decrease in sexual desire or libido. This is not directly due to the treatment unless ADT was used. The reason is that testosterone controls men's interest in sex and none of the other therapies lower this hormone. Most likely, a decreased libido is an indirect effect of treatment due to psychological reasons. To be sure, a testosterone level can be measured. The best time to check it is in the morning because normally it drops in the afternoon. Doctors disagree about how to treat a man with prostate cancer who has low testosterone. Some of them think it is a bad idea to give drugs that will raise the testosterone level because they are worried it might cause growth of the cancer cells that survived the prostate cancer treatment. Others believe that giving testosterone is quite acceptable. They argue that even when the testosterone level is below normal, more than enough is still present to stimulate any remaining cancer cells. Raising the testosterone back to a more normal level will not make things any worse. If having a normal testosterone level truly was bad for men treated for prostate cancer, then all of them would have to be castrated and that is not being done. The bottom line is that no study has shown it as unsafe.

If you are having a problem with your sex drive, be sure to ask the doctor to measure your testosterone level and then discuss getting medication if the level is low. It is treated using a *testosterone gel (Testim, Androgel)* that is applied to the skin on your shoulder or arm once a day. Be careful not to bathe within six hours; otherwise the drug may not be completely absorbed into your body.

Low testosterone is not the only reason for a low libido; stress and certain drugs also can cause it. For example, if you are taking an antidepressant, ask your doctor whether you can stop it, lower the dose, or switch to a different type of medication that is less likely to have that side effect. If you are stressed or depressed, seeing a therapist may help alleviate those problems even if it isn't affecting your sexual function.

Options for Rehabilitation and Treatment of Urinary Problems

The second most bothersome complaint following prostate cancer therapy is problems with urinary control. Men may complain of two types of incontinence: leaking urine when they cough or sneeze, which is called *stress incontinence*, and leakage due to a sudden urge to urinate, which is called *urgency incontinence*. Some men have both complaints. Another problem that may occur is a weak stream, which usually is due to an obstruction.

Changing some behaviors can help reduce the severity of the problem. Reducing fluid intake during the day, avoiding caffeine, alcohol, and spicy foods, and avoiding fluid intake in the evening can lessen the symptoms while waiting for urinary function to improve.

One option to improve stress incontinence is to perform pelvic muscle exercises called *Kegels*. You can learn how to do them by urinating in the shower and practicing tightening of the pelvic muscles until the urine flow stops. Randomized studies have been done to find out whether doing these exercises is worthwhile. One found that men were more likely to regain their normal urinary control and it happened sooner if they started Kegels one month before their prostate was removed rather than waiting until after surgery to begin them. Another randomized study found no benefit if they began 6 weeks after surgery. Doing the Kegels several times each day probably is better than doing them infrequently, although that has not been proven in randomized studies.

Another option for stress incontinence is *electrical muscle stimulation* (EMS). An EMS device produces electrical pulses that are able to stimulate the pelvic floor muscles to contract, which might strengthen them. The stimulation lasts for 4 to 30 seconds. Men are taught to do this at home with a small device they purchase. Unfortunately, a few randomized studies using a Kegel exercise program with or without EMS showed no difference in urinary control at the end of the study compared with Kegels alone. Therefore, the added value of EMS is unproven.

Drugs have also been used to help people suffering from stress or urgency incontinence with varying success. *Duloxetine (Symbalta)* is a drug approved to treat depression that some doctors use to treat urinary leakage. A small, randomized study, done on men given this drug or a placebo for three months after surgery, found some improvement. However, this drug is not FDA approved for this indication, and over 20% of men get bothersome side effects from the drug. Other drugs that have been prescribed by some doctors include *alpha-blockers* or *anticholinergic medications*. However, none of these have been properly tested in men who had their prostate removed to know whether they are helpful.

If your problem is urgency incontinence, the doctor can perform a *urodynamic* test to determine whether you have an overactive bladder. Often men have both stress and urgency incontinence, especially if they received radiation therapy. Anticholinergic drugs can help reduce symptoms but rarely do they completely get rid of them.

Urgency incontinence, urinary frequency, slowing of the urinary stream, burning, and urinating at night, all can occur following seed implantation. The alpha-blockers can improve the urine stream, reduce nighttime urination, and help empty the bladder. In some cases, an operation is needed to open up the urine channel.

Although uncommon, some men have very severe incontinence despite all conservative treatments. Two surgical interventions are available that can greatly improve men's quality of life: a "sling operation" or placement of an artificial urinary sphincter. The sling may be an excellent option for small to moderate leakage and the artificial urinary sphincter is better for larger amounts.

The sling procedure involves increasing the support of the urethra by covering it with a synthetic mesh made of polypropylene. This increases the resistance in the urethra, which reduces or prevents urine from leaking. It is done during a short operation that has few complications. Approximately 60% of men are cured of their incontinence and another 20% are improved.

The "gold standard" approach with the longest track record for treating stress incontinence is placement of an artificial urinary sphincter during a one- to two-hour operation. The device consists of three parts: an inflatable cuff, a balloon reservoir, and a pump. All of them are located inside the body. The cuff is placed around the urethra near the base of the penis. The reservoir, which is filled with water, is located in the lower abdomen. The pump is placed in the scrotum. Silicone tubes connect the three parts. When the operation is completed, the device is inactivated until healing has occurred. The doctor then activates it by pressing the scrotum to squeeze a small button on the side of the pump. This allows the fluid to enter the cuff, which presses against the urethra, preventing urine from leaking out. When a man feels the urge to urinate, the pump is squeezed, which forces the liquid out of the cuff and into the reservoir. He then empties his bladder and within three to four minutes, the fluid automatically returns into the cuff and urine no longer leaks out.

The success of the operation depends in part on how much leakage occurred before the operation. Approximately 25% are completely dry, and more than 50% may use only up to one pad per day. The complication rate is low. The main ones are infection, malfunction of the device, erosion of the cuff into the urethra, and thinning of the urethra. Some men may benefit from a second operation during which two cuffs are placed.

Not all doctors do these operations, so you might not be offered one of them even if you are very bothered by leakage. If your doctor doesn't offer them, then ask for a referral or search for someone who does them. To get the best result possible, you should find a urologist who has a lot of experience.

Another side effect of cancer treatments is the formation of a scar in the urinary channel, which is called a urethral stricture. The symptoms are a slow stream, dribbling, or an inability to urinate. The easiest way to make a diagnosis of a stricture is to do a cystoscopic examination. This involves inserting a telescope into the penis and inspecting the urethral channel. A stricture is treated either by stretching it using special instruments or cutting the scar with a knife attached to the cystoscope or a laser. In most cases, a single treatment will solve the problem, but care is needed to avoid causing stress incontinence.

Treatment Options for Bowel Dysfunction

Some men treated for prostate cancer complain of problems with their bowel function, which includes frequent stools, diarrhea, rectal bleeding, and an inability to control bowel movements. These happen more often after radiation than surgery. Fortunately, the rates are dropping with greater use of the newer equipment. Often these symptoms are only temporary. Drugs and dietary changes can help reduce diarrhea. Avoiding fiber, spicy foods, raw fruits and vegetables, beans, whole grains, and caffeine also can help until the symptoms go away. Drinking fluids is important to avoid dehydration that occurs with chronic diarrhea. Eating smaller, more frequent meals can be helpful. In severe cases, instilling drugs into the rectum or cauterizing bleeding vessels may be needed.

Treatment for Mental Health Problems

Having prostate cancer can be a much more upsetting experience than occurs with most diseases. Usually patients go to the doctor complaining of specific symptoms caused by an illness and the treatment often makes them better. For most men with prostate cancer, however, they have no symptoms when the cancer is found and they often feel worse after the treatment is completed. Their quality of life declines and may never return to where it was before the diagnosis. The urinary and sexual side effects also can affect a man's relationship with his spouse or partner. These changes may be difficult for some men to accept and can lead to clinical depression. The best advice is to get counseling and possibly medication. The worst thing is to ignore your feelings, withdraw from your partner, and try to cope on your own. Fortunately, most men find that they do improve over time.

The Bottom Line on Improving Your Quality of Life

The options available for treating the side effects of prostate cancer therapies keep expanding and improving. There is no reason to ignore the problems and struggle with your symptoms. Some men are reluctant to mention them to their doctor and not all doctors will ask specific questions. Instead they only will ask a general question such as, "How are you doing?" Many men do not want to sound like they are complaining so they simply answer, "OK." The best approach is to be very specific about any problems you are having so you can get the right treatment that will help improve your quality of life.

What to Do If the Prostate-Specific Antigen (PSA) Rises after Local Therapy

In an ideal world, everyone who gets treated for prostate cancer would be cured of his disease. Unfortunately, that does not occur. How do doctors know whether someone hasn't been cured? In almost every case, the first sign will be a rise in the PSA, which occurs long before a man develops any symptoms or changes in scans or x-rays. That is why doctors will continue to recommend PSA tests after someone has been treated. A rise in the PSA can happen within a few months after treatment or even 15 to 20 years later. Fortunately, having a rise in the PSA is not always dangerous. It depends on the interval between the time of treatment and the rise in PSA, and how fast it is rising. Doctors often will use the *PSA doubling time* to decide what to do. This is defined as the time it takes for the PSA to double in value.

If treatment does become necessary, you have many options. The problem is that doctors aren't sure what should be done because few well-done studies have been performed. Therefore, you will again need to learn the "package" of good and bad effects of every treatment so you can share this decision with your doctor. This chapter reviews the options for treating a rising PSA after each therapy.

Managing a Rising PSA for Men on Watchful Waiting

Men who initially chose watchful waiting had decided they did not want to do anything to try to cure the primary tumor. They realized that they would only get treatment to the prostate gland if symptoms developed, such as urinary blockage or blood in the urine. For that reason, many doctors don't check the PSA until symptoms occur or they do it very seldom. After all, why check to see whether the PSA has gone up from 5 to 10 ng/ml if no treatment will be given? Doing the test also can't predict when or if symptoms will develop. Still, an argument can be made to do the PSA test periodically. The reasons are it is easier and less expensive than ordering a bone scan or CT scan every 12 months. These tests rarely show any cancer until the PSA rises above 10 or 20 ng/ml.

The primary treatment used for a rising PSA after watchful waiting is androgen deprivation therapy (ADT), although doctors do not agree on the best time to start it. Some of them believe there are advantages to starting it before a man has metastases. Others recommend waiting until a man has proven metastases or develops symptoms from the disease. Although some studies show an improvement in survival from starting ADT early, many doctors are critical of them and do not think they are good enough to guide treatment. For that reason, they prefer to withhold ADT until cancer is detected in another part of the body. Another argument in favor of starting ADT before symptoms occur is it can decrease the chance of developing serious or permanent problems. That would include a spinal cord compression and possible paralysis, an obstruction to the kidneys leading to permanent kidney damage, or fractures of weight-bearing bones leading to an inability to walk.

The best approach is for you to discuss the pros and cons of starting ADT and share the decision with your doctor. If you think you would want early ADT before symptoms occur, then have your PSA done at least yearly and begin to have a bone scan when the PSA reaches 10 ng/ml. Additional bone scans can be done each time the PSA doubles. If you would rather choose to delay treatment until symptoms appear, then checking your PSA regularly is not worth doing.

Managing a Rising PSA for Men on Active Surveillance

As discussed in chapter 8, active surveillance only has been in use for about 10 years, which means it is a work in progress with many unanswered questions. The most important one is, "When should someone stop active surveillance and get treated?" The PSA doubling time currently is one of the indicators being used to make that decision. Some doctors recommend treating the cancer when the PSA doubles in less than three years. For example, if your PSA was 6 ng/ml in March 2008 and it went up to 8 ng/ml in March 2009 and to 10 ng/ml in March 2010, then you should choose a different approach. Other doctors will do a biopsy and recommend treatment only if the Gleason score increases or much more cancer is found. Until more studies are done, the best approach will remain unknown. In almost all cases of active surveillance, treatment is advised when the cancer is still localized in the prostate. That means all the options discussed in previous chapters can be considered, with no evidence that one is better than another.

Managing a Rising PSA after Radical Prostatectomy

After a radical prostatectomy about 20% to 30% of men eventually will get a rise in their PSA. This can occur within a few months, a few years, or in some cases it can take more than 15 years. In a small percentage of cases, it occurs because the surgeon left some normal prostate tissue behind, which continues to make low levels of PSA. Most doctors do not consider it to be a true recurrence until it rises above 0.2 or 0.4 ng/ml. In most cases, prostate cancer cells that are in the body cause the rise in PSA. Either they were left behind during the surgery or they had already spread to other parts of the body before the operation was done. These cells continue to multiply until they produce enough PSA that can be detected on the blood test.

Fortunately, a rising PSA after the prostate has been removed often is not dangerous. One study found that only 17% of men with a rising PSA died from prostate cancer over the next 10 years. Here too, it depends on when it occurs and how fast it is rising. Doctors at Johns Hopkins Hospital have found a way to predict the odds of dying from prostate cancer using three pieces of information:

- The Gleason score from surgery

- How long after surgery the PSA went above 0.2 ng/ml

- How long it took for the PSA to double

The next table shows the results 15 years after the PSA increased above 0.2 ng/ml. They also determined the results at 5 and 10 years, which can be obtained for free from the Internet at http://urology.jhu.edu/prostate/partintables.php

Table 19.1 Odds of Dying from Prostate Cancer Within 15 Years of Radical Prostatectomy

PSA Doubling Time in Months	PSA Takes More Than 3 Years to Rise Gleason Score Below 8	PSA Takes More Than 3 Years to Rise Gleason Score 8, 9, or 10	PSA Takes Less Than 3 Years to Rise Gleason Score Below 8	PSA Takes Less Than 3 Years to Rise Gleason Score 8, 9, or 10
More than 15	6%	13%	19%	38%
9 –14.9	14%	28%	41%	69%
3– 8.9	41%	70%	84%	99%
Less than 3	81%	98%	99%	99%

To use this table, you must have all three pieces of information. If you do not know the numbers, the easiest way to get them is to call your doctor's office and ask for the results. If you want to avoid any chance of getting the wrong information, then ask for copies of your pathology report and all your PSA levels since surgery. You shouldn't be surprised if your doctor does not know your PSA doubling time because most doctors don't calculate it—they simply do an estimate. The most accurate way to get the doubling time is to use one of the free Internet websites that will figure it out for you. Type "PSA doubling time calculator" in your web browser and several possible sites will appear. The instructions are easy to follow.

Here are some of the key results from the Johns Hopkins study.

- A PSA rising above 0.2 ng/ml within three years of surgery is more dangerous than one rising after more than three years.

- A PSA that takes more than 15 months to double is far less dangerous than one doubling in three months or less.

- A Gleason score below 8 is less dangerous than a score of 8, 9, or 10.

- If no treatment is given, the chance of dying from prostate cancer in 15 years is only 6% if the PSA doubling time is more than 15 months, the Gleason score is less than 8, and the PSA takes more than three years to rise above 0.2 ng/ml.

- A PSA doubling time of less than 3 months, a Gleason score of 8, 9, or 10, AND a PSA rising to 0.2 ng/ml within three years of surgery is very dangerous and should be treated aggressively.

Hopefully you fall into one of the groups with a small chance of dying from your cancer. If so, you may be comfortable playing the odds and not having anything done right away. This partly will depend on your life expectancy when the recurrence happens. The reason is that the odds of dying from prostate cancer are much lower at 10 years for several combinations of PSA doubling time,

Gleason score, and time to PSA recurrence. The benefit of this approach is that you avoid getting a treatment that would have a very small chance of improving your survival. In other words, the treatment wasn't helpful or necessary. You also get to preserve your quality of life that exists following your recovery. The PSA can continue to be monitored unless the tumor begins to cause some problem. At this time, doctors do not agree on what treatment to recommend, when to start it or which men to treat. Some men with less than a 25% risk of dying in 15 years may be willing to roll the dice and not get treated. Others may wish to be aggressive regardless of the side effects that may occur. It is a very personal decision, but you should be aware that doctors do not know the best approach at this time.

Some men may be willing to be part of a study that is comparing different treatments. A search at www.cancer.gov will allow you to find studies that are enrolling patients. If you do not want to do that, your options include:

- Radiation therapy

- ADT

- Radiation therapy + ADT

- Radiation + ADT + chemotherapy

- ADT + chemotherapy

Of course, each option has risks and benefits. The best choice depends on the location of the cancer. It could be in the prostate bed, which is where the prostate was located, some other place in the body, or in both places.

How can your doctor find out where the cancer cells are located? At this time, no test is 100% accurate. The CT scan, MRI, and bone scan are very unreliable, especially when the PSA is below 10 ng/ml. The ProstaScint scan (chapter 2) probably is the best test available, but it also has many false-positive and false-negative results, especially when the PSA is less than 5 ng/ml. *False positive* means the test tells you cancer cells are in some location when they aren't. *False negative* means they are somewhere in the body but the test does not detect them. In either case, the test gives you wrong information and could lead to the wrong treatment. Some studies suggest that a slowly rising PSA with a long PSA doubling time means the cells most likely are only in the prostate bed, but more proof is needed to tell whether that is correct.

A term often used for radiation given to a man with recurrent disease after his prostate has been removed is *salvage radiation*. It is a reasonable option when all the cells are in the prostate bed, and ADT is probably best if the cells are somewhere else in the body. Few doctors recommend getting both treatments because no good studies have been done using that combination. Although doctors do not know for sure whether salvage radiation will help you live longer, some things are known:

- It is more successful if given when the PSA is less than 0.5 ng/ml.

- Men with a Gleason score of 6 and a PSA under 10 ng/ml prior to surgery are more likely to have cancer recur only in the prostate bed.

- More than one-half of men who get salvage radiation will eventually have another rise in their PSA.

- The success of salvage radiation partly depends on the PSA doubling time.

Without a randomized study, doctors cannot tell whether this treatment is beneficial, but it is an aggressive option for you to consider. Your best chance of benefitting is when:

- Your PSA is under 0.5 ng/ml.

- The PSA doubling time is longer than six months.

- The PSA did not rise within three years of your surgery.

- You had a low-risk cancer before surgery was performed.

The side effects of radiation given after a radical prostatectomy were described in chapter 9. Some studies suggest that the complication rates are not much higher compared with men who never had surgery. Another question that has not been answered is what dose of radiation should be given? Different amounts have been used usually ranging from 60 to 70 Gy, but the optimal amount is not known.

Even if you have tumor cells located only in the prostate bed, ADT still is an option, but it does have many more side effects than radiation, as discussed in chapter 14. Also, no information is available about its effect on survival.

Some doctors suggest a different approach. Rather than lowering the testosterone throughout the body, which causes many side effects, they use two drugs that only affect the action of testosterone inside the cancer cells. One drug is called an *antiandrogen* and the other is called a *5-alpha reductase inhibitor*. Both can lower the PSA without causing the same side effects that occur when ADT is given. Here again, not enough information is available to know whether they prevent the cancer from spreading or prolong survival. One advantage, however, is these drugs may delay the need to get other treatments that do have more side effects.

What should be done if you fall into the high-risk group, that is, a PSA rising within three years of surgery, a PSA doubling time less than three months, and a Gleason score of 8, 9, or 10? In that case, you are highly likely to have cancer that has spread to other parts of the body so radiation by itself makes little sense. The options include ADT alone, ADT plus chemotherapy, or both of them plus radiation. Here again, little information is available to guide this decision. Since chemotherapy now is available that improves survival in men with metastatic disease, doctors are testing it in men with a fast PSA doubling time following a prostatectomy. Until results become available, few doctors are recommending this approach. If you are young and want to try everything possible, then at least have a consultation with an oncologist. If chemotherapy is not for you, then ADT using two drugs might be a good choice. One of them lowers testosterone and the second one blocks the action of testosterone. This combination is called *combined androgen blockade* or *CAB* (see chapter 28 for a detailed explanation). Another option to consider is taking part in a research study of some new drug that is being tested.

Managing a Rising PSA after Radiation Therapy

One of the challenges in evaluating the results with radiation therapy is how to interpret the PSA result. After surgery it should reach zero and if it does not, in almost all cases it means some cancer cells remain somewhere in the body. After radiation, however, some normal cells may survive and they continue to make PSA. Therefore, PSA reaching a level of zero is much less common. This persistent PSA makes it harder to tell whether some cancer still is present. For this reason, doctors have used certain values of PSA to indicate recurrent disease. For many years it was thought to be any value above 0.2 ng/ml. Then it was changed to three consecutive increases in the PSA. In 2005, it was modified again. Most doctors now define it as an increase in the PSA by at least 2 ng/ml over the lowest level measured after radiation has been completed. This is called the *"Phoenix"* definition because it was decided at a medical conference that took place in Phoenix, Arizona.

Another reason doctors may have trouble telling whether the cancer is recurring after radiation is because sometimes a rise in the PSA is due to a *PSA bounce*. The value will go above 0.2 ng/ml usually within the first two years after treatment. The reason for it is not really clear. One possibility is that dying prostate cancer cells release the PSA contained inside them, which then gets into the bloodstream. Regardless of the reason, the good news is that *a PSA bounce does not affect a man's survival.* The value will go back down without any treatment.

If the PSA does increase after radiation, how will you know whether it is a PSA bounce or a true recurrence of the cancer? Several indicators can distinguish the two. In most cases, the value does not go above 1.2 ng/ml with a PSA bounce but it can reach up to 1.8 ng/ml. Gradually it will go back down over the next 6 to 12 months without any treatment. For this reason, nothing should be done for several months when the PSA first goes up to see whether it will keep rising or return to its previous level. At this time you need to be aware that a PSA bounce can occur and should be patient rather than panic until you know whether the cancer definitely has returned.

Even a real rise in PSA due to recurrent cancer often is not dangerous. It depends on several factors. One of them is the PSA doubling time. Values of 3, 6, 8, and 12 months have been used to identify the men that are at risk for developing metastatic disease or dying from prostate cancer over the next 10 years. Although more research is needed, finding out that your PSA doubling time is longer than 12 months may provide some comfort that you are not in danger any time soon and immediate treatment is not necessary. This information about PSA doubling times was obtained from men treated by conventional radiation. At this time doctors do not know whether the same is true for men treated with proton beam radiation or stereotactic radiation.

Another factor determining a man's risk is the timing of the PSA rise. If the value is less than 1.5 ng/ml two years after radiation, only 8% may develop metastatic disease over the next 10 years without any treatment. Also, if it rises above 0.2 ng/ml beyond 18 months after radiation, it is less dangerous than if it rises sooner.

The options for treating a true recurrence after radiation depend not only on when it occurs and how fast the PSA is rising, but also on where the cancer cells are located. They could be located:

- In the prostate gland.

- Or outside the prostate in some other part of the body.

- Or both inside the prostate and in other parts of the body.

How will the doctor make that determination? A prostate biopsy is the most accurate way to find out whether cancer cells still are in the prostate gland. Most doctors only will recommend it if a man would consider having his prostate removed, which is called a *salvage radical prostatectomy*. Otherwise, there is no reason to do this test because it will not help you decide what to do. The operation is performed using the same method as described for a standard prostatectomy. If a biopsy does show cancer then most doctors will order a bone scan, an ultrasound, and a CT scan or MRI. They are done because removing the prostate makes no sense if cancer has already spread to other parts of the body. PET-CT scans are also being used in some cases although their true value has not yet been established. If a biopsy is not being considered, these tests are usually done; however, they rarely find any cancer when the PSA is less than 5 ng/ml. For this reason the tests should be delayed until that value is reached.

If you do decide to get treated for a rising PSA your options include:

- Salvage radical prostatectomy

- Brachytherapy

- Salvage cryotherapy

- High-intensity focused ultrasound (HIFU)

- ADT by itself or combined with one of the other options

Once again, no well-done studies have been performed, so the best treatment is not known. The most aggressive option is to undergo a salvage radical prostatectomy. You should only consider it if your life expectancy is at least 10 years and you can safely undergo an operation. Of course, the prostate biopsy should definitely show cancer cells and you should have no evidence of cancer in other parts of your body. Salvage surgery appears to give better results if it is done when the PSA is under 4 ng/ml and the PSA doubling time is greater than six or eight months. The obvious problem here is the tests to detect distant cancer are not reliable at that low level. That means some men may undergo the operation even though the cancer has already spread. Other methods are needed to accurately find out which patients are best suited for this treatment.

If you do select a salvage prostatectomy, have it done by someone who has considerable experience. Radiation makes the operation more difficult and increases the risk of complications, particularly incontinence and impotence. Don't hesitate to ask your surgeon how many salvage prostatectomies he or she has performed before you schedule the operation.

Salvage cryotherapy and brachytherapy also are options when the cancer is only in the prostate and the gland is smaller than 50 g. In 2008, a consensus panel stated that salvage cryotherapy was a reasonable option for men with a PSA less than 10 ng/ml, a PSA doubling time of greater than 16 months, and at least a 10-year life expectancy. So far, long-term survival rates are not available. One way to measure the success of this treatment is to do another prostate biopsy, which has resulted in cancer being found in 0% to 37% of men after this procedure. Since false-negative biopsies can occur, the actual failure rate probably is a little higher. In other words, many men are not being cured by this treatment.

The PSA level also can tell how well the cryotherapy worked. If it begins to increase, this means some cancer is present. One large study found that the PSA increased again in 66% of patients. Another study found that at five years, the PSA increased again in 27% of men with low-risk cancers, 55% of men with intermediate-risk disease, and 89% of those with high-risk cancer. That either means the treatment did not kill all the cells in the prostate or the men had cancer cells in other parts of the body when the cryotherapy was done.

If you are considering salvage cryotherapy, be aware that many men will get worsening urinary and sexual function. One study that used written surveys two years after the treatment found urinary problems were a moderate or big program in 29% and sexual dysfunction was a moderate or big problem in 56% of patients. The bottom line on salvage cryotherapy is it may get rid of cancer remaining in the prostate in carefully selected patients, but it can significantly affect a man's quality of life.

High-intensity focused ultrasound also has been used to treat recurrent cancer after radiation. However, all the information comes from studies done outside the United States and none of them have been well designed to permit a valid assessment of this treatment. One study found that 57% of men had a rising PSA within two years of this treatment. For now, patients should consider salvage HIFU after radiation as an unproven therapy that is not yet available in this country.

In many cases, ADT may be the best option. The reason is that a large percentage of men with a recurrence after radiation have cancer cells that are outside the prostate gland and only ADT can treat them. Treatment directed solely at the prostate gland will be inadequate. The best candidates may be men with a short doubling time. Good studies show better survival in men initially diagnosed with locally advanced disease that get immediate rather than delayed ADT. It seems logical then that the same benefit may occur from treating men with a rising PSA after radiation. Of course, randomized studies are needed to prove whether this is true. Until then, it is a very reasonable option to consider.

Some doctors are using ADT intermittently instead of continuously. Drugs are given to lower the testosterone in the body and then after several months the drugs are stopped. They are restarted again when the PSA reaches a specific level. This cycle is repeated until the PSA stops responding, which could take many years. Getting a "drug holiday" gives men a chance to get rid of some of their side effects and improve their quality of life.

A randomized study was recently completed in men with a PSA level greater than 3 ng/ml after radiation therapy. One group was given continuous combined androgen blockade using a drug to lower testosterone and another drug to block the action of testosterone produced in the adrenal glands. The second drug was given for at least four weeks. The other group was given this treatment for eight months and then it was stopped until the PSA increased above 10 ng/ml. It was then restarted for another eight months. The treatments continued until they were no longer effective. At seven years, overall survival was similar for the two groups regardless of whether the PSA increased in the first three years of radiation or after that time. However, about 18% of the men on intermittent therapy and 15% on continuous therapy died of prostate cancer. In other words, the chances of dying from prostate cancer was 3% higher for men on intermittent therapy. The trade-off was that men on intermittent therapy had fewer hot flashes, better desire for sexual activity, and less urinary symptoms. Based on this study, intermittent ADT should definitely be offered to anyone faced with a rising PSA after external radiation therapy. The bottom line on treating a recurrence after external radiation is several options are available depending on the location of the disease but all of them can affect a man's quality of life.

Managing a Rising PSA after Brachytherapy

A PSA bounce also can occur in up to 80% of men after brachytherapy. Just like with external radiation, it may take eight months or more before it drops back down to the original level. For that reason, doctors will wait after the PSA begins to rise before starting another treatment. If the PSA continues to go up or it drops and rises again, then the cancer probably has recurred. The treatment options for these men are identical to those for men failing external radiation. At this time, however, no information is available about long-term survival with any of them.

The Bottom Line on Treating a Rising PSA after Radiation

Regardless of the type of radiation used, the following is a way to think about the different treatments available. Observation is the most conservative choice because many men with a rising PSA won't get any symptoms or problems from their cancer for many years, if ever. Avoiding the other therapies allows someone to maintain their quality of life and avoid getting additional or worsening side effects. If the cancer continues to grow and symptoms do develop, ADT can be started. Treatment at that time will not get rid of all the cancer cells, but it does slow down their growth and reduces symptoms. It also may delay the appearance of cancer in other parts of the body. Salvage prostatectomy is the most aggressive way to eliminate the cancer, but it comes with a higher risk of complications compared with having no prior radiation. Salvage cryosurgery may also eliminate the cancer but more men will probably get a recurrence than if they had the prostate removed. Lastly, ADT may be the best approach for men who are less likely to have cancer limited to the prostate gland. It too has potentially bothersome side effects, which can be reduced by using ADT intermittently rather than continuously. It offers the same survival as continuous treatment while enabling men to have a better quality of life.

Managing a Rising PSA after Androgen Deprivation Therapy (ADT)

If you have been on ADT and your PSA begins to rise, what do you do next? The first thing to do is make sure your testosterone is in the proper range because sometimes the drug being used stops controlling it properly. A blood test should show that it is less than 50 ng/dl. If it is above that level, then switching to a different drug having the same effect or removing the testicles should be done. If a different drug is used and it also does not result in the testosterone reaching the right level, then it should be stopped and the testicles should be removed. This will be the most reliable way to lower testosterone.

If the testosterone is in the right range, then the next approach depends on whether you are taking an antiandrogen. Studies have found that sometimes the cancer initially responds well but then eventually it gets worse when one of these drugs is taken. Stopping it may result in a drop in the PSA over the next one to two months in about 40% of patients, which is called *antiandrogen withdrawal*.

If an antiandrogen is not being used, then a bone scan and CT scan or MRI should be done next. Doctors vary in their recommendations when cancer is not found outside the prostate. Currently, the FDA has not yet approved any of the newer therapies for men with a rising PSA who don't have evidence of cancer outside the prostate. Many doctors will suggest you continue on ADT without doing anything else and undergo periodic tests to search for more cancer. When cancer is detected elsewhere, several options are available as discussed in chapters 26 through 28.

Sometimes, doctors will use drugs "off-label" meaning they are approved for use in humans, but not specifically for men with a rising PSA, who don't have metastases. Many insurance companies will not cover the cost of a treatment when it is used "off-label." In those cases, the patient will have to pay for it out of pocket.

Managing a Rising PSA after High-Intensity Focused Ultrasound (HIFU)

If you have been treated with HIFU and your PSA rises, all the same options are available as for radiation failures. Outside the United States, some doctors are repeating HIFU before trying something else, provided that a prostate biopsy shows cancer and it has not spread to other parts of the body. The downside is that patients will have to pay another out-of-pocket fee and there is no long-term survival information. A reasonable question is, why repeat a treatment when it failed to eliminate the cancer the first time it was used?

The Bottom Line on Managing a Rising PSA after Local Therapy

You may have found reading this chapter to be a little frustrating, wondering, "Why isn't there better information about each treatment?" The main reason is that not enough studies have been conducted and too few men were willing to participate when one was started. Until more is known, the best approach is to weigh the pros and cons of each choice and then tailor the decision to suit your specific situation and your willingness to accept the possible side effects.

III

MANAGING LOCALLY ADVANCED PROSTATE CANCER

Overview of Treating Locally Advanced Prostate Cancer

Locally advanced prostate cancers are defined as tumors growing outside the prostate capsule. They are staged at a clinical level of T3 or T4. Stage T3 tumors have grown outside the prostate capsule or they have spread into the seminal vesicles. Stage T4 tumors have grown into the bladder or the pelvic sidewall. They may extend into the seminal vesicles, the bladder, or the pelvic sidewall. Before widespread PSA testing, locally advanced prostate cancers were very common. Fortunately, this is no longer the case; fewer than 15% of all new cases have a clinical stage T3 or T4 tumor.

Locally advanced tumors are harder to treat than localized cancer for several reasons. First, surgery may not be able to remove all the cancer cells in and around the prostate, and radiation may not kill all of them. Even if those treatments are successful, some men still develop recurrent disease because cancer cells had already spread to other parts of the body by the time the cancer was first detected. They couldn't be detected at that time because there weren't enough of them. In other words, the true location of the tumor was not known.

The options for treating locally advanced disease are:

- Radical prostatectomy

- External radiation

- Androgen deprivation therapy (ADT)

- External radiation + ADT

- External radiation + brachytherapy + ADT

To date, few randomized studies have been done. Therefore, patients should understand the pros and cons of each treatment so they can share the decision with their doctor. The next several chapters will provide this information.

Radical Prostatectomy

Good arguments can be made for and against doing a radical prostatectomy to treat locally advanced disease. First, removing the prostate can reduce the chances of getting urinary or kidney obstruction in the future. This happens to 15% to 25% of men when the prostate is not removed. If either problem does occur, it is treated by either a surgical procedure to relieve the obstruction, radiation, androgen deprivation therapy (ADT), or some combination of these options.

A second reason for having surgery is to find out whether cancer has spread to the lymph nodes. One randomized study in men with lymph node metastases showed that performing a radical prostatectomy followed by immediate ADT gives a better survival rate than just performing the prostatectomy and delaying the use of ADT. The only reliable way to know whether cancer has spread to the lymph nodes is to remove them.

Another reason to perform a prostatectomy is that the digital rectal examination (DRE) is not always correct. About 15% to 25% of men thought to have cancer growing outside the prostate turn out to be overstaged. This means their cancer really was localized rather than locally advanced. If surgery had not been done, they most likely would have been treated with radiation plus ADT for at least 18 months. The side effects of the ADT might be more bothersome than the side effects of surgery and there is no proof that the survival would be better.

The arguments against radical prostatectomy also are valid. First, removing all the cancer is more difficult when cancer is growing outside the prostate gland. Although it is true that some men are overstaged by the DRE, the vast majority of men are staged correctly. Normally, the goal of surgery is to remove a margin of normal tissue surrounding the tumor; otherwise the chances for recurrence are greater. Getting a clear margin can't be done with most locally advanced prostate cancers because the rectum is very close to the prostate gland and it might be injured. This means some cancer cells often will be left behind after the prostatectomy. If that occurs, radiation will be recommended even though it increases the risk for complications and only helps a small percentage of men. Some doctors believe that a better approach is to do radiation plus ADT without removing the prostate. Many people question why a man should undergo a major operation only to then need radiation when he could have been treated initially with radiation and avoided the surgery altogether with a similar survival.

A second reason for not doing surgery is that doctors do not know whether men really benefit from taking out the prostate when cancer is in the lymph nodes. The survival rate might be the same if the prostate was left in place and instead ADT was given alone. So far, no well-done study has compared these two options.

Lastly, surgery is a poor choice for a man who is concerned about his sexual function. The few studies reporting results show more than 80% have problems with erections. Nerve-sparing surgery is a bad idea for these men because it increases the chance that cancer will be left behind. In contrast, more men treated with ADT and external radiation will get back to their baseline sexual function after the ADT has stopped.

What Are the Results with Radical Prostatectomy?

Several studies have reported survival results following radical prostatectomy. The most helpful results are part of two randomized studies that compared radical prostatectomy alone with radical prostatectomy plus postoperative radiation therapy. In the first study done in the United States, about 39% of the men not receiving radiation developed metastatic disease and 26% died by 10 years after surgery. At 13 years, 54% had either died or their cancer had spread to other parts of the body.

In the second study, done in Europe, 59% of the men had a rise in their prostate-specific antigen (PSA), 11% had developed metastatic disease, and 23% had died at 10 years. As you can see, the survival at 10 years was very similar despite having very different groups of men in each study.

Some uncontrolled studies have followed men for many years with results being estimated using statistical methods. Five of these studies have been combined together in the next table. Since these are only estimated results, the true results may be 15% lower or 10% higher.

Table 21.1 15-Year Estimated Results after Radical Prostatectomy for Locally Advanced Disease

No Increase in PSA	Did Not Die from Prostate Cancer	Overall Survival
38%–51%	32%–84%	37%–53%

The results are very variable and most importantly, the survival appears lower than observed in the two randomized studies. Some of the differences can be explained by differences in:

- The Gleason score

- The PSA

- The health of the patients

- The percentage of men with localized disease or cancer in the lymph nodes

- The percentage of men also getting external radiation, ADT, or both

Similar to treating localized prostate cancer, the success of treating locally advanced disease depends on the tumor grade and the PSA. The worst results occur in men with Gleason 8, 9, or 10 cancers and a PSA over 10 ng/ml; at 10 years, only 29% did not die of their disease. That group in particular may be more suitable for radiation plus ADT. Men with a lower-grade tumor and a PSA under 10 ng/ml appear to do much better with surgery compared with those with a higher PSA and Gleason score of 8, 9, or 10. There is a challenge in selecting these men, however. More than 30% of men thought to have Gleason 8, 9, or 10 actually have a score below 8 based on the final pathology report after the prostate has been removed. This means that some men who might benefit from surgery will not get it. The bottom line is that some men with locally advanced disease will benefit from radical prostatectomy and may not need additional therapy.

Is There a Benefit from Postoperative Radiation Therapy?

Since many men develop recurrent disease after radical prostatectomy for extracapsular tumors, studies have been done to improve the results. The best studies have been done using external radiation, but the results have been inconsistent. One randomized study compared men getting no radiation with those receiving 60 to 64 Gy. With one-half of the men followed for about 12.5 years, the overall survival was 52% in the men getting radiation compared with 41% in men who did not get it. This means that one man avoided dying out of every nine men getting the radiation. The true benefit could be a little higher, however. The reason is that one-third of the men assigned to the surgery-only group ended up getting delayed radiation when their PSA began to rise, which probably helped some of them. In other words, it made the results in the "nonradiated" group look better. Although the improvement in survival wasn't that high, better results might occur if a higher dose of radiation is used.

In the second randomized study, 50% of the men have been followed for nearly 11 years. Although the radiated men had a lower chance of the PSA rising (39% with radiation vs. 59% without it), so far they have not had a higher survival rate or lower chance of developing metastatic disease. You may wonder why the results differ. The answer may be because some men benefit from postoperative radiation and others do not. As explained above, men with higher Gleason scores have more dangerous cancers, and perhaps radiation has a different effect on them compared with men with lower-grade tumors.

The bottom line on postoperative radiation is that the benefit appears to be small. More work is needed to identify which patients are most likely to benefit so the others can be spared from this treatment. One way to help some men avoid getting radiation that doesn't help them is to delay giving it to them until the PSA begins to rise. That way, those men who will never have a rise in their PSA can avoid getting radiation and avoid the added side effects. Randomized studies are needed to prove whether this will work. Before you agree to have the surgery to treat your locally advanced cancer, make sure to discuss the possibility of needing radiation after you recover so you know what to expect.

What Are the Side Effects following Radical Prostatectomy?

The side effects that can occur after radical prostatectomy are the same as those occurring after surgery for localized disease (see chapter 9). Most studies have not used written surveys, so it is difficult to give the exact odds of whether they will occur or whether it is any different compared with men with localized disease. More information is needed about the impact of surgery on quality of life. In general, it should be very similar to the results from treating men with localized disease except for sexual function. That is likely to be worse because one or both pelvic nerves will be removed during the operation. There also may be a higher chance of getting blood clots in the legs because an extensive dissection should be done to remove the pelvic lymph nodes.

Who Is a Good Candidate for a Radical Prostatectomy?

Despite the lack of good studies in men with locally advanced disease, radical prostatectomy may be a good option for you. The most important consideration is your life expectancy. Surgery is not a good choice unless you expect to live more than 10 years. Your general health also is a factor; you must be able to safely undergo anesthesia and the rigors of a major operation.

The type of tumor you have will affect the results. The best patients are those with a PSA less than 20 ng/ml, a Gleason score less than 8, and a clinical stage of T3a. Men with these tumor traits are less likely to have cancer in the lymph nodes or need additional treatment in the future. If you are hoping to have only one treatment for your cancer, then don't choose surgery unless you have the optimal PSA, Gleason score, and tumor stage. This does not guarantee that surgery will cure you but your odds are better. Another factor is how fast your PSA has been rising. If it has been going up slowly, surgery alone may be able to get rid of all your cancer.

Another factor to consider is how the side effects of treatment will affect your quality of life. Surgery would be the wrong choice if you are sexually active now and hope to regain that ability after treatment. If both pelvic nerves are removed, there is no chance of regaining normal erections. Even if one nerve is spared, the odds are only half as good as when both are preserved. Urinary problems are also higher with surgery compared with radiation; so if you wish to minimize this problem, then don't choose surgery. Lastly, if bowel function is a concern, then you might choose surgery because radiation is more likely to cause a problem.

How Is a Radical Prostatectomy Performed?

Any of the four surgical methods described in chapter 9 can be used to treat locally advanced disease because no study has shown that one method gets better results. The operation is done exactly in the same way as for men with a localized tumor except for the decision about doing a nerve-sparing operation. Leaving the nerves in place greatly increases the odds of leaving cancer behind. For that reason, a nerve-sparing operation usually is not advised. In some cases, the surgeon may feel that the cancer is limited to one side of the gland and decide to preserve the nerve on the opposite side. That will give the patient at least a chance to regain sexual function.

Unlike surgery in men with localized disease, the pelvic lymph nodes should be removed routinely because the risk of lymph node invasion is high. This should be an extensive rather than a limited dissection to avoid missing cancer-containing lymph nodes. The side effects and details about the operation are contained in chapter 10.

The Bottom Line on Radical Prostatectomy for Locally Advanced Disease

Good arguments can be made for and against performing a radical prostatectomy. Removing the entire tumor can be done safely, but the odds of getting a complication probably are higher. Another disadvantage is that surgery by itself often will not cure the disease. That means you are highly likely to need additional therapy. You still might decide it is right for you after learning about the other options.

If you choose to take this option, be sure to find an experienced surgeon because the operation is more difficult than for localized disease. Your best chance for a good result is to choose a surgeon who has operated on many men with locally advanced disease. Don't hesitate to ask how many operations have been done and how often complications occurred. Radical prostatectomy is a reasonable option for locally advanced prostate cancer but you must understand the risks and benefits.

Radiation Therapy

In the 1980s, doctors recognized that prostate cancer progressed in many patients with locally advanced disease who were treated only with external radiation therapy. One explanation is that the dose of radiation was too low to kill all the cancer cells. At that time, higher doses could not be used because it would have caused too much damage to surrounding tissues. The development of three-dimensional conformation therapy (3D-CRT) and intensity-modulated radiation therapy (IMRT) made it possible to deliver higher doses safely. Also, studies were done combining the following therapies to determine whether better results could be obtained.

- External radiation + androgen deprivation therapy (ADT)
- External radiation + brachytherapy
- External radiation + brachytherapy + ADT
- Brachytherapy + ADT

External Beam Radiation

What Are the Results of External Radiation Alone Compared with External Radiation Plus Androgen Deprivation Therapy (ADT)?

A number of randomized studies have been done to determine whether combining ADT with radiation would give better results than radiation alone. Each of these studies used an injection to lower testosterone for different lengths of time. The earliest study compared immediate versus delayed ADT in men getting radiation therapy. The ADT was continued indefinitely in the first group and it resulted in a 10% higher survival at 10 years. The problem was that men had to endure the side effects of ADT for most of their lives.

In an effort to reduce side effects, another study compared external radiation alone and external radiation plus 36 months of ADT. About 80% of the men in this study had cancer outside the prostate and the others had high-risk localized disease. The most important results are shown in the table.

Table 22.1 Estimated Results of External Radiation Compared with External Radiation + ADT

Result	Radiation + ADT	Radiation Alone
Overall survival at 5 years	79%	62%
Overall survival at 10 years	58%	40%
Dying from prostate cancer	11%	31%

This study showed a large benefit from adding hormone therapy even by five years after the treatment was started. By 10 years, the estimated survival rate improved by 18%. The treatment also prevented many men from getting widespread disease and it lowered the chance of dying from prostate cancer by 20%. This means that nearly one out of every five men benefitted from getting hormone therapy for three years. The reason that the results are estimated is that not all men were followed for the full 10 years. The true benefit might be slightly different, but doctors can't know for sure without a longer follow-up.

This study had some weaknesses. Nearly 10% of the men in both groups did not follow their assigned treatment. They either refused radiation or ADT or did not complete a full 36 months of treatment. Fortunately, the results are unlikely to have been affected very much.

Lowering the testosterone did cause some added side effects. About 62% of the men noticed hot flashes with one-third of them having more than three per day. Overall, the side effects were not very severe, but quality-of-life surveys were not used, meaning that more side effects probably occurred. This study gave doctors an opportunity to examine the effect of ADT on overall health. Uncontrolled studies have suggested that hormone therapy increases a man's chance of dying from heart disease. This study showed that ADT did not increase this risk. The bottom line is that ADT improves survival in men with locally advanced disease who are treated with external radiation without harming their heart.

Another randomized study compared 4 months to 28 months of ADT. Although the study showed a benefit to the men with high-risk disease, the conclusion is not as reliable as the study using 36 months of ADT.

In an effort to reduce the duration of side effects from ADT, other well-done studies have tested three, four, and six months of ADT and none of them has shown an improvement in survival compared with external radiation alone. Then, in 2013, the results of another study were reported that compared 18 and 36 months of ADT. With half of the men followed for at least 77 months, there is no difference in overall survival, cancer-specific survival, or the odds of developing metastatic disease. A longer follow-up still is needed to be sure that the shorter course of treatment is truly as good. If that does occur, men will benefit greatly by having to endure the side effects of ADT for a shorter time. Until then, any man with locally advanced disease should discuss these results with his doctor and consider the shorter course of therapy.

These studies are an excellent example of the proper way to find the best therapy. We can conclude from these studies that 6 months of ADT is not enough while 36 months offers the best improvement in survival. Hopefully, a longer follow-up will result in finding that 18 months of ADT gives the same survival as longer treatment because it results in a better quality of life.

After discovering that men benefit from adding ADT to external radiation, doctors then asked whether the radiation really is necessary or would the same benefit occur with ADT alone? A randomized study was done to find the answer. Men with locally advanced or high-risk localized prostate cancer were assigned to get ADT alone or in combination with external radiation. The study is not yet over, but so far survival is much better if men get both treatments rather than hormone therapy alone. The estimated difference in survival is about 20%, which means one out of every five men is benefitting from the combined treatments.

Some doctors think that the results would have been even better if a higher dose of radiation had been used, while others have questioned whether the reason the ADT improved survival is because the dose of radiation used in these studies is too low to kill all the cancer cells. Now that higher doses are given using 3D-CRT or IMRT, maybe the ADT won't be needed. To answer this question, additional studies will be needed.

What Are the Results of External Radiation Plus Brachytherapy?

Brachytherapy also has been combined with external radiation for locally advanced disease because it can deliver a very high dose to the prostate without delivering dangerous amounts to the surrounding tissues. One small, randomized study assigned men to receive external radiation or external radiation plus a temporary implant using iridium-132. About 40% of the men had locally advanced tumors. The total dose of radiation was only 66 Gy for the external radiation group and 75 Gy for the group getting both treatments. About two years after the radiation, prostate biopsies were performed. More men receiving external radiation alone had a positive biopsy (51%), compared with those having the combination therapy (24%). At eight years, the results show no difference in survival, but more men receiving external radiation alone had a rising PSA. Unfortunately, this study has several weaknesses that prevent any valid conclusions. First, the study is not valid because the dose of external radiation was too low to adequately kill the cancer. Secondly, the study should have been done using a combination of external radiation plus ADT rather than external radiation alone because the combination has already been shown to result in a better survival. Without better information, the value of combining external radiation plus brachytherapy cannot be determined.

Nonrandomized studies do provide some information about the side effects that occur with this combination but it is quite limited. In one study of men having external radiation with permanent brachytherapy using iodine-125 (I-125), 15% of men developed significant urinary and/or intestinal side effects by eight years. This included urinary frequency, burning during urination, and inflammation of the anus or bowel. About 42% of men complained of significant problems with erections during the eight years. Men with urinary problems before treatment appear to be at a higher risk for complications after the treatment is completed. Uncontrolled studies of external radiation plus brachytherapy suggest morbidity may not be higher compared with external radiation alone; however, validated surveys are rarely used and without a randomized study, the true difference in side effects is difficult to assess. At this time, the information is insufficient to determine whether combining brachytherapy with external radiation offers patients a significant benefit over external radiation plus ADT, and it may cause more side effects.

What Are the Results with External Radiation Combined with ADT and Brachytherapy?

Another option for treating locally advanced disease is to combine brachytherapy with external radiation and ADT. So far, no randomized studies have been done to know how it compares with external radiation plus ADT without the brachytherapy. A few uncontrolled studies using iridium-192, palladium-103 or cesium-131 have been published. So far, none of them prove that the results are superior to external radiation plus ADT.

Doctors who have a special interest in temporary or permanent brachytherapy usually are the ones promoting this combination, but they have an obvious bias because the treatment is more profitable for them while being more costly to the patient and to the insurance company. Nevertheless, men who want to take a very aggressive approach to their treatment can consider it, but a second opinion is probably worth doing before signing up. If you see a doctor who does recommend this combination, you should consider getting answers to the following questions.

- What is the evidence that it is better than external radiation plus ADT?

- What complication rates have occurred in your practice using this combination?

- Does it matter whether temporary or permanent seed implantation is used?

- What are the advantages of using palladium-103, cesium-131, or iodine-125?

- How long will ADT be used with this combination?

As has been mentioned throughout this book, no valid conclusions can be made from uncontrolled studies. Until more information is available, the value of combining brachytherapy with external radiation and ADT is unclear.

The Bottom Line on External Radiation Therapy for Locally Advanced Disease

If you have been diagnosed with locally advanced prostate cancer, external radiation is a reasonable option, but it definitely should be combined with ADT to get the longest survival. The ADT should begin when radiation starts and continue for 36 months, although the latest ongoing study *suggests* that 18 months may be just as good. If bothersome side effects occur, medications are available to reduce them or make them more tolerable. Do not expect all doctors to be aware of the studies discussed in this chapter. A recent study showed that at least for the years between 2004 and 2007, ADT was often used improperly in men getting external radiation. If your doctor does advise a different amount of ADT other than those discussed in this chapter, be prepared to ask about the studies cited here so you can get the best result. If you want to take the most aggressive approach possible, then consider combining temporary or permanent brachytherapy with external radiation plus ADT. At this time, however, there is little evidence that it improves survival compared with external radiation plus ADT.

One of the remaining unanswered questions is, what amount of radiation should men receive? Several randomized studies are in progress with short-term results showing a lower chance of the PSA rising when more radiation is given. So far, however, none of these studies has shown an improvement in survival and some show an increase in side effects. Even so, many doctors in the United States routinely are recommending that higher doses be used. Hopefully the ongoing studies will mature soon in order to know whether more radiation is better when combined with ADT.

Brachytherapy without External Radiation

Little information is available about using permanent or temporary brachytherapy to treat locally advanced disease. Since the seeds are not placed outside the gland, this treatment may not be able to kill all the cells in that location. Several uncontrolled studies have been performed in high-risk localized disease but not in men with locally advanced disease. Also, at this time no good information is available comparing brachytherapy plus ADT to external radiation plus ADT. For now, the impact of treating locally advanced disease with brachytherapy alone cannot be determined.

Other Methods for Delivering Radiation Therapy

Newer methods of delivering radiation therapy include proton beam radiation and stereotactic guided radiation therapy, or SGRT. Both have potential advantages, but long-term results are not available for localized disease and even less is known about treating locally advanced tumors. There is nothing wrong with choosing one of them, but again, be aware that you don't know what to expect about their ability to cure locally advanced prostate cancer or the frequency and severity of side effects. If you do choose one of these treatments, ADT probably should also be given for at least 18 months, although no studies have been done to know its effect on survival. More information is needed to provide men with a better idea of what to expect.

Summary of Radiation Therapy for Locally Advanced Disease

Much better information is available about treating locally advanced disease with radiation than other options. Studies clearly show that a higher rate of survival can be achieved by combining external radiation with ADT for at least 36 months and possibly for only 18 months. This combination has the advantage of treating cancer that is both inside and outside the prostate, which is harder to do with surgery. How this treatment compares to radical prostatectomy cannot be determined at this time. Clearly, more information is needed to provide men with better counseling.

Androgen Deprivation (ADT)

The next option for men with locally advanced prostate cancer is androgen deprivation therapy (ADT). This is a general term used to describe treatments that lower testosterone, the male sex hormone. ADT can be undertaken either with drugs injected into a muscle or under the skin, or taken by mouth. An alternative treatment is to remove the testicles, which are the organs that produce most of this hormone. The advantage of injections is that side effects will usually go away once the drugs are stopped, which is not the case with removal of the testicles. A detailed explanation of the different methods for delivering ADT is provided in chapters 14 and 26 through 28.

The reason to consider this treatment for locally advanced disease is that often the cancer is more extensive than revealed by the digital rectal examination or the bone scan and CT scan. Some cancer cells already may have spread to other parts of the body, but doctors have been unable to detect them. Both surgery and radiation do not treat these cells, so they keep growing. Both treatments initially will cause the PSA to decline, but eventually it will increase again as the cells keep dividing. ADT is a better option because it can affect cancer cells located anywhere in the body.

What Are the Benefits and Risks of ADT?

The benefits of ADT are the opportunity to avoid the side effects of surgery or radiation. If some cancer cells have already spread, no study has proven that either of those treatments is helpful, so why bother having them? Although ADT will rarely cure a man with locally advanced disease, often it will do the following:

- Slow down the growth of the cancer.

- Delay its appearance in the bones.

- Reduce the chance of getting urinary blockage or kidney damage.

- Allow a man to live out his life without being harmed by the cancer.

The risks of ADT are that the cancer may have not yet spread to other parts of the body and could have been cured either by surgery or radiation plus ADT. By choosing ADT instead, the cancer may not be cured and eventually can spread to other parts of the body. In addition, this treatment often causes bothersome side effects that can affect a man's quality of life. The odds of that happening depend in part on how long a patient is treated. A list of potential side effects is shown in the next table.

Some of these side effects may be very bothersome, particularly if a man is very active. The most common one is hot flashes. Drugs can be given to reduce them, but sometimes they will persist, and stopping the treatment doesn't always make them go away. The loss of a man's sex drive may affect his relationship with his partner. For those who spend time at the beach or local swimming pool, breast enlargement, gaining weight, and a decrease in muscle mass may be major concerns. Over time, a loss of memory also can be very troubling. Another risk is the possibility of developing a fracture due to thinning of the bones. Your take-home message is

Table 23.1 Potential Side Effects of ADT

Hot flashes

Decreased sex drive

Weight gain (increase in body mass index)

Anemia

Difficulties with memory

Osteoporosis

Fatigue

Changes in body composition including weight gain, breast enlargement, and decrease in muscle mass

Increase in lipids (cholesterol, triglycerides, low-density lipoprotein)

that ADT has many side effects that may be as troubling as those following surgery or radiation. Chapter 14 discusses ways to manage these side effects.

What Are the Results with ADT?

In the previous chapter, a well-done study was reviewed that compared ADT alone or in combination with external radiation for men with locally advanced prostate cancer. It found that men lived longer if they received radiation with ADT. A randomized study has never been done comparing ADT to surgery in men with locally advanced disease, so doctors do not know whether one of them gives better results.

One question that has been asked and studied is, when is the best time to give ADT? Should it be started immediately or delayed until the cancer causes symptoms? The reason to do it immediately is the cancer cells may respond better. One good study found that men who were given ADT right away were less likely to develop metastatic disease and less likely to develop bone pain compared with delaying the therapy. Although the effect on survival was unclear, the other benefits of early ADT outweighed its disadvantages. The study has received some criticism, but it still does provide useful information about the best timing of hormone therapy.

Another study enrolled men who either weren't suitable for surgery or radiation or they refused those treatments. Nearly one-half of them had locally advanced disease. They were assigned to receive ADT either immediately or when the disease caused pain or other symptoms. The study has several important results. First, survival at 10 years was 11% higher in men treated immediately. That means the treatment helped about one out of every nine men live longer. The results are estimated because not everyone was followed for 10 years. The actual benefit could be slightly different and more time is needed to know for sure. Still, it does demonstrate a survival benefit from getting treated right away. This means the best approach for men who do not want to have either surgery or radiation is to begin ADT when their locally advanced cancer is diagnosed.

Who Is a Good Candidate for ADT?

Although anyone with locally advanced disease can be given ADT, some people may be more suitable for it. Men with a life expectancy less than 10 years may not live long enough to benefit from surgery or radiation. ADT may be better for them because it can slow down the growth of the tumor and reduce the chances it will cause harm. That will enable those men to avoid the side effects of surgery and radiation and possibly live out their lives without suffering from prostate cancer.

Men with a high risk of developing progressive disease also are good candidates. One study suggested that the most dangerous tumors are those with a PSA between 8 ng/ml and 50 ng/ml and a

PSA doubling time of less than 12 months. Having a PSA over 50 ng/ml, regardless of the PSA doubling time, also puts men at a high risk for progression. Surgery and radiation may be less likely to help them, although this needs to be tested in a proper study. Of course, delaying therapy has the advantage of delaying the onset of symptoms. This option may be best for a man who is sexually active, is not being bothered by any symptoms from the cancer, or has a short life expectancy.

Continuous, Delayed, and Intermittent ADT

ADT therapy can be used in three ways:

- Continuously, when locally advanced disease is diagnosed

- Delayed until the cancer begins to cause problems

- Intermittently

These three choices are all about the trade-offs of quality of life and survival. Based on the studies described above, using it continuously after locally advanced disease is diagnosed rather than delaying it may be the best way to prolong survival and prevent or delay the harmful effects of the cancer. Of course, the side effects of treatment can be troubling to some men.

Intermittent therapy, or intermittent androgen deprivation therapy (IADT), means undergoing treatment until the man's testosterone drops and becomes stable, then stopping it to allow the testosterone to rise (see chapter 14). This cycle is repeated over and over again until it is no longer working. The advantage of IADT is it will give a person "rest" periods during which some of the side effects may go away. One randomized study was done in men with a rising PSA of greater than 3 ng/ml after either surgery or radiation therapy. In other words, they were not cured by their initial treatment, but the cancer had not spread to other parts of the body.

So the men included were not really the same as those with newly diagnosed locally advanced disease. Even so, it does provide important and helpful information about the effects of IADT. With half of the men followed for at least 7 years, the following results occurred:

- Overall survival of men on intermittent therapy was not significantly different from those on continuous therapy (8.8 years on IADT vs. 9.1 years on continuous ADT).

- At 7 years, 18% of men on IADT died from their disease compared with 15% of those treated continuously. This means IADT resulted in a 3% higher chance of dying from prostate cancer.

- Those receiving IADT were about 3% less likely to die from other causes.

- IADT resulted in significantly fewer hot flashes, better desire for sexual activity, better urinary symptoms, and less fatigue compared with continuous treatment.

What do these results mean? For many years, doctors had thought that IADT might result in better survival and better quality of life compared with continuous treatment. This study shows that is not the case. Although one cannot know whether the same results would apply to men with untreated locally advanced disease, it is a reasonable assumption. Until a study is done in men with locally advanced disease, the information from this study should be discussed with anyone having this tumor stage who is considering IADT. Some men will clearly favor this treatment because the improvement in their quality of life during the drug holiday will outweigh the slightly higher risk of dying from prostate cancer. Others may be willing to accept the side effects to have a lower chance of dying from this disease even though it does not prolong their survival. Each man should share this decision rather than let the doctor decide.

One of the ongoing challenges regarding IADT is how it should be done. That means doctors are not sure how long it should be given before it is stopped, when it should be restarted, and whether one or two drugs should be given to affect the testosterone. Although ADT was restarted when the PSA reached 10 ng/ml in the study described earlier, better results might have occurred if treatment was resumed at a lower PSA. Another alternative would be to restart the treatment when the testosterone rises back to a certain level. Without additional studies, these questions cannot be answered.

The Bottom Line on ADT for Locally Advanced Disease

Unlike localized prostate cancer, doctors have better information about the effects of different treatments in locally advanced disease. Based on good studies, ADT is not the best choice if you want to maximize your survival. The best way to achieve that goal is to combine ADT with external radiation. ADT is a better choice for men who are more concerned about avoiding the side effects of surgery or radiation or have a tumor that has a low chance of being cured by either of those options.

Choosing a Therapy for Locally Advanced Disease

24

Now that you have read about different options, how do you decide which one is right for you? Find the treatment that best fits your goals of treatment, the type of tumor you have, and your health concerns.

The place to start is with your treatment goals. Is curing this cancer your top priority or are you comfortable with just keeping it under control? Have you thought about which side effects you can live with and which ones are completely unacceptable?

Next, consider the details about your tumor. Did the doctor tell you how big it was when the rectal examination was done? Was it growing just outside the capsule or extending into the seminal vesicles or pelvic wall? What about your protate-specific antigen (PSA), is it under 20 ng/ml or over 50 ng/ml? Has it been going up rapidly over the last few years or has it changed very little? How high is your Gleason score? Is it above 7 or not?

Finally, how is your health? Do you have serious illnesses such as heart disease or are you as "fit as a fiddle"? Are you urinating without any problems or getting up several times each night to urinate? Do you have any bowel difficulties such as chronic diarrhea or blood in the stool? Lastly, how good is your sexual function? Have your erections largely gone away or are you still performing like a 40-year old? The answers to all of these questions will influence which treatment you choose.

Let's begin with your goals. If survival is your overwhelming priority, then androgen deprivation therapy (ADT) will not be the right choice because it rarely cures prostate cancer. Although no studies have compared surgery against radiation, doctors now know that ADT combined with radiation is better than either of them alone. Doctors have some evidence that 18 months of ADT may be as good as a longer course of therapy although a longer follow-up is needed to be sure. Until then, men wanting to be safe should get ADT for 36 months unless the side effects become intolerable. The radiation either can be three-dimensional conformation therapy (3D-CRT) or intensity-modulated radiation therapy (IMRT) to a dose above 70 Gy. If you really want the most aggressive approach, then you might consider adding brachytherapy. Be aware, however, that no studies have shown it will deliver a better result and it will increase your risk of side effects.

What about having surgery instead? It might be reasonable provided your tumor is not too extensive. That means it is not growing into the seminal vesicles, the PSA is not above 20 ng/ml, it hasn't been rising rapidly, and your Gleason score is under 8. Otherwise surgery is unlikely to get rid of the cancer and more therapy will be needed. No information is available to tell you how surgery compares with radiation and hormones. Certainly, if you want to be cured and you hope to have some chance of regaining your sexual function, the odds are probably better with radiation and hormones. To get rid of your cancer with an operation, your doctor will have to remove one or both pelvic nerves, which will greatly reduce or eliminate your chances of regaining erections.

Suppose you are more comfortable just keeping the cancer from spreading. Your life expectancy may be less than 10 years either because of your age or some other illness. In that case, either immediate or delayed ADT would make more sense than surgery or radiation. It could be done intermittently rather than continuously to reduce side effects, but that could result in a slightly higher chance of dying from prostate cancer and a slightly lower chance of dying from other causes.

Which treatment is best for your quality of life? Without the right studies, the answer is unclear. External radiation will be the wrong choice if you have bowel problems and brachytherapy will not be good if you have urinary difficulties. The biggest challenge is deciding what to do if maintaining sexual function is your highest priority. Surgery and ADT could be excluded and external radiation might achieve your goals, but many men still will lose their normal sexual function. You should realize that many good options exist to help improve erections if that becomes necessary. The only safe way to maintain your sexual function is to delay all treatments until it becomes absolutely necessary. This might be reasonable if you are fortunate enough to have a slower growing cancer with a long PSA doubling time and maximizing your survival is not your primary goal.

Two treatments not discussed are cryotherapy and high-intensity focused ultrasound, or HIFU. At this time, limited information is available about their effect on locally advanced disease. On a theoretical basis, neither makes good sense because the cancer is growing outside the gland and attempting to kill those cells with either of these treatments exposes patients to rectal injury or a high risk of leaving cancer behind. Perhaps studies will be done to find out whether either has a role in men with this stage of disease.

The bottom line is that your choice should take many factors into consideration. The best advice is to try to find the right fit for your type of cancer and what you hope to achieve.

What Happens If the PSA Rises after Treatment Is Completed?

Chapter 19 discussed the options for treating a rising PSA after local therapy. The same options apply here except neither salvage cryotherapy nor high-intensity focused ultrasound would be good choices. A PSA bounce can also occur after radiation therapy, so patience is needed before reacting to the first change in PSA. In most cases, the best option is ADT. A search for metastatic disease probably should be done beginning when the PSA is 10 ng/ml even if no symptoms are present. The treatment options for managing metastatic disease are discussed in the next section.

IV

MANAGING METASTATIC PROSTATE CANCER

Overview of Metastatic Prostate Cancer

25

Some people get confused about what to call a cancer that appears in a new location. They think it is a new cancer. For example if prostate cancer cells spread into the bones, they incorrectly call it bone cancer. It is still prostate cancer. The correct thing to say is the patient has *metastatic prostate cancer* or the cancer has *metastasized*. Prostate cancer most commonly metastasizes to the bones, lymph nodes, liver, lungs, and brain. The bones and lymph nodes are far more common than the other sites. Prostate cancer metastases can cause many symptoms such as:

- Bone pain

- Fractures

- Compression of the spinal cord with paralysis

- Urinary obstruction

- Kidney failure

- Weakness

- Weight loss

- Decreased appetite

- Leg swelling

- Blood clots

- Anemia

Each year about 29,000 men die from this disease in the United States. Throughout the 1990s and early 2000s, only 50% of men with metastatic prostate cancer survived longer than three years. Since then several new therapies have been approved that have extended this survival to over five years and other therapies are showing great promise that are likely to extend it even further. Hopefully, they also will be available in the near future.

How the Male Sex Hormones Affect Prostate Cancer

Male sex hormones are chemicals produced in the body that are responsible for a man's secondary sex characteristics such as sperm production, hair growth, and muscle strength. These hormones are also responsible for a man's sexual desire, called libido, and his ability to have erections. The following table shows a list of these hormones.

Table 25.1 Male Hormones

Testosterone
Dehydroepiandrosterone (DHEA)
Androstenedione
Androstenediol
Androsterone
Dihydrotestosterone

The most abundant of these is testosterone. About 95% is produced in the testicles and 5% is produced in the adrenal glands.

Another property of these hormones is they stimulate the growth of prostate cancer cells located anywhere in the body. Many years ago, two doctors discovered that lowering the testosterone level in men with metastatic disease significantly improved their symptoms. It reduced pain, improved urinary function and increased appetite, which helped men regain some weight. Today it is still the *first and best* treatment for metastatic prostate cancer. As mentioned in chapter 14, several terms are used to describe this treatment including *hormone therapy, androgen ablation, androgen suppression therapy (AST), hormone deprivation, androgen deprivation therapy (ADT), and medical* or *surgical castration.* Although they all mean the same thing, androgen deprivation therapy, or ADT, has become the preferred term. When ADT was first discovered, two options were available. One was to do a minor operation called a *bilateral orchiectomy* or *bilateral orchidectomy.* Another name for it is *surgical castration.* The other option was to give men a female hormone pill called *diethylstilbestrol* or DES. Over the last 30 years, other ways of affecting testosterone have been developed giving men more options as described in the next few chapters.

When Should Androgen Deprivation Therapy (ADT) Begin?

When ADT was first discovered, its main effect was to reduce the symptoms caused by widespread cancer, but its effect on survival was unclear. Since then, most men are being diagnosed with metastatic disease before any symptoms develop. Since ADT can cause many side effects, doctors disagree on the best timing for this treatment. Some of them believe treatment should be delayed because the small increase in survival is more than offset by a worsening of men's quality of life. Others believe it should start when metastases are first discovered because delaying treatment allows more cancer cells to *mutate* or change and become resistant to ADT.

Two randomized studies have been done aimed at solving this debate. In the first one, patients were assigned to get immediate or delayed ADT. It found that the group getting delayed ADT was more likely to:

- Die from prostate cancer.

- Develop urinary blockage requiring surgery.

- Develop spinal cord compression, kidney blockage, fractured bones caused by cancer, and new metastases.

Initially the survival rate also was better, but over time that benefit disappeared. Even so, the advantages outweighed the disadvantages and early treatment was advised.

A second study enrolled men who refused the treatments or weren't suitable for surgery or radiation. Many of them probably had very early metastatic disease but the cancer was not causing many symptoms. Nearly one-half of them had locally advanced disease. They were randomized to receive ADT either immediately or when the disease caused pain or other symptoms. At 10 years, survival was about 11% higher in men treated immediately. Although this study does not prove that men with metastatic disease will also live longer, it does support that possibility.

The bottom line is the advantages of early ADT appear to outweigh the disadvantages. Therefore, your best approach to avoid being harmed by the disease and living as long as possible is to begin treatment when metastases are first detected. This should be done even if no symptoms are present. Also, every effort should be made to prevent or treat the side effects of this treatment as discussed in chapter 14. The next several chapters explain different ways to do ADT.

Bilateral Orchiectomy

Dr. Charles Huggins is credited with discovering the effect of testosterone on prostate cancer growth. This led to the first anticancer therapy when both testicles were removed to reduce this hormone, which reduced the symptoms caused by the disease. Bilateral orchiectomy was the primary therapy for advanced prostate cancer until the discovery of medical therapies that had a similar effect.

What Are the Results with Bilateral Orchiectomy?

Probably the most reliable source of information about this treatment comes from a randomized study that evaluated combined androgen blockade (CAB) in men undergoing bilateral orchiectomy. CAB will be described in detail in the next chapter, but it involves using two treatments that interfere with the male hormone rather than only one. In the study, all the men with metastases to the bones or other organs underwent this operation and then they received either a placebo or a drug called an antiandrogen. The results with bilateral orchiectomy plus the placebo are shown in the following table.

Table 26.1 Results of Bilateral Orchiectomy Plus Placebo

Outcome	Results
Overall survival	29.9 months
Survival with minimal disease	51.0 months
Survival with extensive disease	27.5 months
Time until disease progressed	18.6 months
Minimal disease	46 months
Extensive disease	16 months

Many men with newly diagnosed disease may look at these results and be discouraged seeing that only 50% of the men live more than 29.9 months. Keep in mind that these results were obtained before any of the new therapies discovered since 2000 became available. Current estimates are that more than half of the men survived at least 5.5 years and it is continuing to increase.

Overall, the treatment was well tolerated. The most serious side effect was anemia, which occurred in 5.4% of the men having surgery plus the placebo. No deaths occurred as a result of the treatment. Other side effects and their management were discussed in chapter 14.

What to Expect from the Operation

The operation can be performed under a local, spinal, or general anesthetic. If a spinal or general anesthetic is to be used, your doctor will send you for a preoperative evaluation to make sure it is safe for you to have the anesthetic.

For at least one week before surgery, *do not take* over-the-counter medications that might increase the risk of bleeding. That includes any drug belonging to a group called nonsteroidal anti-inflammatory drugs, or NSAIDs, such as aspirin, Motrin, Advil, naprosyn, Aleve, and Celebrex. Also vitamin E should be avoided. If you take one of these by mistake within seven days of surgery, notify your surgeon right away. Also, you should not eat or drink anything after midnight the day before surgery.

When you arrive for surgery, you will change into a surgical gown and an intravenous line will be started. When it is time for surgery, you will be brought into the operating room and transferred onto the operating table. The anesthetic will be started and then someone will wash and shave your scrotum, coat the scrotum with an antiseptic, and then put sterile drapes around the area where the incision will be made.

The operation begins with the surgeon making about a three-inch cut in the middle of the scrotum. It is continued through the tissues until one testicle is reached. The blood vessels supplying the blood supply to the testicle are tied off with sutures and then the testicle is removed. The other testicle can be reached without making another cut in the scrotal skin by continuing the cut through the tissue separating the two testicles. The same method is used to remove the second testicle. The scrotum is then closed with sutures placed under the skin, which eventually will dissolve. The skin is covered with bandages and often a man is given a scrotal support or "jock strap" to wear. This keeps some pressure on the scrotum and may lessen the chance for bleeding. Ice is applied over the bandages to reduce swelling.

The patient is then brought to the recovery room and discharged when he is able to drink liquids, urinate, and his vital signs are stable. Physical activity should be limited for several days to reduce the chance of bleeding. A shower usually is permitted after 24 to 48 hours. Patients usually have minimal pain after the operation, which usually can be controlled with an NSAID or a Tylenol with codeine. Rarely is the pain so severe as to warrant stronger narcotics. The doctor will recheck the wound about 10 to 14 days later.

A bilateral orchiectomy has few risks. Besides the risk of anesthesia, the most common complication is bleeding under the skin. This sometimes results in a blood clot, which is called a *hematoma*. It occurs in less than 5% of patients and eventually will go away within a few weeks without any treatment. Rarely, the hematoma must be drained during a small operation. Although an infection also is possible, it is much less common.

What Happens to Testosterone following a Bilateral Orchiectomy?

Normal adult men have testosterone levels ranging from 250 to 800 ng/dl. The amount in the blood stream changes over the course of the day; it is highest in the morning and lowest late in the afternoon. After the testicles are removed, the testosterone level begins to drop rapidly, reaching its lowest level, called the *nadir*, within a few days. In most cases the level drops to 15 to 20 ng/dl as shown in the following table.

Table 26.2 Changes in Testosterone Level after Bilateral Orchiectomy

	Testosterone Level
Highest testosterone	30 ng/dl
Lowest testosterone	10 ng/dl
Median testosterone (50% of patients are above and 50% are below this level)	15 ng/dl
75% of testosterone values below	20 ng/dl
20% of testosterone values below	10 ng/dl

After a bilateral orchiectomy, the drop in the testosterone level is permanent. This can cause a number of side effects. Chapter 14 explained them and the different treatment options for improving a man's quality of life.

The Bottom Line on Bilateral Orchiectomy

Bilateral orchiectomy is a simple, easy alternative for achieving androgen deprivation therapy. Its primary advantage over medical therapy is convenience because men do not need specifically timed visits to receive an injection. Also, bilateral orchiectomy is much less costly than medical therapy, which may be important to men without good insurance.

Nonsurgical Options for Androgen Deprivation Therapy (ADT)

Fortunately, bilateral orchiectomy is not the only way to affect testosterone; nonsurgical options are also available, which many men prefer. About the same time the benefits of removing the testicles were discovered, doctors also found that giving men a female hormone called diethylstilbestrol (DES) had a similar result. This was called medical castration. Unfortunately, DES had one very serious side effect. About 5% of men had a heart attack when given 5 mg per day. A less serious side effect was breast enlargement. Studies were done using smaller doses, which did lower the heart risk, but didn't always drop the testosterone low enough to benefit all patients. Eventually, some doctors prescribed 2 or 3 mg of DES per day, but even at those doses, men still had an increased risk of heart attacks. The bottom line is that any dose of estrogen taken by mouth carries this risk. For this reason, DES is rarely used today. In fact, few pharmacies now carry it.

Doctors eventually learned why this drug is harmful. When taken by mouth, the drug is absorbed in the stomach and it then passes through the liver where it is changed to a slightly different drug. This modified drug was the cause of the heart attacks. Doctors then discovered that this side effect could almost be eliminated if estrogen was given *parenterally*, which means either through a vein, into a muscle, or placed on the skin. Today, this approach is sometimes used to treat metastatic disease. Fortunately, other safer drugs have been developed so that estrogen is no longer used as a first-line or second-line treatment.

How Does the Body Control Testosterone?

In the 1970s, researchers discovered a protein produced in a part of the brain called the *hypothalamus* that helped to regulate the testosterone level in the body. It is called *luteinizing hormone releasing hormone* (LHRH). It acts on another part of the brain called the *pituitary gland* where it attaches or binds to LHRH *receptors*. You can think of LHRH and LHRH receptors as two pieces of a jigsaw puzzle that "fit" together. When this binding occurs, the pituitary gland releases a protein called *luteinizing hormone,* or LH. It enters the blood stream and goes to the testicles where it stimulates the production of testosterone. As the testosterone level in the body drops, LHRH production increases leading to more release of LH and more production of testosterone. When the body has enough testosterone, LHRH goes down, less LH is released and less testosterone is produced.

Medical Castration Using LHRH Agonists

The discovery of LHRH led doctors to experiment with ways to interfere with its normal action. They developed drugs called LHRH *agonists* with a slightly different chemical structure and different action than LHRH. After entering the body, these drugs circulate throughout the bloodstream and go to the pituitary gland. There, they bind to the same receptors as LHRH. Initially, this binding causes the testosterone to rise, which occurs between 10 and 20 days after the first injection. Gradually, the LHRH agonist prevents the release of LH and the testosterone level goes down. By 28 days after the injection, the testosterone reaches its nadir or lowest level.

Sometimes this short-term rise in testosterone causes an increase in cancer symptoms such as more pain in the bones or more difficulty urinating. It even can cause a spinal cord compression leading to paralysis. Any worsening of symptoms that occurs when an LHRH agonist is first injected is called a *flare response*. Today, this is very uncommon because most men are being diagnosed with only small amounts of metastatic disease.

Fortunately, drugs are available that can reduce the chance of getting a flare response. The most commonly used ones belong to another group of drugs called *antiandrogens*. They prevent the testosterone from stimulating the growth of prostate cancer cells. Although antiandrogens are helpful, they are not 100% effective in preventing a flare response. In the best study done, a flare response occurred in 6% of men taking a placebo compared to only 3% of men receiving an antiandrogen called *flutamide*.

Three antiandrogens currently are on the market in the United States. In alphabetical order they are *bicalutamide (Casodex)*, *flutamide (Eulexin)*, and *nilutamide (Nilandron)*. Bicalutamide and nilutamide are taken once a day and flutamide is taken every eight hours. All three usually are given when an LHRH agonist is first injected and then continued for about three weeks. Side effects are very uncommon with this short course of therapy, but some men complain of diarrhea when taking flutamide. Although no good studies have shown that one antiandrogen works better, bicalutamide is used most commonly because it has fewer side effects. Since antiandrogens interfere with prostate cancer cell growth, they also have been tested as a treatment for metastatic disease. Unfortunately, randomized studies found that they were inferior to an LHRH agonist, so it is rarely recommended.

Another drug that can prevent the flare response is *ketoconazole*. The U.S. Food and Drug Administration (FDA) has approved it for treating fungal infections but not for prostate cancer. A secondary effect of this drug is that it rapidly lowers testosterone levels within 24 hours. Although no randomized study has been done using this drug to block the flare response, it is widely used "off label" for this purpose because of its rapid effect on testosterone. Ketoconazole is taken by mouth at a dose of 200 to 400 mg three times a day for about 10 to 14 days starting with the first LHRH agonist injection. Most men tolerate it without side effects, although some have nausea at the higher doses. It should be taken on an empty stomach. Anyone at risk for developing a flare response when starting an LHRH agonist should discuss getting one of these drugs.

Which LHRH Agonist Should You Receive?

The FDA has approved several LHRH agonists for men with advanced prostate cancer. The main difference between them is how they are administered and their chemical structure. They are given either subcutaneously, which means underneath the skin, or intramuscularly, which means into a large muscle. The names (in alphabetical order) and dosing intervals are shown in the next table.

Table 27.1 LHRH Agonists Available in the United States

Drug Name	Chemical Name	Dosing Intervals in Months	Made By
Eligard	Leuprolide	1, 3, 4, 6 months	Sanofi-Aventis
Lupron	Leuprolide	1, 3, 4, 6 months	Takeda
Trelstar	Triptorelin	1, 3, 4, 6 months	Watson
Viadur	Histrelin	12	Endo
Zoladex	Goserelin	1, 3, 4 months	Astra-Zeneca

Since no randomized study has shown a difference in survival, all of them are a reasonable choice if you have metastatic disease. However, some uncontrolled studies suggest that leuprolide may be inferior. One benefit of all the options is being able to select an interval that best fits your lifestyle and circumstances. For example, if you migrate south for the winter or live hundreds of miles away from your doctor, a longer-acting medication will be more convenient. If you want more frequent contact with your doctor, then you can have a shorter-acting drug. Since most doctors want to follow the prostate-specific antigen (PSA) level every three months, usually they will give the drug at the same time. Since there is no proof that one gives better results, any one of the drugs can be used.

Although you can choose the interval, you probably will be unable to choose which drug is to be used. Most doctors carry products made by only one or two companies for business reasons. Normally, they buy the drug and then get reimbursed from insurance with a small profit. The more they buy, the less they will pay and the greater is their profit. Some doctors will switch to a different drug if the profit increases. For these reasons, do not be surprised or alarmed if your doctor changes your LHRH agonist from time to time even if your PSA is stable. So far, no study has shown any problem from switching drugs.

The discovery of LHRH agonists to lower testosterone was very important for men with metastatic prostate cancer. It was safer than DES and more acceptable to men than having a bilateral orchiectomy. When a study was done to see which treatment patients would choose if given a choice, 80% selected an LHRH agonist instead of the operation. Men prefer not to have their testicles removed even though the chances for side effects are the same as with the injections. How you are affected mentally and emotionally by a treatment is an important part of deciding which treatment is right for you.

The Importance of Monitoring Testosterone

You should be aware that unlike bilateral orchiectomy, LHRH agonists are not 100% effective in keeping the testosterone at low levels. Each drug was approved because it lowered the male hormone into the *castrate range*, which was defined by the FDA as less than 50 ng/dl. The reason they selected that value was the tests available when these drugs were developed couldn't reliably detect lower levels. Since then, more sensitive tests have been developed that have shown much lower testosterone levels than achieved with ADT. As explained in the last chapter, the testosterone level following a bilateral orchiectomy is no higher than 30 ng/dl and most of the time it is closer to 20 ng/dl. Many doctors believe that lower is better because even small amounts of testosterone can cause prostate cancer cells to grow. So, how good are these drugs at controlling testosterone? Well-done studies show that:

- Approximately 1% to 7% of men starting an LHRH agonist do not drop their testosterone level below 50 ng/dl.

- Anywhere from 3% to 27% of men will have at least one increase in their testosterone above 50 ng/dl even when the drug is given properly. This is called a *testosterone escape* or a *breakthrough response.*

For these reasons, the FDA recommends regularly checking the testosterone level in all men receiving one of these drugs. Unfortunately, many doctors do not follow this advice and instead, they just monitor the PSA. If it does rise, they will recheck the testosterone level and if it still is above 50 ng/ml then they will consider other therapies. What should be done if a man's testosterone level is above this level? All the following options are reasonable:

- Repeat the test one month later.

- Switch to a different LHRH drug.

- Recommend a bilateral orchiectomy.

- Add an antiandrogen.

No studies have shown which approach is best. For now, discussing the options with your doctor makes the most sense.

One question needing a good answer is whether the testosterone level really does matter. A few weak studies do suggest that it is important. One study measured at least three testosterone levels over at least 18 months in patients who had been on an LHRH agonist for several years. The study divided men into three groups: Group I never had a testosterone higher than 20 ng/dl, Group II had levels between 20 and 50 ng/dl, and Group III had at least one value above 50 ng/dl. The first group did the best, Group II was second, and Group III had the poorest result. This study only *suggests* but does not prove that always keeping the testosterone below 20 ng/dl is best for men with advanced disease. The reasons are that the study was retrospective, it contained a small number of patients, and it did not report the impact on survival. A better study is needed to confirm whether this finding is correct.

Another study measured testosterone levels in men with metastatic disease who were receiving an LHRH agonist. It found that men with a higher testosterone level at six months were more likely to die from their cancer compared with those with lower levels. This study also *suggests* but does not prove that keeping the testosterone level very low is best. Perhaps new studies will appear that provide more information. Be aware that many doctors do not routinely check the testosterone level even though the FDA recommends it.

If you do decide to get treated with an LHRH agonist, then the following are key points to follow:

- All LHRH agonists cause an initial rise in testosterone following the first injection. This may cause a flare response in some men, depending on the location and extent of the cancer. Taking an antiandrogen can reduce the odds.

- Make sure your doctor checks the testosterone level about two or three months after starting an LHRH agonist. If it does not drop below 50 ng/ml, consider trying a different drug or having surgical castration, even if your PSA level drops.

- Have the testosterone rechecked once or twice each year. If the testosterone rises above 50 ng/ml during your treatment, then discuss with your doctor about switching drugs or having surgical castration even if your PSA is stable.

- If the testosterone level is under 50 ng/ml but much higher than 20 ng/dl, you can talk to your doctor about the pros and cons of switching your treatment to see whether you can get the testosterone level closer to that achieved following a bilateral orchiectomy.

- At a minimum, talk to your doctor about this controversy when you start an LHRH medication and make a shared decision.

Medical Castration Using a GnRH Antagonist

In 2009, the FDA approved another drug for the treatment of men with advanced prostate cancer called *degarelix* (*Firmagon*). That includes men with metastatic disease and those with a rising PSA after one of the other treatments. This medication is called a GnRH antagonist. It works a little differently from an LHRH agonist. Degarelix also binds to the receptors in the pituitary gland but unlike the LHRH agonists, it does not cause an increase in testosterone after the first injection. The testosterone drops more rapidly, usually by 90% within three days of starting the drug. Therefore, the primary advantage of this drug is it will not cause a flare response. Despite this difference, there is no proof that the antagonist results in a higher survival, although an uncontrolled study suggests it may be better and possibly safer than leuprolide. In randomized studies, the PSA was less likely to rise with the antagonist compared with the LHRH agonist, leuprolide. For now, the GnRh antagonist and the LHRH agonists are equally reasonable options for men with advanced prostate cancer.

Degarelix is given by a subcutaneous injection. When the treatment first begins, men get two injections, each one containing 120 mg. Additional doses of 80 mg are then injected once every 28 days. One disadvantage of degarelix compared with the LHRH agonist is only a four-week preparation is available, which some men may feel is more inconvenient. Another disadvantage is that about one-third of men complain of pain at the injection site when the drug is started. This complaint is less common with the other drugs.

The FDA also recommends measuring testosterone regularly with this drug because 3% of men do not keep their testosterone in the castrate range. If testosterone is not maintained at that level, then you should switch to an LHRH agonist or have the testicles removed to get the testosterone into the proper range.

LHRH Agonist or Antagonist: Which One Is Best?

None of the FDA-approved drugs controls the testosterone level in 100% of men, which means testosterone levels must be checked regularly. Degarelix has the advantage of dropping the testosterone and PSA more quickly than an LHRH agonist, which eliminates any chance of a flare response. It may be the preferred drug for men who have symptoms from their metastatic disease or are at the risk of developing them. However, no randomized study has shown a significantly better survival, and at one year after treatment, both groups of drugs did not differ in their ability to control testosterone. Recent uncontrolled studies suggest that the antagonist may have fewer cardiovascular side effects and a lower failure rate than leuprolide, but this must be confirmed before any conclusions can be made. Also, there are no data comparing degarelix and triptorelin. One disadvantage of degarelix is that it must be given every four weeks because no long-acting preparation is available. Another difference is that more men complain of pain and discomfort at the injection site on the first day of injections.

Intermittent Androgen Deprivation Therapy (IADT)

In chapter 14, intermittent androgen deprivation therapy (IADT) was discussed for men with localized disease. One randomized study of IADT also has been done in men with metastatic disease. The results were reported in April 2013 and are confusing to interpret. The question to be answered by the study was whether IADT was not inferior to continuous therapy. So far, one-half of the men on continuous therapy lived 5.8 years compared with 5.1 years for men on IADT. The only conclusions possible so far are that IADT is not better and could be inferior by 20%. More time will be needed to make a final determination. Until then, men should not assume that the two treatments have similar survival. However, some men did have an improved quality of life on IADT with stronger libido and better erections. Other studies have shown that men on IADT also have higher energy levels and less weight gain. Even if IADT turns out to result in a worse survival, some men will feel that the small improvement in their quality of life is worth it. These results are very important because so many men have been placed on IADT, believing it was no worse than continuous therapy. Based on this new study, all men now should be carefully counseled about the trade-offs with IADT; there may be a lower survival rate but a better quality of life.

One of the uncertainties about IADT is how to do it; how long should the hormone therapy be given before it is stopped and when should it be restarted? Although the study described above showed that the approach used might be inferior compared with continuous therapy, perhaps doing IADT in a different way would work better. For now, that question cannot be answered.

The Bottom Line on ADT Using an LHRH Medication

The development of alternatives to surgical castration was an important innovation in the treatment of advanced prostate cancer. It has given men more options with an opportunity to avoid surgery and the psychological distress of losing their testicles. At the same time, the drugs do not always work as well at controlling testosterone and closer monitoring is needed. A frequent question among patients is what they should do if the PSA begins to rise. Unlike many other cancer treatments, keeping the testosterone low should be continued even when the cancer begins to progress. The reason is that some prostate cancer cells will grow faster if the testosterone is allowed to rise. That will happen in most, but not all men if the drugs are stopped. Sometimes the body loses its ability to produce testosterone and in those cases, continued drug treatment would not be necessary. The options for treating men who progress while on an LHRH drug are described in later chapters.

Combined Androgen Blockade (CAB) and Triple Drug Therapy

As explained previously, about 95% of the body's testosterone is produced in the testicles and 5% is produced in the adrenal glands. Removing the testicles or giving an LHRH agonist or antagonist only will affect the testosterone from the testicles. However, even the small amount coming from the adrenal glands can stimulate prostate cancer cell growth. This was proven years ago when castrated men with prostate cancer improved after their adrenal glands were surgically removed. Since then, drugs called *antiandrogens* have been developed that have almost accomplished the same goal—they block the action of testosterone coming from the testicles and the adrenal glands.

Since antiandrogens are taken by mouth, some doctors thought they would be a convenient alternative to medical or surgical castration for treating metastatic disease. Unfortunately, when the treatments were compared, men treated with an antiandrogen had a lower survival rate. However, doctors also asked the question whether patients might do better by being treated with a combination of an antiandrogen and medical or surgical castration rather than either one alone. That way *all* the testosterone produced in the body could be affected.

What Is CAB?

Several names have been used when medical or surgical castration is combined with an antiandrogen including *combined androgen blockade (CAB), maximum androgen blockade (MAB)* or *total androgen blockade (TAB)*. Many randomized studies have been done comparing CAB with medical or surgical castration and three showed a significant improvement in the average survival ranging from three to six months. Several good reasons can explain why more studies didn't show a benefit or the benefit was not greater.

Perhaps the most important one is doctors were unaware that antiandrogens sometimes *stimulate* rather than *prevent* the growth of prostate cancer cells. When an antiandrogen is stopped in men with progressive prostate cancer, 20% to 40% of them have an improvement in their cancer symptoms and the prostate-specific antigen (PSA) level goes down. This is called the *antiandrogen withdrawal phenomenon (AAW)*, which lasts an average of four to six months before patients begin to progress again. AAW wasn't discovered until several years after the CAB studies were completed, which means that men participating in them stayed on their antiandrogen too long. This made their cancer progress more quickly. Had the drug been stopped when the patients began to get worse, they likely would have had a better survival. Now, the standard practice for *everyone* taking an antiandrogen is to stop it when the PSA begins to rise, recheck it after one to two months, and not begin any other therapy until the PSA goes up again.

Doctors who do not recommend CAB believe that the benefit of this combined treatment is at best very small and the side effects are significant:

- **Breast Tenderness and Gynecomastia:** These side effects occur in approximately 33% to 67% of men on these drugs but few men are very bothered by them. Breast enlargement (gynecomastia) but not breast tenderness can be prevented using one to three doses of radiation delivered to the breasts before starting the drugs. Radiation is not effective after the breast enlargement has occurred. The dose of radiation needed has no side effects so men should strongly consider it before starting one of these drugs. Studies are in progress to reverse gynecomastia, but the U.S. Food and Drug Administration (FDA) has not yet approved any drug for that purpose.

- **Liver Changes:** All three antiandrogens can cause damage to the liver, but only very rarely is it life-threatening. The drugs should be used very cautiously in men with liver disease. In well-done studies, less than 1% of men had to stop the drug due to liver damage. Anyone taking one of these drugs should have liver function tests done every few months. If they become abnormal, the drug should be stopped for several months and the tests repeated. If the tests improve, the drugs can be started again to see whether the problem recurs. If it does, then the drug should be stopped.

- **Diarrhea:** This happens much more often in men taking flutamide compared with the other two drugs. In one well-done study, 24% of men getting flutamide had diarrhea compared with only 10% taking bicalutamide. Lowering the dose may reduce or eliminate the diarrhea, but studies have not been done to find out whether the drug is still as effective. A safer approach is to switch to a different antiandrogen. The diarrhea usually will go away when the drug is stopped.

- **Night Blindness:** An unusual side effect of nilutamide is having difficulty driving at night when the light is low. It happens to about 12% to 14% of men taking this drug and the only treatment is to stop taking it.

- **Interstitial Pneumonitis:** This is an inflammation in the lung that results in fever, coughing, shortness of breath, and chest pain. It has been reported with all three antiandrogens, but is about 10 times more common with nilutamide. For that reason, this drug should not be used in men with lung disease. The chances of this happening are about 17% in Japanese men, but only 2% in other ethnic groups. Usually it goes away when the drug is stopped.

Another reason many doctors do not recommend CAB is they believe the antiandrogen can be delayed until the PSA begins to rise while on androgen deprivation therapy (ADT) and the same benefit will occur. However, no study has ever shown that delaying the antiandrogen is as effective as starting it immediately and one randomized study suggested that delayed therapy results in a lower survival.

Another approach used by some doctors is to start the antiandrogen along with ADT and then stop it after one month. In other words, it is being used only to reduce the chance for a flare response. Here again, no study has shown that short-term use is as effective as prolonged therapy in men with advanced disease.

Which Antiandrogen Is Best for You?

The most commonly used antiandrogen in the United States is bicalutamide (Casodex). It may be the best choice when one of these drugs is needed because:

- It is taken only once per day.

- Less frequent diarrhea occurs compared with flutamide.

- Both night vision problems and interstitial pneumonia are avoided.

- The drug is a generic, which should drive down the cost to patients not covered by insurance.

The next table summarizes the differences among the three FDA-approved antiandrogens.

Table 28.1 FDA-Approved Antiandrogens

	Chemical Name		
	Flutamide	**Bicalutamide**	**Nilutamide**
Drug name	Eulexin (125 mg)	Casodex (50 mg)	Nilandron (150 mg)
Dosing	Two pills every eight hours	One pill per day	Two pills a day for 30 days, then one pill daily
Most common side effects	Breast tenderness and enlargement Liver changes Diarrhea	Breast tenderness and enlargement Liver changes	Breast tenderness and enlargement Liver changes Night blindness

The Bottom Line on CAB

Since more studies of CAB probably will never be done in the United States, the decision about its use must be made using those completed many years ago. Although this combination showed on average only a three- to six-month increase in survival, it is still significant. In fact, many therapies in wide use today for treating other cancers have a similar improvement in survival and they are used routinely. CAB may not be for everyone, but all men with metastatic disease should be informed about the pros and cons when beginning ADT so they can have a chance to decide what to do.

CAB is the right thing to do for men who want to do everything possible to prolong their survival. The antiandrogen should begin when ADT begins and be continued until the PSA starts to rise. At that time it should be stopped. Patients should wait about

one month to recheck the PSA if they were on flutamide or nilutamide and two months if they were on bicalutamide before beginning the next therapy. During that time, men are encouraged to be
patient. If the PSA does drop after stopping the antiandrogen, then
no other treatment is needed until the PSA begins to rise again.
Doctors are not sure at what PSA level the antiandrogen should be
stopped, but an increase by 1 or 2 ng/ml on at least two tests is
probably a reasonable indication.

What Is Triple Hormone Blockade?

Another treatment promoted by a few doctors is triple hormone
blockade. It consists of combining CAB with a drug called a 5-alpha
reductase inhibitor, or 5-ARI, which is normally used to treat men
with symptoms from prostate enlargement. The FDA has approved
two drugs for men with these complaints, finasteride (Proscar) and
dutasteride (Avodart). The drugs work by preventing normal prostate
cells from converting testosterone to a more potent hormone called
dihydrotestosterone or DHT. They both shrink the size of the prostate.

Some doctors thought these drugs also might help men with
prostate cancer. Several years later, this idea was supported by two
randomized studies that showed these drugs could reduce the
chance of men being diagnosed with prostate cancer. Also, laboratory studies showed that these drugs stopped cancer cells from
growing in a plastic dish. However, little evidence exists to show
that prostate cancer patients who are taking either of these drugs
have any clinical benefit.

Recently, a follow-up report of one of these studies showed
men who received finasteride to reduce their chance of being diagnosed with prostate cancer did not have any improvement in survival compared with those taking a placebo. Despite lowering the
chance of being diagnosed with prostate cancer, the FDA has
decided not to approve either drug for preventing this disease
because they also may increase the risk of developing more aggressive tumors.

So, what is known about triple hormone therapy for men with metastatic disease? The answer is, not very much. A small, uncontrolled study has been done in men with localized disease from which no conclusions can be made. Even less information is available for men with advanced disease.

Without proper studies, what should men do? Since finasteride and dutasteride have few side effects, taking one of them with CAB is an option, but don't be surprised if your doctor doesn't encourage it. As for any doctor who strongly recommends them, you should be aware that it is only his or her personal opinion and it lacks good scientific proof. Taking triple hormone therapy is an option with few side effects, but you should understand that doctors do not know whether it will help you. It also could be harmful if somehow it delays the use of other drugs that have been shown to improve survival.

The Bottom Line on Triple Hormone Blockade

At this time, evidence is lacking that triple drug therapy is helpful, but it is an option for motivated patients and is unlikely to cause problems. Hopefully, studies will be done to find out whether it is a good thing to do.

Treatment Options for Bone Metastases

When prostate cancer spreads into the bones it can cause pain and fractures. In rare cases it may cause a spinal cord compression leading to temporary or permanent paralysis. The net result is a worsening of a man's quality of life and possibly decreased survival. Fortunately, improvements in treatment have made these events less common.

How Are Bone Metastases Monitored?

The bone scan continues to be the most sensitive way to detect or monitor bone metastases. After bone metastases are diagnosed, additional bone scans are ordered based on the prostate-specific antigen (PSA) test. There is little reason to repeat the bone scan when the PSA is stable. However, when it is rising, doctors vary on when they recommend doing another scan. New onset or worsening of previous bone pain usually will lead to another scan regardless of the PSA result. If the PSA is rising and a bone scan shows no new or progressive disease, additional scans will be ordered, but here too doctors vary in how they come to that decision.

After a bone scan is performed, it is compared with the previous one to see whether old "spots" of cancer have gotten worse or new ones have appeared. Your doctor should determine whether cancer has spread into your weight-bearing bones like the hip, femur, or spine. In those cases, plain x-rays, a CT scan, or MRI of those bones are recommended. They are done to see whether a fracture has occurred or a bone is at risk for fracturing in the near future. These additional tests are needed because not all the spots seen on a bone scan are due to metastases. They could be caused by a previous fracture or arthritis, or other noncancerous conditions. Rarely, a biopsy of a bone must be performed to find out why a scan is abnormal. If your PSA is rising and new spots are seen, most likely it means your cancer has gotten worse. After confirming that a weight-bearing bone could fracture, or if it is causing pain, the next step is to arrange for a consultation with a radiation therapist and possibly an orthopedic surgeon.

What Are the Options for Treating Bone Metastases?

In addition to taking drugs to relieve the pain, several bone-specific treatments can also be given including:

- External radiation

- Radioactive isotopes (radiopharmaceuticals)

- Bisphosphonates

- Other bone-protecting agents

External Radiation for Bone Metastases

Some doctors call external radiation to the bones, *spot radiation*. The number of treatments needed is much smaller than when the entire prostate is treated. Randomized studies have shown that *a single treatment is as effective as 30 of them*. You may be surprised to learn that the number of treatments and total dose given to the bones are quite variable throughout the United States. A large survey found that about one-half of the radiotherapists give 10 treatments. If you are going to receive this treatment for your pain and are told it will take one to two weeks, then ask, "Why is more than one dose needed when there is no proof it is better?" You might consider a second opinion also. More radiation will be given if a bone has been severely damaged. About a fourth of men get complete relief of pain. Another 41% can expect more than one-half of their pain to decrease within one month of receiving radiation. It is well tolerated and causes no side effects.

Radiopharmaceuticals (Radioisotopes)

Radiopharmaceuticals are drugs that contain a radioactive compound. When injected into a vein they circulate throughout the body, find their way into bones invaded by cancer, and then give off their radiation. They can kill cancer cells and relieve pain or protect the bone from fracturing in the future. The radiation only extends a short distance away from the radioactive material so the whole body is not affected. Small amounts do stay in some normal parts of the body. They include the bone marrow, the wall of the colon, the bladder, the testicles, and the kidneys.

The most common side effects are a lowering of the white blood cells and platelets. For that reason, monitoring with frequent blood tests is needed, especially if you are also getting chemotherapy. Blood products may be needed if the cell counts drop too low.

Eventually, the radiation goes away or decays depending on its *half-life*, which is the time required for one-half of the radiation to disappear. The amount of the radiopharmaceutical given will depend on your weight. Most of the radioactivity gets out of the body through urine. Although caution is advised when urinating, a few drops of urine missing the toilet bowl are unlikely to harm anyone. Several radiopharmaceuticals are available to treat painful bone metastases including:

- Radium-223

- Strontium-89

- Samarium-153

- Rhenium-186

Radium-223 (Xofigo)

Of these options, radium-223 appears to offer the greatest benefit. It has been studied in a randomized trial of men with symptoms from bone metastases. Men enrolled in the study had either failed chemotherapy or were not good candidates to receive it. The study found that radium-223 improved symptoms and increased survival. The results are summarized below:

- Overall survival was improved by 2.8 months (14 months for radium-223 compared with 11.2 months for the control group).

- Time until the first skeletal related event (SRE) was delayed by 5.2 months (13.6 months for radium-223 compared with 8.4 months for the control group).

- Fewer men reporting bone pain (43% for radium-223 against 58% for the control group).

- The drug significantly prolonged the time until the PSA increased.

The differences in the side effects were:

- Nausea (34% in radium-223 group and 32% in the control group)

- Diarrhea (22% in radium-223 group and 13% in the control group)

- Vomiting (17% in radium-223 group and 13% in the control group)

Based on this study, the U.S. Food and Drug Administration (FDA) approved this drug in May 2013 under the trade name Xofigo. It is the only radiopharmaceutical that has been shown to improve survival.

Strontium-89 (Metastron)

This radioisotope has been used for bone metastases for more than 15 years. It has a half-life of 55 days in bones containing cancer, but only 14 days in normal bones. That means the radiation is almost completely gone from the body in about eight months. Pain usually will be improved in one to three weeks after the injection. Older studies showed that about 65% of men receiving strontium-89 plus external radiation had a significant drop in bone pain in six months compared with only 35% receiving external radiation alone. Blood counts drop in two to four weeks. Over the following 12 weeks they gradually return to their baseline level. At that time, another dose can be given if needed.

In randomized studies comparing external radiation alone to radiation plus strontium, the combination showed a delay in progression of pain, a decrease in the amount of pain medication being used, and a better quality of life. Based on these results, strontium-89 would be a good option if radium-223 is no longer effective or cannot be used for some reason.

Samarium-153 (Quadramet)

This agent has a half-life of only 46 hours. It is excreted in the urine so precautions should be used when urinating. It will disappear from your body much faster than strontium-89. Men are advised to drink plenty of fluids and urinate often to minimize the amount of radiation affecting the bladder. Studies show that by three weeks, 53% of patients getting samarium-153 had significant improvements in pain compared with 25% getting placebo. The treated group reduced their intake of narcotics also.

Samarium-153 caused about a 50% drop in white blood cell counts and platelets, but serious complications occurred in very few patients. If you get this treatment, your blood counts should be measured every two weeks.

The Bottom Line on Spot Radiation and Radiopharmaceuticals

Doctors have different opinions about whether to use spot radiation or one of these radiopharmaceuticals. Spot radiation may be safer and more convenient if only a few bones are treated. However, it may cause more permanent damage to the bone marrow if multiple bones need treatment. In that case, a radiopharmaceutical is a better choice. Sometimes both are used.

Bisphosphonates

A two-step process called remodeling is constantly renewing the bones in our body. In the first step, old bone tissue is broken down and removed, and in the second step, new bone is formed. Prostate cancer that has spread to the bones can interfere with this remodeling. Bisphosphonates work by stopping the breakdown of bone, which makes them useful when someone has bone metastases or osteoporosis.

A randomized study was done in men on hormone therapy who had metastatic disease and a rising PSA. They were assigned to get a bisphosphonate called zoledronic acid (Zometa) or a placebo. The drugs were given intravenously every three weeks for 15 months. Zoledronic acid was tested at two doses, 4 and 8 mg.

The goal of the study was to compare quality of life, pain, and the frequency of SREs (skeletal related events), which includes:

- Bone fractures caused by prostate cancer

- Compression of the spinal cord

- Radiation treatment to involved bones

- Surgery on a bone affected by the cancer

- A change of therapy because of worsening cancer

The results are shown in the next table.

Table 29.1 Comparison of Skeletal Related Events (SREs) with Zoledronic Acid and Placebo

Result	Zoledronic Acid (4 mg)	Placebo
SRE	38%	49%
Fracture due to cancer	13%	22%
Median time to first SRE	488 days	321 days

The study showed a significant benefit from the 4-mg dose of the drug. For every nine men getting treated, one avoided getting an SRE. The drug also delayed the time until the first SRE occurred by six months. Pain scores and quality of life measurements did not differ at 15 months. Based on this study, the FDA approved the drug in February 2002 for men with bone metastases who were getting worse during hormone therapy.

The drug did not cause many significant side effects as shown in the next table.

Table 29.2 Comparison of Side Effects of Zoledronic Acid and Placebo

Side Effect	Zoledronic Acid (4 mg)	Placebo
Fatigue	33%	26%
Anemia	27%	18%
Decreased kidney function	15%	12%

Doctors have learned that worsening of kidney function is partly due to how fast the drug is given. Now, the safest approach is to give it over a minimum of 15 minutes. Also, kidney function should be measured by a simple blood test before each treatment. If your kidney function is not normal, then the dose should be reduced or the treatment delayed until the kidneys improve.

Since the study was done, another complication was discovered that occurs with any bisphosphonate. It is called *osteonecrosis of the jaw* (ONJ). It is defined as the development of pain, swelling, and decreased healing following a dental procedure such as removing a tooth. ONJ is more common in men getting intravenous treatment compared with those taking a bisphosphonate by mouth. Also, the longer the drug is used, the greater is the chance it will occur. One study found that ONJ occurred in about 1% of men after 12 months, 7% after 24 months, and 21% after four years of taking zoledronic acid. For that reason, if you need oral surgery, make sure your dentist knows you are taking this drug.

The Bottom Line on Bisphosphonates (Zoledronic Acid)

This drug is another good example of the importance of weighing risks and benefits. Zoledronic acid does help a small number of men who have cancer in the bones avoid radiation to the bones in the future. The question for you to decide is whether having a one in nine chance of benefitting from the drug is worth the risk of side effects and the need to get a treatment every three weeks.

Denosumab (Xgeva)

Denosumab is the latest agent for helping men with painful bone metastases. Two types of cells are involved in remodeling bone, *osteoblasts* and *osteoclasts*. The osteoblasts release a protein called RANK, which activates the osteoclasts to reabsorb bone, and then the osteoblasts produce new bone. In prostate cancer patients with bone metastases, however, the cancer cells stimulate osteoblasts to produce an increased amount of RANK, which stimulates the osteoclasts to absorb more bone. This also results in stimulating the cancer cells to grow. Eventually this process results in an SRE as more bone is broken down but not replaced. Denosumab is an *antibody* that works by attaching to RANK, greatly reducing its ability to stimulate the osteoclasts, which reduces the risk for an SRE.

The FDA approved this drug in November 2010 under the trade name Xgeva based on a randomized study comparing it with zoledronic acid in men with symptomatic bone metastases. Both drugs were given every four weeks. Patients were monitored for the development of an SRE. The study showed that the time until the first SRE was longer with denosumab compared with zoledronic acid. Half of the men had their first SRE within 17.1 months of starting the zoledronic acid compared with 20.7 months for denosumab. In men not receiving either treatment, 50% of patients have an SRE by 10.7 months. The study also found that the total number of SREs was significantly lower in men receiving denosumab.

The overall number of side effects was similar for the two treatments as shown in the next table.

Table 29.3 Comparison of Side Effects for Denosumab and Zoledronic Acid

Side Effect	Denosumab	Zoledronic Acid
Anemia	36%	36%
Back pain	30%	32%
Decreased appetite	29%	28%
Nausea	26%	29%
Fatigue	23%	27%
Constipation	27%	25%
Bone pain	26%	25%
Low calcium	6%	13%

Many of these side effects occurred because of the disease itself and the other treatments patients were receiving rather than being caused by the drug. In the first three days after treatment, fever was more common in the zoledronic acid group (20.2% vs. 8.7%). The most significant difference between the two treatments was the development of a low calcium level, which occurred more often in men receiving denosumab. For that reason, calcium levels should be checked regularly and men should take calcium supplements (500–1000 mg per day) and vitamin D (400–800 International Units per day). ONJ occurred in 1% of men on zoledronic acid and 2% of men on denosumab. Most of them had poor oral hygiene, used a dental appliance, or had a recent tooth extraction. Men taking denosumab should be counseled about this risk and they should alert their dentist when they are taking this drug if any dental work is needed.

The Bottom Line on Denosumab

Based on this study, denosumab appears to be a better drug to prevent SREs than zoledronic acid, with the following advantages. It is more effective; easier to administer; not necessary to monitor kidney function; and not necessary to lower the dose if kidney functions are slightly impaired.

The usual dose is 120 mg given by a subcutaneous injection once every four weeks. All patients should also take daily calcium and vitamin D as described above.

Focused Ultrasound for Painful Bone Metastases

Another very new treatment uses ultrasound waves to treat painful bone metastases. A recent randomized study found a significant percentage of men had improvement with a small incidence of side effects but more data are needed to determine its exact role for these patients.

The Bottom Line on Managing Bone Metastases

Bone metastases are an unfortunate development for men with progressive prostate cancer that can lead to a number of problems and decrease their quality of life. Fortunately, many options are available to reduce the odds that they will happen and treat them if they occur. Anyone with advanced disease should make sure to discuss these options with their doctor to minimize morbidity from this disease.

V

MANAGEMENT OF CASTRATION-RESISTANT PROSTATE CANCER (CRPC)

Overview of Castration-Resistant Prostate Cancer (CRPC)

Although androgen deprivation therapy (ADT) helps most men for several years, its benefits rarely last forever. At some time, the cancer begins to progress again. The first sign is a rise in the prostate-specific antigen (PSA) level and later symptoms appear. Doctors call this *androgen-independent prostate cancer (AIPC), hormone refractory prostate cancer (HRPC), or castration-resistant prostate cancer (CRPC).* The last term is becoming the term of choice by most experts.

Do You Really Have CRPC?

Before getting treated for CRPC, the testosterone level should be measured to be sure it is still below the castrate level of 50 ng/ml. A higher level may make the cancer grow and reducing it may help delay progression of the disease or the need for other treatments. The term CRPC only applies if the testosterone is below this level. As discussed in chapter 27, the LHRH agonists and the LHRH antagonists do not always keep the testosterone level under 50 ng/ml. When it is above that level, the best treatment is to either switch to a different drug that lowers testosterone or have surgical castration. The PSA and testosterone then can be rechecked and no additional treatment is needed if they go back down. If the testosterone remains above 50 ng/dl, then another treatment should be considered.

Assuming the testosterone level is in the castrate range, doctors have three ways to tell whether someone has CRPC.

- The PSA increases.

- Symptoms from the cancer get worse.

- The bone scan or CT scan shows new metastases or the existing ones get worse.

In almost every case, the PSA will rise weeks or months before the symptoms or scans get worse. How much must the PSA level increase to diagnose CRPC? Many people now define it as three consecutive increases in PSA by at least 50% each time. Another indication is the appearance of new spots on the bone or CT scans.

When Should Men with CRPC Consult an Oncologist?

Urologists most often are the doctors responsible for treating men with ADT. At present, however, most of them are not prescribing the newer therapies. Medical oncologists usually are the doctors administering them. This may gradually change, but even if it does, men can still benefit from a consultation with an oncologist to hear about the pros and cons of the latest advances for managing CRPC to make sure they are properly informed.

Management Options for CRPC

One of the most significant changes in the treatment of prostate cancer has been the development of new therapies for men with CRPC. Before 2004, only one FDA-approved therapy was available. The good news for patients is that several are now available and more are expected within the next several years. The approved options as of June 2013 include:

- Sipuleucel-T (Provenge) (chapter 31)

- Abiraterone acetate (Zytiga) (chapter 32)

- Docetaxel (Taxotere) + prednisone (chapter 34)

- Enzalutamide (Xtandi) (chapter 35)

- Cabazitaxel (Jevtana) (chapter 36)

- Mitoxantrone (Novantrone) and prednisone (chapter 36)

Other options used by many doctors include second-line hormonal therapies even though none of them are FDA approved for this disease nor have they been shown to improve survival. Their main benefit appears to be that they lower PSA and reduce some cancer-related symptoms. One of the newer challenges for doctors is to decide the best sequence for some of these therapies because few studies have been done to make this determination. As a result, opinions vary widely. For that reason, the pros and cons of these options will be reviewed in chapter 33 with some guidance provided that you can use when being counseled by your doctor.

Immunotherapy Using Sipuleucel-T (Provenge) for Castration-Resistant Prostate Cancer (CRPC)

The immune system is your body's defense against things that may harm you such as bacteria, viruses, wounds, and even cancer. It is a complicated interaction between certain organs, cells, and chemicals made by your body. They work together when threatened by something "foreign." Your immune system is much better at defending against germs than against cancer cells. Germs are very clearly foreign, but cancer cells have some things in common with normal cells in your body so they are not easily recognized as being foreign. Cancer cells also release certain chemicals that protect them from being destroyed by the body. Using the immune system to fight disease is called immunotherapy.

How Your Immune System Works

An immune response can be stimulated by any substance your body thinks is foreign. These foreign substances are called antigens. Usually they are present on the surface of invading cells. When an antigen enters the body, several types of normal cells work together in a complicated way to kill foreign cells directly or help the body get rid of them. One of them is called a dendritic cell. These cells are very effective but not many of them are present in the body at any one time.

For years, doctors have searched for ways to improve the ability of the immune system to fight cancer cells, but with little success.

All that changed when studies showed that the survival of men with advanced prostate cancer could be improved by a treatment named *sipuleucel-T*.

What Is Sipuleucel-T and How Is the Treatment Done?

This is a vaccine therapy that stimulates the body's own immune system. The treatment involves several steps that include:

- Collecting a man's blood and separating the dendritic cells and other lymphocytes by a process called *leukopheresis*.

- Sending them to a special laboratory for processing where the dendritic cells are combined for 40 hours with an antigen located on the surface of most prostate cancer cells called *prostatic acid phosphatase*. This results in the formation of "activated" cells called *sipuleucel-T*.

- Three days after the cells have been collected and activated they are given back to a patient by injecting them into a vein, which stimulates other normal cells to kill prostate cancer cells. Each injection contains at least 50 million cells.

- The process is repeated two more times over the next six weeks.

What Are the Results with Sipuleucel-T?

Considerable controversy has surrounded this treatment. The initial study was designed to determine whether sipuleucel-T would delay the progression of the cancer in men with metastatic disease. Although it did not achieve that goal, longer follow-ups showed that men receiving the active treatment lived longer compared with men in the control group. Despite this result, the U.S. Food and Drug Administration (FDA) did not approve the treatment and instead required that another study be done.

In the next study over 500 men with castration-resistant prostate cancer (CRPC) and few or no symptoms received either sipuleucel-T or dendritic cells that were not combined with prostatic acid phosphatase. The study found that one-half of the men getting sipuleucel-T lived 4.1 months longer than the men in the control group (25.8 months compared with 21.7 months). Thirty-six months after enrolling in the study, 32% of the men receiving sipuleucel-T were still alive compared with only 23% of men in the control group. This means that about one person benefitted out of every 11 men treated. Based on this result, the FDA approved this treatment in April 2010 under the trade name *Provenge*.

Additional evaluations have been done to identify which men were most likely to benefit from sipuleucel-T. After the study was completed, the results were reanalyzed. Patients were divided into four equal groups according to their prostate-specific antigen (PSA) level, from lowest to highest, as shown in the next table.

Table 31.1 Impact of PSA Level on Overall Survival with Sipuleucel-T

	PSA Less Than 22.1 ng/ml	PSA Between 22.1 and 50.1 ng/ml	PSA Between 50.1 and 134 ng/ml	PSA Over 134 ng/ml
Placebo	28.3 months	20.1 months	15 months	15.5 months
Sipuleucel-T	40.3 months	27.1 months	20.4 months	18.4 months
Difference in survival	13 months	7 months	5.4 months	2.9 months

Those men in the lowest PSA group, which ranged from 0 to 22 ng/ml, lived about 13 months longer than men in the control group. In contrast, the difference was only 2.9 months for men with a PSA over 134 ng/ml. This analysis suggests that using sipuleucel-T at lower PSA levels offers the best chance to help men with CRPC.

What Are the Side Effects of Sipuleucel-T?

Almost everyone in the randomized studies reported having some side effects as shown in the next table.

Table 31.2 Frequency of Side Effects of Sipuleucel-T Compared with Controls

Side Effects	Sipuleucel-T Group	Control Group
Chills	53%	11%
Fatigue	41%	35%
Fever	31%	10%
Back pain	30%	29%
Nausea	22%	15%
Joint ache	20%	21%
Headache	18%	7%
Vomiting	13%	8%
Pain	12%	7%
Muscle ache	12%	6%
Weakness	11%	7%
Diarrhea	10%	11%
Flu-like illness	10%	4%

(continued)

Table 31.2 Frequency of Side Effects of Sipuleucel-T Compared with Controls (continued)

Side Effects	Sipuleucel-T Group	Control Group
Musculoskeletal pain	9%	10%
Shortness of breath	9%	5%
Hypertension	8%	5%
Sweating	5%	1%

These side effects need little explanation. How severe were they? When clinical studies are done, side effects are graded on a scale of one to five. For this study, the following descriptions were used.

- Grade 1 = Mild side effects
- Grade 2 = Moderate side effects
- Grade 3 = Severe side effects
- Grade 4 = Life-threatening or disabling side effects
- Grade 5 = Fatal side effects

Mild and moderate side effects are not serious and do not require much treatment. Treatments are needed, however, when side effects are severe. The study found about 25% of the men had severe side effects, and in 4% they were life-threatening. Chills, fatigue, and fever were most common. You may wonder why so many side effects occurred in the control group. One reason is because blood cells were removed from the body, kept in a laboratory for 40 hours, and then given back to those men three days later. Another reason is that the cancer may have caused some of them.

Who Is a Candidate for Sipuleucel-T?

This study was specifically designed to treat men with CRPC who had few or no symptoms from their cancer and had not yet received chemotherapy. For that reason, only those men are eligible to get treated at this time because that is the way the FDA gave its approval. If you are interested in this treatment and your doctor doesn't use it, you can visit the company website to find a physician near you who can treat you (www.Provenge.com).

The treatment is quite expensive, costing about $93,000, but fortunately Medicare and most insurance companies will cover it.

The Bottom Line on Sipuleucel-T

Many critics of sipuleucel-T argue that the treatment is too expensive and improving survival by an average of only four months may not be worth the expense. Although spending that much money for an average of about four extra months of survival may seem overly expensive, it is in line with other cancer therapies. Others are skeptical that sipuleucel-T truly works because it does not lower PSA nor prevent progression of the disease. For those reasons, they will not offer it until the patient fails one or two of the other therapies available, if at all. Despite these concerns, however, the improvement in survival is real and perhaps improving the body's immune system works differently against prostate cancer than the way traditional drugs work. The approval of Provenge is a major advance in treating CRPC, and all men with CRPC and few or no symptoms should consider getting it as one of their next options. Keep in mind that men with lower PSA levels may get a much greater increase in survival so if it is going to be used, earlier is better. Although side effects may be common, they are less serious compared with chemotherapy. If you do get sipuleucel-T, be aware that you will be unable to tell whether it is working because the PSA, scans, and x-rays are not affected. For that reason, many experts are proceeding to add the next therapy after completing the administration of sipuleucel-T without much delay.

Abiraterone Acetate (Zytiga) for Castration-Resistant Prostate Cancer (CRPC)

32

As previously explained, the adrenal glands make only a small percentage of the body's testosterone. Even so, it is enough to stimulate prostate cancer cells when a man is on androgen deprivation therapy (ADT) and his testosterone is below 50 ng/dl. Treatment with an antiandrogen interferes with the adrenal testosterone and helps some men with metastatic prostate cancer. Support for this comes from the finding of a higher survival with combined androgen blockade compared with ADT alone (chapter 28).

In recent years, doctors made another discovery about testosterone: tumor cells also are able to make it. For that reason, even when the testosterone coming from the testicles and adrenal glands is reduced, prostate cancer cells still can be stimulated by the testosterone they produce.

After doctors learned that a certain enzyme was necessary to make testosterone in the adrenal glands, they began to develop drugs that could block it, hoping that it would help slow down tumor growth. One of them was named *abiraterone acetate*. It comes in a tablet containing 250 mg. Four of them are taken once a day by mouth. Patients taking this drug also must take prednisone because the adrenal gland makes other chemicals that are important for normal body function. Abiraterone acetate may reduce those chemicals when it lowers testosterone and the prednisone is a good substitute to keep the body functioning properly. The initial studies suggested that this drug could help men with advanced prostate cancer.

How Effective Is Abiraterone Acetate?

Based on the early test results, studies were conducted in men with metastatic disease who failed a chemotherapy drug called *docetaxel* (see chapter 34). This group was chosen because a shorter time would be needed to complete the studies compared with testing it in men with less advanced disease.

In the initial randomized study, men were assigned to receive 5 mg of prednisone twice each day plus 1000 mg of abiraterone per day or prednisone plus a placebo. The study showed a significantly higher survival in the abiraterone group; one-half of the men receiving this drug lived 15.8 months compared with only 11.2 in the placebo group. Based on this 4.6 months' increase in survival, the FDA approved the drug in April 2011 in combination with prednisone for men with castration-resistant prostate cancer (CRPC) *after* they progress on chemotherapy. The commercial name of abiraterone acetate is Zytiga. In 2013, the results were updated with a longer follow-up showing very similar results. Other patient benefits included a reduced intake of narcotics for pain relief and a delay in the need for chemotherapy.

The next goal was to find out whether men would benefit from getting abiraterone *before* being treated with chemotherapy. This was determined in another randomized study in which men again received 1000 mg of abiraterone and 10 mg prednisone per day or prednisone plus a placebo. A preliminary analysis showed that the active drug resulted in fewer men developing progressive disease based on changes in their x-rays, bone scans, CTs, and MRI; one-half of the patients on abiraterone progressed in 16.5 months compared with only 8.3 months for those getting the placebo. It is too early to tell the impact of this drug on overall survival, although the preliminary analysis suggests it has increased. Based on the delay in disease progression, in December 2012, the FDA approved the drug for use in men with CRPC and few or no symptoms prior to receiving docetaxel.

The abiraterone must be taken on an empty stomach; otherwise too much drug will be absorbed, leading to more side effects. Patients are advised to avoid any food intake for two hours before and one hour after each daily dose. Patients take all four pills together at the same time each day. They should be ingested whole with some water, without crushing or chewing them. Because of potential dangers to a fetus, any man considering impregnating a woman should wear a condom during sexual intercourse. There are no restrictions for taking the daily doses of prednisone.

What Are the Side Effects of Abiraterone Plus Prednisone?

Overall, the drug was well tolerated. The most severe side effects in the randomized study were an elevation in blood pressure and a decrease in the amount of potassium in the blood stream. High blood pressure occurred in 3.9% of men on abiraterone compared with 3.0% for men on the placebo. A low potassium level occurred in 2.4% of the abiraterone group compared with 1.9% of the control group. Another side effect was elevated liver enzymes, which occurred in 5.4% of men taking abiraterone compared with less than 1% of the controls.

Optimal Sequencing of Abiraterone in Men with CRPC

With the approval of sipuleucel-T and abiraterone acetate, patients with few or no symptoms from metastases now have the following treatment options before getting chemotherapy:

- Sipuleucel-T followed immediately by abiraterone + prednisone

- Abiraterone + prednisone followed by sipuleucel-T when the disease progresses

- Simultaneous treatment with Sipuleucel-T and abiraterone + prednisone

Chapter 31 explained that sipuleucel-T has no effect on the prostate-specific antigen (PSA) level so there is no way to determine whether a patient is benefitting. It also means there is no reason to delay starting another treatment shortly after the sipuleucel-T infusions have been given. In addition, a recent study suggested that using sipuleucel-T when the PSA is low (less than 22 ng/ml) results in a 13-month improvement in survival compared with the control group. The overall survival benefit is less at higher PSA levels. Another factor affecting the best sequence of treatments is that when men receive abiraterone, they also must be given prednisone, which may have a negative effect on the body's immune system. For these reasons, sipuleucel-T might be best if given before abiraterone is started. However, preliminary studies have found that men still get a good immune response when the two treatments begin at the same time. More information is needed before this can be resolved. Until then, sipuleucel-T should be given first if both therapies are going to be used.

This sequencing may change if another new drug called enzalutamide (see chapter 35) gets approved prior to chemotherapy. If that occurs, many doctors may choose it before abiraterone because it does not need to be given with prednisone. That would likely result in sipuleucel-T and enzalutamide being given at the same time, followed by abiraterone if the disease progressed. Studies will be needed to determine if patients do better getting enzalutamide followed by abiraterone or whether the reverse sequence is better.

The Bottom Line on Abiraterone for CRPC

For now the most logical approach for a man with asymptomatic or minimally symptomatic metastatic CRPC is to first take sipuleucel-T followed by abiraterone plus prednisone soon after the third injection of sipuleucel-T. The two drugs should be continued until the PSA begins to rise. If that happens, the next option currently is chemotherapy or second-line hormonal therapies, but this may change in the near future based on new results with enzalutamide.

Second-Line Therapies for Castration-Resistant Prostate Cancer (CRPC) that Affect Male Hormones

33

Before abiraterone and sipuleucel-T were approved for castration-resistant prostate cancer (CRPC), the only other option for men before chemotherapy was another group of drugs that affected male hormones. None of them have been tested in randomized studies nor approved by the Food and Drug Administration (FDA) for this indication. Doctors use them anyway, however, because many patients want to delay chemotherapy or avoid it altogether. Now that new drugs are available, these other second-line options are likely to be used much less often. Even so, they are explained so that you can be aware of their strengths and weaknesses. They may still be an option if abiraterone (and enzalutamide if it gets approved) stops working and a man doesn't want to go on chemotherapy. The reasons to use these agents are:

- They lower the PSA.
- They can reduce symptoms caused by the cancer.
- They may delay the time until chemotherapy is needed.
- The side effects are usually milder and occur less often than those caused by chemotherapy drugs.

- Men still respond to chemotherapy and immunotherapy even if one or two of these second-line hormone therapies are used first.

The argument against using these drugs is that doctors don't know whether any of them improve survival because the necessary studies have not been done. Although it seems logical that lowering the prostate-specific antigen (PSA) level and reducing symptoms should improve survival, the fact is that no one knows for sure. This means that the benefit of these drugs is more uncertain than the benefit of chemotherapy or immunotherapy. Still, you may feel that the package of risks and benefits is more acceptable than for chemotherapy.

The Risks and Benefits of Second-Line Treatments Affecting Male Hormones

Understanding the potential risks and benefits of each second-line hormone therapy will help you discuss the options with your doctor and decide whether any one of them is right for you. Studies have shown that 10% to 40% of men will respond to the drugs listed in the next table, although they were all studied before abiraterone and sipuleucel-T were available. They may not be as effective if used after a patient is treated with one or both of them.

Although the best case is for the PSA to go down when these agents are used, stopping it from rising still may be helpful because it will often delay the need for other therapies. The challenge for patients considering these options is no study has been done comparing them to know which one is best or in what order they should be used. Without better studies, each doctor has her or his own personal approach. Fortunately, if you try one medication and it does not help or it helps and then stops working, another one can be tried. At any time you can consider switching to chemotherapy. The available options are shown in the next table.

Table 33.1 Second-Line Hormonal Therapies

Options for Second-Line Hormone Therapy	Major Side Effects	Frequency of Side Effects
Ketoconazole + hydrocortisone	Nausea Upset stomach Liver injury	10%–30% 10%–30% Less than 0.1% All depend on dose used
Antiandrogens a. Bicalutamide (Casodex) b. Flutamide (Eulexin) c. Nilutamide (Nilandron)	All three cause: Breast tenderness Breast enlargement and liver injury Diarrhea (flutamide) Difficulty with night vision Interstitial pneumonia (nilutamide)	60%–80% 60%–80% Less than 0.01% 20%–24% 13% 1%–3%
Steroids A. Dexamethasone B. Prednisone C. Hydrocortisone	All three cause: Fluid retention Diabetes Hypertension	5% 20% 12%

Estrogens
A. Parenteral
  —Polyestradiol phosphate
  —Estradiol patch
B. Oral
  —Diethylstilbestrol
  —Estramustine (Emcyt)
	Fluid retention
	Hypertension
	Breast enlargement
	Breast tenderness
	Heart attacks
	Blood clots
	Breast tenderness
	Breast enlargement
	Myocardial infarction
		17%–22%
		NA
		18%–60%
		70%
		2%–5%
		7%
		66%
		7%–65%
		3%

NA = No information available.

Ketoconazole

Many years ago, the FDA approved ketoconazole to treat fungal infections. It also was found to help some men with CRPC by blocking the production of male hormones in the adrenal gland and testicles. Although it has some of the same action as abiraterone, ketoconazole is 10 times less effective. The daily dose of ketoconazole ranges from 200 to 400 mg taken by mouth every eight hours. Doctors recommend taking it on an empty stomach because food decreases the absorption. Antacids also should be avoided within two hours of each dose. Most men tolerate the low and middle dose quite well but the higher dose may cause too much nausea. Three approaches are generally used when doctors prescribe ketoconazole.

- **Option 1:** Start with the lowest dose (200 mg every eight hours) and repeat the PSA in one month. If it drops, then the same dose can be continued. If the PSA does not change, then the dose can be increased. The PSA should be repeated one month later to see whether the higher dose has helped. If the PSA still does not drop, then the drug should be stopped and a different treatment should be selected.

- **Option 2:** Start with the highest dose (400 mg every eight hours) for one month and recheck the PSA. If it declines without bothersome side effects occurring, then that dose is continued until the PSA goes up. If this dose causes side effects, then it is reduced and the PSA is checked again after one month. The drug should be discontinued if the PSA does not go down.

- **Option 3:** Start with the middle dose (300 mg every eight hours). The PSA is monitored monthly and if it begins to rise, then the higher dose can be tried for one month. If it goes up again, then the drug should be stopped.

This last option may make the most sense because it is more easily tolerated, but without good studies they all are reasonable options. Although most men tolerate ketoconazole very well, particularly at the low or intermediate dose, about 10% to 30% will get an upset stomach. A potentially serious and life-threatening side effect is liver toxicity. Although it occurs in only 1 out of 10,000 individuals taking the drug, doctors are advised to do a blood test for liver function every few months.

This drug also can cause a drop in blood pressure in about 10% of patients. *Hydrocortisone* usually is prescribed along with the keto-conazole to avoid this problem. The dose is 20 mg in the morning and 10 mg in the evening.

Antiandrogens

Antiandrogens were previously discussed in chapter 28 as part of combined androgen blockade (CAB) and triple hormone therapy, but many doctors do not prescribe it for metastatic disease. Instead, they prefer to delay giving the antiandrogen until the PSA rises. About 20% of men with CRPC will respond to one of these drugs. Of the three antiandrogens available, the best choice probably is bicalutamide (Casodex) because:

- It is taken only once a day, whereas flutamide (Eulexin) is taken three times per day.

- Flutamide causes diarrhea in more than 20% of men, whereas it is very uncommon with bicalutamide.

- Nilutamide (Nilandron) can cause difficulty with night vision and interstitial pneumonia, but neither side effect occurs with bicalutamide.

The dose of bicalutamide approved by the FDA for use with CAB is 50 mg per day. Some doctors recommend a dose of 150 mg a day (three 50 mg tablets taken at the same time). Without any studies to support the higher dose, 50 mg once a day is adequate. If this dose is not effective, then men should switch to a different drug rather than use a higher dose.

Some studies have shown that men can respond to a different antiandrogen after one of them fails. Of course, the first one should be stopped and the PSA is repeated in one to two months.

For a man who fails bicalutamide and wants to try a different anti-androgen, which one should be next? Both flutamide and nilutamide are reasonable because no studies have shown either is better. You can make the choice based on which of the possible side effects you find more acceptable. Diarrhea happens in about 20% to 24% of men on flutamide and the problem with night vision occurs in 90% of men on nilutamide. If you must drive at night then flutamide is obviously a better choice. If you are not driving at night, then nilutamide may be a better choice because it is only taken once a day and does not cause diarrhea. Nilutamide also is a better choice if you have loose bowel movements from previous radiation. Except for breast enlargement, the side effects usually will go away when you stop the drug. The dose of nilutamide is two 150 mg tablets per day taken at the same time for one month and then one pill a day thereafter. The FDA-approved dose of flutamide is two 125 mg tablets taken every eight hours. Some doctors use a lower dose to avoid the diarrhea, but it is not known whether it works as well.

Regardless of which drug you choose, try it for one month and then recheck the PSA level. If it has declined, then you can continue the drug. If the PSA does not go down, then either try the other antiandrogen or change to a different treatment. Remember, you must wait at least four weeks after stopping an antiandrogen before trying a different treatment. Your liver function should be tested every two or three months.

Corticosteroids

Steroids are a group of chemicals produced in the body that control many bodily functions. *Corticosteroids* are steroids that are produced in the adrenal glands. Several synthetic corticosteroids have been developed that are used to treat inflammation. They also lower the PSA and reduce pain in some men with CRPC. Corticosteroids are thought to work by reducing the male hormones produced in the adrenal glands.

The names of the corticosteroids used for prostate cancer are prednisone, hydrocortisone, and dexamethasone. They are all taken by mouth and are well tolerated. The medicine is best taken in the morning with some food, which makes it more tolerable and less likely to cause stomach irritation. No studies have compared the three drugs to know whether one is more effective. The doses that have been found to lower PSA are shown in the table below.

Table 33.2 Doses of Corticosteroids

Drug	Dose
Prednisone	5–10 mg per day
Hydrocortisone	20–40 mg per day
Dexamethasone	0.75 mg 1–2 times per day

Prednisone and hydrocortisone have been used more often than dexamethasone for CRPC, which is the only reason to try one of them first. As with the other second-line hormone drugs, you try one and follow the PSA in one month. If your PSA drops or remains stable then it is reasonable to continue the drug. It should be stopped if the PSA level goes up. Most doctors will repeat the PSA every one to three months. It is unknown whether using a second corticosteroid is helpful after the initial one fails. Therefore, a better idea would be to try a different drug if your PSA is increasing. The most common side effects of these medications include fluid retention, called edema, increased blood pressure, and the development or worsening of diabetes.

If you do take a corticosteroid for several weeks, it is very important that you don't stop it abruptly, otherwise your blood pressure could suddenly drop. These drugs stop your adrenal glands from working properly and it takes time for them to function normally again. Your daily dose is gradually reduced over five to seven days. Most, but not all doctors know this, so don't hesitate to ask questions if you are told to stop a corticosteroid all at once.

Estrogens

When ADT was first discovered in the 1940s, Dr. Huggins also discovered that estrogen helped men with advanced prostate cancer. A drug called diethylstilbestrol (DES) initially was given by mouth at a dose of 5 mg per day. Unfortunately, this drug caused severe side effects. Many men died from a heart attack or they developed blood clots. Even when a lower dose was used, those side effects still occurred, but less often. Some doctors recommended taking a blood thinner such as coumadin or aspirin to reduce the risk of blood clots. Another suggestion was to drink plenty of fluids to keep well hydrated. Neither treatment has been well studied to know whether they lower the side effects.

Despite these risks, some doctors still recommend using 1 mg of DES per day but few pharmacies carry it. For that reason it must be specially ordered. If you have a history of heart disease it would be best not to use this drug without first getting approval from your cardiologist or family doctor. Since no studies show that DES is better than other second-line hormonal therapies, it is not the best option. If you and your doctor decide to use it, the PSA should be monitored every one or two months. The drug can be continued if you tolerate it well and the PSA declines. Switching to a different drug is a safer choice than raising the dose.

Fortunately, when estrogens are given parenterally these complications are much less common. Parenteral routes for this drug include placing them on the skin, or injecting them into a vein, a muscle, or under the skin.

An approved estrogen is called estramustine (Emcyt). It actually is a combination of estrogen and a chemotherapy drug, which is taken by mouth at a dose based on each man's weight. It has almost the same frequency of side effects as 3 mg of DES. Few doctors choose it for CRPC because better and safer choices are available.

Both parenteral and oral estrogens do have one advantage over other second-line hormonal therapies. They can potentially protect against *osteoporosis* and fractures, which occur more often in men on ADT, but no study has determined whether they are effective. Also, safer ways are available for treating osteoporosis.

If you decide to be treated with parenteral estrogen, which route is best for you? Placing patches on your skin may be easier and more convenient than getting an injection every two weeks. Each patch contains 0.1 mg of *estradiol*. It is placed usually on the abdomen and changed approximately every three to four days. The location of the patches does not appear to influence how well they work. No studies have determined the optimal number of patches to use for CRPC. Weak studies found a drop in the PSA level from using two patches changed every three or four days. That seems like a reasonable approach until better studies are done. The PSA can be measured after one month and the symptoms can be assessed before deciding what to do. This dose can be continued if the PSA declines and/or you feel better. If neither occurs, then the dose can be increased to three or four patches twice a week or a different treatment can be tried. Following the testosterone level is not very helpful because already it should be less than 50 ng/dl from the bilateral orchiectomy or one of the luteinizing hormone-releasing hormone (LHRH) drugs.

The other parenteral estrogen is an intramuscular injection of *polyestradiol phosphate* or (PEP). Good studies have compared this drug with an LHRH agonist in men getting primary ADT for advanced prostate cancer. The results showed a similar survival. The dose given was 240 mg injected into the muscle every two weeks for two months followed by 240 mg every month. This dosing schedule was able to lower testosterone to a castrate level as often as an LHRH medication when given as "first-line" treatment.

No studies have been done using polyestradiol phosphate as a second-line treatment. Until studies become available, the best advice is to use the same dosing schedule for second-line therapy as was used for primary therapy. The PSA should be checked after one month and the medication can be continued until the PSA increases.

What Happens to Androgen Deprivation Therapy (ADT) When a Second-Line Hormonal Agent Is Started?

What should be done about the LHRH drug when starting a second-line hormonal drug? Should it be stopped because it is no longer controlling the cancer or does it still help in some way? Although no good studies have been done, most experts recommend continuing the treatment to keep the testosterone below 50 ng/dl. If the treatment is stopped and the testosterone rises, then the cancer is likely to grow faster.

Some doctors do suggest a different approach. Studies have shown that the testosterone level will remain low in about 20% to 30% of men when an LHRH drug is stopped. The reason for it is unclear, but it appears that the body loses its ability to start producing testosterone again. For that reason, the drug may be stopped when CRPC occurs and the testosterone is rechecked. It does not have to be restarted provided that the testosterone stays low. The test must be repeated every few months because many months may go by before the testosterone begins to rise again. The main advantages of stopping the drug are avoiding the need for injections and reducing costs. The one downside is the possibility of a new flare response if the testosterone rises and an LHRH agonist is restarted. This can be avoided by using the LHRH antagonist, *degarelix* (see chapter 27).

The Bottom Line on Second-Line Therapies Affecting Male Hormones

Doctors are still not sure whether any second-line therapy that affects male hormones will help men live longer. They do seem to reduce cancer symptoms and lower PSA in approximately 10% to 40% of men. The good news is that some men respond for more than a year. Those benefitting are able to delay receiving chemotherapy, which would be the next treatment, assuming they already have received abiraterone and/or sipuleucel-T. Since no one can predict which patient will benefit, all second-line agents should be discussed as options for treating CRPC.

First-Line Chemotherapy for Castration-Resistant Prostate Cancer (CRPC) Using Docetaxel (Taxotere)

34

Chemotherapy is a broad term that means using chemicals to treat a disease. *Cytotoxic chemotherapy* uses drugs that kill cells. Many cytotoxic chemotherapy drugs have been discovered over the years for treating cancer, and several have been approved to treat castration-resistant prostate cancer (CRPC). They are used when a patient is no longer responding to androgen deprivation therapy (ADT) or the newer agents approved within the past few years. Some important facts you may not know about cytotoxic chemotherapy drugs are:

- Some cancers respond very well to certain chemotherapy drugs but are totally unaffected by others.

- They also can kill normal cells, which can lead to serious side effects.

- These drugs rarely kill all the cancer cells in a person's body because some are resistant or become resistant and they can continue to grow.

What Are the Results with Docetaxel ?

The first chemotherapy drug that improved survival in men with CRPC was docetaxel. It belongs to a group of drugs called taxanes that come from yew trees. In 2004, two good studies reported that docetaxel could improve survival in these patients. It is given intravenously (through a vein) over about one hour.

In one study, men with CRPC were assigned to one of three groups. One was given docetaxel and prednisone weekly; the second group was given these two drugs every three weeks; and the control group was given mitoxantrone and prednisone every three weeks. Mitoxantrone is another approved chemotherapy for prostate cancer that improves symptoms of advanced disease, but it does not improve survival. The study found that the group getting the docetaxel and prednisone every three weeks had a significantly better survival rate than men getting mitoxantrone and prednisone. One-half of the men survived about 18.9 months compared with only 16.9 months for the control group. That means one-half of the men getting docetaxel lived about two months longer than the men getting mitoxantrone. They also were more likely to have their pain reduced, which occurred in 35% compared with only 20% in the control group. This means about one out of every six men felt better while taking the drug. Weekly docetaxel did not improve survival when compared with mitoxantrone. The frequency of side effects is shown in the table on the following page and the side effects not described in previous chapters are explained following the table.

Table 34.1 Side Effects of Docetaxel Compared with Mitoxantrone

Side Effects	Docetaxel + Prednisone Every Three Weeks	Mitoxantrone + Prednisone Every Three Weeks
Anemia	5%	2%
Neutropenia	32%	22%
Worsening heart function	10%	22%
Fatigue	53%	35%
Alopecia	65%	13%
Nail changes	30%	7%
Nausea, vomiting	42%	38%
Diarrhea	32%	10%
Neuropathy	30%	7%
Anorexia	17%	14%
Dysgeusia	18%	7%
Stomatitis	20%	8%
Myalgia	14%	13%
Dyspnea	15%	9%
Tearing	10%	1%
Peripheral edema	19%	1%
More than one serious event	26%	20%

Anemia: A decrease in the number of red blood cells in the body. Red blood cells deliver oxygen to the body. When the number of red blood cells drops, men may feel weak, tired, and short of breath during exertion. Advanced prostate cancer often causes anemia and mitoxantrone may make it worse. Blood transfusions are needed if the red blood cells drop very low. Another option is to give drugs that help the body make more red blood cells.

Neutropenia: A decrease in the number of white blood cells in the body, which increases the risk for developing infections.

Alopecia: Many chemotherapy drugs cause hair loss, which usually grows back if the drug is stopped.

Nail Changes: This includes a change in the color of the nail bed, or the nail breaks easily.

Neuropathy: A feeling of burning or tingling in the fingers and toes.

Dysgeusia: A change in the taste of food.

Myalgia: Pain in the muscles.

Dyspnea: Difficulty catching your breath or feeling short of breath during physical exertion.

Tearing: The eyes easily water.

Peripheral Edema: Collection of fluid in the body usually occurring in the lower part of the legs.

Despite the higher incidence of side effects in the men getting docetaxel, they still had a better overall quality of life. Also, their frequency of serious side effects was only 6% higher compared with the control group.

The second randomized study combined docetaxel with another chemotherapy drug called *estramustine* (Emcyt). These two were compared with mitoxantrone and prednisone. The docetaxel and the mitoxantrone were given intravenously every three weeks. Estramustine is an estrogen-containing pill that was approved many years ago to reduce symptoms of men with advanced prostate cancer. It is now used infrequently because of its side effects.

This study also found that men getting docetaxel and estramustine lived longer than those getting mitoxantrone and prednisone. One-half of the men survived 17.5 months compared with only 15.6 months in the control group, a difference of about two months. Another advantage of the docetaxel was that it delayed the time before the patient's condition worsened. That occurred in 6.3 months in the docetaxel group but in only 3.2 months in the control group. Side effects were common, but some probably were caused by the estramustine.

Based on these two studies, the U.S. Food and Drug Administration (FDA) approved this drug in May 2004 for men with progressive metastatic prostate cancer under the trade name Taxotere.

The Bottom Line on Docetaxel

Although the improvement in survival was not very large, it still represented a significant advance in the treatment of CRPC. Presently, men have several good options before they need to consider chemotherapy, but if those stop working, docetaxel is another option that can help them live longer.

Treatment Options for Men with Progressive Disease after Docetaxel

In recent years, more research has been done on the way prostate cancer progresses after testosterone is reduced. Many believed this hormone no longer played a role in cancer growth; however, this has turned out to be not true. Not only have doctors found new ways to block the hormones produced in the adrenal glands, they also have discovered that prostate cancer cells can make their own testosterone. So far this has led to the approval of two new therapies that affect prostate cancer cell growth: abiraterone acetate and enzalutamide.

Abiraterone Acetate (Zytiga)

Abiraterone was previously discussed in chapter 32 as a first-line treatment for castration-resistant prostate cancer (CRPC). Before it was approved for that indication, it was tested in men with CRPC who had failed docetaxel chemotherapy. All of them had their testosterone level maintained below 50 ng/dl during the study. Men were randomly assigned to receive abiraterone 1000 mg per day plus prednisone 5 mg twice per day, or prednisone plus a placebo. The study found that abiraterone significantly improved survival; one-half of the men receiving abiraterone plus prednisone lived for 14 months compared with only 10.9 months for the control group, an improvement of 3.1 months. Several other benefits were also observed, as shown in the next table.

Table 35.1 Secondary Benefits of Abiraterone Acetate Compared with Placebo

Outcome	Abiraterone + Prednisone	Placebo + Prednisone
Time until PSA increased	10.2	6.6
Time until worsening; scans or x-rays	5.6	3.6 months
Decrease in PSA by at least 50%	29.1%	5.5%

Men treated with abiraterone were more likely to have at least a 50% drop in their prostate-specific antigen (PSA), a longer time until the PSA increased, and a longer time until their x-rays and scans showed progressive disease.

Fatigue, nausea, back pain, constipation, and bone pain occurred in nearly the same percentage of patients in the two groups. The side effects related to adrenal gland function including hypertension, fluid retention, edema, and a low potassium level in the blood were more common in men receiving abiraterone (see table).

Table 35.2 Side Effects Related to Adrenal Gland Function

	Abiraterone + Prednisone	Placebo + Prednisone
Low potassium in blood	17%	8%
Fluid retention and edema	31%	22%
High blood pressure	10%	8%

Based on this study, the U.S. Food and Drug Administration (FDA) approved abiraterone (Zytiga) in April 2011. This was used in combination with prednisone for men with CRPC who progressed on docetaxel. The dose is the same as used before docetaxel—four 250 mg tablets once per day on an empty stomach-plus 5 mg prednisone twice per day.

Enzalutamide (Xtandi)

The next new drug was developed based on a better understanding of the way prostate cancer grows in men with low testosterone. In order for this hormone to stimulate cancer growth, it must first get inside the nucleus of a cancer cell. It does this by binding to a protein called the *androgen receptor*. The following changes can occur to this receptor as the cancer gets worse:

- More of the androgen receptor is produced, making it possible for very small amounts of testosterone to help the cancer grow.

- It can stimulate the cancer even without first binding to testosterone.

- The structure of the androgen receptor changes or mutates, making it possible for other chemicals besides testosterone to cause the cells to grow.

Enzalutamide has some of the same properties as the antiandrogens described in chapter 28. One important difference, however, is that it does not appear to stimulate the cancer to grow as was found for bicalutamide, flutamide, and nilutamide. It also binds much more strongly to the androgen receptor, which makes it more effective at blocking the growth of cancer cells than those other drugs.

After the initial studies showed promise in men with CRPC, a randomized study was done. All the participants had progressive disease after being treated with docetaxel. They were given either 160 mg of enzalutamide or a placebo once a day by mouth. The study showed that the drug significantly improved survival. One half of the men taking enzalutamide were still alive at 18.4 months compared with 13.6 months for those on placebo. Based on this 4.8-month longer survival, the study was stopped and all the men on placebo were offered enzalutamide. Several other benefits also occurred, as shown in the next table.

Table 35.3 Secondary Benefits of Enzalutamide Compared with Placebo

Outcome	Enzalutamide	Placebo
Drop in PSA by at least 50%	54%	25%
Improvement in tumor, not in bone	29%	4%
Improvement in quality of life	43%	18%
Time until PSA increased	8.3 months	3 months
Time until scans, x-rays worsened	8.3 months	2.9 months
Time until first skeletal related event	16.7 months	13.3 months

The drug was well tolerated, but several side effects were more common in men taking enzalutamide as shown in the next table.

Table 35.4 Side Effects of Enzalutamide Compared with Placebo

Outcome	Enzalutamide	Placebo
Fatigue	34%	6%
Diarrhea	21%	1%
Hot flashes	20%	0%
Musculoskeletal pain	14%	1%
Headache	12%	1%

The one side effect that has received some attention is the development of seizures, which occurred in 0.6% of men taking enzalutamide but in none of the men on placebo. Several of these events can be explained by factors other than the drug but it is being closely monitored in other men on this treatment. For now, there is no major concern. Based on this study, the FDA approved this drug in August 2012 under the name of Xtandi for men with CRPC who failed docetaxel. Studies currently are underway in men who have not yet received chemotherapy and many experts expect it also will get an approval for that indication.

How to Select the Next Drug When Docetaxel Is No Longer Effective

As more drugs get approved for advanced prostate cancer, doctors face an increasing challenge to decide which drug to use first, second, and third. Currently, cabazitaxel, enzalutamide and abiraterone are approved for men with CRPC who have already progressed after receiving docetaxel. Sipuleucel-T and abiraterone are approved for men prior to chemotherapy. This means that in most cases men with CRPC will already have received sipuleucel-T and/ or abiraterone, followed by docetaxel, and then they most likely will be offered enzalutamide. In chapter 32, sequencing of the various drugs was discussed based on the possibility that enzalutamide will become available for men before chemotherapy. For now, the best approach for treating metastatic disease based on FDA approvals is as follows:

- For men with newly diagnosed metastatic disease, combined androgen blockade offers the best chance for survival. If the PSA begins to rise, the testosterone should be checked. If it is below 50 ng/dl, the antiandrogen should be stopped and the PSA repeated in one to two months.

- If the PSA continues to rise, sipuleucel-T should be considered and after that is completed, abiraterone + prednisone can be offered if neither one has been used before. Patients stay on these drugs until the disease again begins to progress. At that point they are stopped and docetaxel is the next option. It is continued as long as the patient is responding, meaning the PSA does not increase and x-rays and scans show no disease progression.

- If the disease does progress, then enzalutamide should be given until the disease shows further progression. At that time men can receive second-line chemotherapy drugs starting with cabazitaxel or they can try one of the secondary hormonal therapies. Patients who continue to get worse then can be offered palliative chemotherapy with mitoxantrone and prednisone. These second-line chemotherapy drugs are discussed in the next chapter.

Second-Line Chemotherapy

Men failing docetaxel followed by abiraterone and enzalutamide still have the option of trying other chemotherapy drugs including:

- Cabazitaxel (Jevtana)

- Mitoxantrone (Novantrone)

- Estramustine (Emcyt)

Cabazitaxel (Jevtana)

Cabazitaxel is a chemotherapy drug that has a chemical structure similar to docetaxel. It also is given through a vein over one hour. Preliminary studies suggested it could benefit men who no longer were responding to docetaxel. A randomized study was done in these men comparing cabazitaxel plus prednisone with prednisone and mitoxantrone (the control group). The treatment was given monthly for up to 10 months. The study showed that men getting cabazitaxel and prednisone lived longer than men in the control group; one-half of them were alive at 15.1 months compared with only 12.7 months in those getting mitoxantrone and prednisone. Based on this study, cabazitaxel was approved by the Food and Drug Administration (FDA) in June 2010 under the commercial name *Jevtana*.

The trade-off with this drug is the type, frequency, and severity of the side effects. About 1 out of 20 men (5%) died from getting cabazitaxel. This partly occurred because medications that would have protected most men could not be used during the first month of treatment. Therefore, anyone now starting cabazitaxel is advised to receive them to reduce the risk of a life-threatening event. Another caution is that the drug can cause severe allergic reactions. The frequency of the most common and significant side effects occurring during this study is shown in the next table. Grade 1 (mild) and Grade 2 (moderate) side effects are somewhat annoying and bothersome but not dangerous; Grade 3 (severe) and Grade 4 (life threatening) are much more dangerous. The side effects not described in previous chapters are explained below the table.

Table 36.1 Frequency and Severity of Side Effects of Cabazitaxel

Side Effects in Men Receiving Cabazitaxel + Prednisone	Grade 1 or 2	Grade 3 or 4	Percent of Men Having Side Effect
Leukopenia	27%	69%	96%
Anemia	87%	11%	98%
Thrombocytopenia	44%	4%	48%
Neutropenia	12%	82%	94%
Nausea	32%	2%	34%
Vomiting	20%	2%	22%
Diarrhea	41%	6%	47%
Constipation	19%	1%	20%

(continued)

Table 36.1 Frequency and Severity of Side Effects of Cabazitaxel (continued)

Side Effects in Men Receiving Cabazitaxel + Prednisone	Grade 1 or 2	Grade 3 or 4	Percent of Men Having Side Effect
Abdominal pain	15%	2%	17%
Fatigue	32%	5%	37%
Pyrexia	11%	1%	12%
Asthenia	15%	5%	20%
Urinary tract infection	6%	2%	8%
Anorexia	15%	1%	16%
Back pain	12%	4%	16%
Peripheral neuropathy	12%	1%	13%
Dysgeusia	11%	0%	11%
Hematuria	15%	2%	17%
Dysuria	7%	0%	7%
Alopecia	10%	0%	10%
Dyspnea	11%	1%	12%

Leukopenia: A drop in the number of white blood cells in the blood stream, which increases the chance of developing infections.

Thrombocytopenia: A drop in the number of platelets in the blood stream, which increases the chances of bleeding.

Pyrexia: The development of a fever.

Asthenia: Muscle weakness.

Peripheral Neuropathy: A feeling of burning or tingling in the fingers and toes.

Hematuria: Means blood is present in urine. Depending on the amount, it can turn the urine red. Rarely, blood clots may appear. Treatment is unnecessary unless a clot blocks the flow of urine.

The Bottom Line on Cabazitaxel

Until this drug was approved, men getting worse while receiving docetaxel had no other good options that could improve their survival. The treatments that were available only could provide some pain relief and improve men's quality of life. Cabazitaxel definitely is an important advance, but it does have significant risks. For that reason, it is best to delay its use until men have at least been offered sipuleucel-T, abiraterone, and enzalutamide. Men receiving cabazitaxel need careful monitoring to minimize the side effects caused by this drug.

Mitoxantrone (Novantrone)

Mitoxantrone is a chemotherapy drug that has been used to treat men with progressive, symptomatic prostate cancer. It is given intravenously every three weeks in combination with prednisone. The drug was tested in a randomized study in which men received mitoxantrone plus prednisone or prednisone plus a placebo. Patients completed written surveys that asked about their quality of life and their use of drugs to treat pain. The study found that quality of life improved in about 30% of the men getting both drugs compared with only 12% getting prednisone. One-half of the men in the mitoxantrone group responded for about 7.6 months compared with only 2.1 months in the control group. The drug also delayed the time until the disease progressed. One-half of the patients on mitoxantrone progressed after 4.4 months compared with 2.3 months in the control group. The men in the control group eventually could receive mitoxantrone after six weeks if their symptoms got worse. About 20% of those men responded, which means the drug may be slightly more effective when used sooner rather than later. The drug did not improve survival.

Another randomized study was conducted and it too showed that mitoxantrone plus placebo was more effective at improving pain and other symptoms. Based on these two studies, the drug was approved by the FDA in 1996 for men with symptomatic advanced prostate cancer.

The following table shows a comparison of the important side effects occurring in the first study followed by an explanation of the medical terms. They were far more common in the group getting mitoxantrone. The side effects not described earlier are explained below the table.

Table 36.2 Side Effects of Mitoxantrone Plus Prednisone Compared with Prednisone Alone

Side Effect	Mitoxantrone + Prednisone	Prednisone Alone
Impaired heart function	4%	0%
Neutropenia	87%	4%
Anemia	75%	39%
Nausea	26%	8%
Fatigue	34%	14%
Alopecia	22%	1%

Table 36.2 Side Effects of Mitoxantrone Plus Prednisone Compared with Prednisone Alone (continued)

Side Effect	Mitoxantrone + Prednisone	Prednisone Alone
Anorexia	22%	14%
Infections	17%	4%
Edema	10%	4%
Stomatitis	8%	1%
Vomiting	11%	5%
Night sweats	9%	2%
Hematuria	11%	6%
Dyspnea	15%	8%

Impaired Heart Function: This drug weakens the muscle of the heart, resulting in permanent heart damage. Regular monitoring of heart function is required.

Stomatitis: This is an inflammation in the mouth that can lead to open sores. It may be very bothersome because chewing is painful and some foods or liquids can be quite irritating.

The Bottom Line on Mitoxantrone

When you read the long list of side effects, your first thought might be, "Why would I ever consider taking this drug?" Keep in mind that despite all of them, men taking the drug still felt that overall it improved their quality of life and reduced their use of pain medication. The trade-off seemed worthwhile to these men. Clearly, if your pain from the cancer is only mild, then this drug probably is not for you. But if you require narcotics or you have trouble moving around or sleeping, then the benefits of the drug may outweigh its side effects. Since this drug does not improve survival, it should be delayed until men are no longer responding to abiraterone, enzalutamide, and cabazitaxel.

Estramustine (Emcyt)

This drug is an unusual combination of a chemotherapy agent and estrogen. It is given by mouth and is used primarily in very advanced disease. The clinical studies showed that it improves symptoms but does not improve survival of men with metastatic prostate cancer. The major problem with estramustine is that it has some of the same side effects as estrogen including cardiovascular morbidity, fluid retention, and breast enlargement. It is rarely used now in the management of advanced disease.

The Bottom Line on
Second-Line Chemotherapy

Of the three chemotherapy drugs available for men failing docetaxel, cabazitaxel clearly is the one to use first because it does improve survival. It must be used carefully because of the risk of life-threatening side effects. Mitoxantrone plus prednisone would be the next best option for men with symptoms caused by metastatic disease. The final option is estramustine, but other treatments directed at the bone metastases may be more appropriate as discussed in chapter 29.

New Treatments on the Horizon for Castration-Resistant Prostate Cancer (CRPC)

37

After so many years without new therapies, now the treatment of castration-resistant prostate cancer (CRPC) is changing very quickly. So far, sipuleucel-T, abiraterone, and enzalutamide have been approved and the following list contains other new therapies showing promise that are in the advanced phase of clinical testing.

- Enzalutamide (Xtandi) (see chapter 35)

- Orteronel (Tak-700) + prednisone

- Tasquinimod

- Other immunotherapies

Enzalutamide (Xtandi) was discussed in chapter 35. It has some of the same properties as other antiandrogens such as casodex, flutamide, and nilutamide but it is more potent. Also, the three earlier drugs sometimes stimulated prostate cancer cells to grow, but that does not appear to happen with this drug. Enzalutamide has already been approved in men failing chemotherapy, and studies are in progress using the drug for men prior to chemotherapy. Based on the preliminary studies, it is likely to get approved with the same indication as sipuleucel-T and abiraterone, which is for asymptomatic or minimally symptomatic men with CRPC prior to chemotherapy. If that occurs, increased uncertainty will occur for which treatment should be used first, second, and third. Once again, sipuleucel-T may be the best treatment to use first for the same reason given before: it has no effect on prostate-specific antigen (PSA), but it does prolong survival. In the absence of any new studies, many doctors may argue that enzalutamide should be used second because it does not need to be given with prednisone, which can cause some side effects. Next will be abiraterone plus prednisone. Information is definitely needed about whether one drug works much better if used first and whether the other drugs work equally well if used after another drug is no longer effective.

Currently, Tasquinimod has no data in men failing chemotherapy, so its optimal sequencing isn't clear. A randomized study of Orteronel in men failing chemotherapy was recently stopped because it was ineffective; if effective when given earlier, it must be given with prednisone.

The Future of Managing CRPC

Over the next several years, patients with CRPC could have five or six more options that improve survival, allowing them to further delay the need for chemotherapy. If and when they are approved, the entire management of CRPC will present doctors and patients with difficult choices and it could take many years before the optimal sequence is identified. At this time, little guidance can be offered. Some doctors will make their decision based on the number of months survival was increased compared with placebo. However, comparing results from unrelated studies is not really valid because the patients aren't identical. All of these new options will be taken by mouth making them easy for patients. However, for that reason, cost is very likely to be an issue, because most insurance companies may be reluctant to cover the expense and few patients will be able to pay out of pocket. For now, the best news for patients would be to have too many options rather than too few, and ultimately men will be living even longer even if androgen deprivation therapy (ADT) no longer controls the disease.

Other Therapies in Development

From reading the last few chapters you can see that significant progress has occurred in the treatment of men with metastatic disease. Other new drugs are showing encouraging results in earlier phases of clinical testing and you may hear or read about them. They are listed below in alphabetical order.

- **Cabozantinib:** Attacks certain proteins that stimulate prostate cancer growth. It has shown activity against bone metastases and is now undergoing a Phase III randomized study.

- **Galaterone:** Works in several ways; it blocks an enzyme that is needed to make testosterone; it decreases the amount of androgen receptor that is needed to help cancer cells grow and inhibits its function.

- **ODM-201:** Works against the androgen receptor.

- **OGX-011 (Custirsen):** Blocks the production of a protein called clusterin, which is needed to keep cancer cells alive. It is being tested in combination with docetaxel and prednisone in men who have failed hormone therapy.

- **ProstAtak:** Another form of immunotherapy that is injected into the prostate where it kills prostate cancer cells. It is then followed by radiation treatment. The ongoing phase III studies are aimed at treating intermediate- and high-risk localized disease.

- **PSMA/ADC:** This is a combination of an antibody that targets prostate cancer cells and a chemotherapy drug called monomethyl auristatin E, or MMAE.

- **Prostvac:** Another immunotherapy that is being tested in men with CRPC.

- **Toremifene (Acapodene):** An FDA-approved drug under the name Fareston for use in women with advanced breast cancer. Studies show it also may reduce fractures in men on hormone therapy for prostate cancer.

Many other drugs not described here also are being tested in Phase I and Phase II studies. Hopefully, the initial results will be positive, leading to their continued development and eventual approval by the FDA.

VI

WHAT YOU CAN DO TO HELP YOURSELF

The Pros and Cons of Enrolling in a Clinical Research Study

38

Progress in treating prostate cancer can only occur if proper research studies are done and that requires men who are willing to volunteer. To help you decide whether a research study is right for you, a basic understanding is needed of the four types of studies that are performed.

After a drug or treatment has been tested in the laboratory and in animals, clinical studies then begin. It starts with a Phase I study in which everyone is given the experimental treatment but the dose and timing will vary. Initially, little is known about the optimal dose and schedule that will give the best response. The goal of a Phase I study is to determine whether a treatment is safe for patients and the maximum dose patients can receive without causing too many side effects. Also, the drug is tested in more than one type of cancer to see which one might be suitable for further testing. It is not intended to find out whether a drug is effective; that happens in Phase II and Phase III studies. Usually only small numbers of participants are needed for a Phase I study.

After reading this description, you may wonder why anyone would join a Phase I study because patients have no idea whether the drug works or the dose being given is really safe. Participating in a Phase I study does make sense for people who have few other options, meaning all approved therapies have already been used for them, and they are no longer effective. Although there is little information about whether the treatment will help you, it certainly is possible. Also, it is the only way you can get this treatment without having to wait many years until the Food and Drug Administration (FDA) approves it. At the end of a Phase I study, a dose and frequency for giving the drug will be selected for use in the next study.

A Phase II study is done to find out whether a treatment may be effective against a particular disease. The goal is to search for some evidence that patients are responding such as reduction in symptoms or improvement in blood tests or x-rays. Also, more information is gained about potential side effects. In a Phase II study, everyone still gets the experimental treatment but some may receive a dose that may be too low to be helpful. The results of a Phase II study will be used to determine whether the treatment should be tested in a Phase III study and which individuals should be enrolled.

The Phase III study is the most important one because the FDA uses the results to decide whether a drug is safe and effective and should be approved for patient care. These studies must be prospective, randomized, and controlled, which means only some people are assigned to get the experimental treatment. Participants cannot choose their therapy. Be aware that many individuals who want to enroll may not be permitted to do so because they don't satisfy all the necessary requirements. For example, a person may be required to have certain tumor characteristics, a certain stage of disease, or certain findings on blood tests, x-rays, or scans. Some people are excluded if they have certain medical problems that would increase the chances of having complications.

In most cases participants who meet the entry requirements have a 50% chance of getting the new treatment, but sometimes the odds are better than that. If a study has a two-to-one randomization, it means that 67% of the participants will get the experimental drug and 33% will get the standard therapy. Some studies are designed that way to help get the study done sooner; more people are likely to sign up knowing that their odds of getting the new treatment are better. Another reason to join a Phase III study is that even if someone is assigned to the control group, he still will be getting the standard therapy in use at that time and probably more intense monitoring of his disease. *No one joining a randomized study will be deprived of the best treatment known at that time.* Also, if the study is stopped because the new treatment is found to be better, then in most cases the patients in the control group will be offered the experimental treatment before it is approved by the FDA. So the bottom line is that joining a randomized study offers a chance to get the newest treatment earlier than the general population.

The final study design is called a *Phase IV* trial. It is done after the FDA has already approved that treatment. The goal is to learn more about longer-term risks, side effects, and benefits. It will include many more individuals than the Phase III study but everyone will be receiving the new drug at the dose approved by the FDA.

Should You Join a Research Study?

Nothing is wrong with feeling reluctant to sign up for a research study. After all, it may seem like you would be a "guinea pig" and you may be concerned about your safety. Fortunately, strict guidelines exist in the United States and many other countries that regulate how research studies are performed. They require that everyone joining a study be protected by certain rules and good clinical practice is followed. The rules do vary slightly for studies that test drugs rather than medical devices. Another way individuals are protected is having all clinical research studies reviewed and approved by an oversight committee before they can begin. This is done to make sure the studies are ethical and they protect a patient's safety. Also, physicians who conduct research on new drugs are monitored to ensure they are complying with the rules governing research.

Another reason you may not want to enroll is because many studies require that the treatments be randomized. This means neither you nor your doctor gets to decide whether you will receive the "standard" or "experimental" treatment. You must understand that doing a randomized study is the only way to find out whether a new treatment is as good as, or better or worse than the standard treatment in use at that time.

The following reasons may make you less reluctant to sign up.

- As mentioned above, participants will never be deprived of a treatment that has been shown to be beneficial. That will be the treatment used in the "control" group.

- If you are randomized to the control group, you are no worse off than if you never joined the study because you are getting the same treatment you would have normally received.

- Often, new treatments generate some excitement during the preliminary studies and the only way someone can get it without having to wait for several years is to enroll in a study.

- You will be more closely monitored with tests and examinations than if you just received routine care.

- You get the satisfaction of knowing you may be helping others by contributing to medical research.

- If you do not have good health insurance you may be able to get access to doctors and treatments that would not be possible without enrolling.

Of course there are potential risks.

- You may get side effects from the experimental treatment, which were not known at the time you signed up.

- The study could be time consuming, requiring you to undergo extra tests or see a doctor more often than if you weren't in the study.

- There is always a chance that the experimental treatment is inferior to the standard treatment.

How Can You Find Out about Ongoing Studies?

Most doctors treating prostate cancer do not participate in clinical studies nor are they aware of ones that you might consider joining. Therefore, you should not rely on your doctor to discuss ongoing studies or find one for you. In some cases, they may not encourage you to join for financial reasons; they will lose out on the revenue they might have earned by taking care of you. The sad truth is that most clinicians do not seem interested in their patients joining a research study. Fortunately, many clinical trials are registered. You can find studies that are on the lookout to recruit volunteers by visiting www.ClinicalTrials.gov or www.cancer.gov/clinicaltrials. The second site allows you to search for a study according to the extent of your cancer and where you live.

The Bottom Line on Joining a Research Study

Although joining a research study is not for everyone, the best thing you can do is get all the information about ongoing studies for your medical condition and then make a decision. There definitely are potential advantages that outweigh the disadvantages. If you find a study that interests you, do not hesitate to call one of the doctors conducting the study to learn more about the details. Your family doctor also may be a good resource to discuss whether you should sign up. You should be able to make a decision after you are fully informed.

The Role of Complementary and Alternative Medicine

39

People who are ill often search for things they can do to help their condition, and men with prostate cancer are no exception. Surveys have found that more than one-quarter of men with this disease do something on their own. This includes modifying their diet or taking unconventional therapies such as herbs, vitamins, or dietary supplements. Other approaches include yoga, exercise, massage, meditation, spiritual healing, and group counseling.

Eastern medicine has used herbs for thousands of years, with abundant testimonials from physicians, patients, and holistic caregivers praising their value. Laboratory and epidemiologic studies often are cited to support them. Many people make the argument that, "Even if there is no proof they work, they are certainly not harmful and maybe they will help."

Unfortunately, that argument may be incorrect. Randomized studies of vitamins, supplements, and some unconventional therapies have found that *sometimes they do cause harm.* For example, vitamin A increases the risk of dying from lung cancer in people who smoke and vitamin E can cause bleeding in the brain. Those results alone should make you think twice about claims that supplements are never harmful. Many more examples are available. Since the goal of this book is to tell you the strengths and weaknesses of all the things you can do for your cancer, the same will apply for these unconventional treatments. To aid in your decision about what to do, each intervention discussed in this chapter will be assigned to one of the following four groups based on the best available scientific information.

- **Group I:** Well-done studies show they *are definitely helpful* meaning you *should strongly consider using them.*

- **Group II:** Uncontrolled studies show they *could be helpful* and more importantly they *do not cause serious harm.* Using anything in this group is *reasonable* if you are highly motivated to do something on your own.

- **Group III:** Studies show there is *some biological activity against cancer cells in the laboratory,* but there is no way to tell what they would do to men with prostate cancer. Also, there is insufficient information to know what dose is safe or whether they might be harmful in some way. This means you *probably should avoid them* until better information becomes available.

- **Group IV:** Well-done studies show they *do not help and/or they cause harm,* which means you *should definitely not use them.*

The National Cancer Institute puts the various interventions into one of five categories:

- Biologically based, which uses things occurring in nature such as diet, foods, herbs, and vitamins.

- Whole-medical systems such as Chinese medicine, homeopathy, or naturopathic medicine.

- Mind–body medicines such as meditation, yoga, or hypnosis.

- Body-based practices such as massage.

- Energy medicines such as tai chi.

Biologically Based Alternative Interventions

Diet definitely plays an essential role in our health. Certain nutrients are required to function properly. Heart disease, diabetes, and obesity are clearly on the rise, in part because of poor nutrition. Diet is often used as one explanation for the much lower incidence of prostate cancer in Japan compared with the United States; they ingest more fresh fruits and vegetables and less meat and fried foods. Uncontrolled studies *suggest* but do not prove that foods such as tomatoes, soy, red wine, and green tea reduce the chance of getting this disease. Other foods such as fat and red meat *may* increase the risk of developing it or *may* make prostate cancer progress more quickly.

Many men are motivated to change their diet after they have been diagnosed with this disease. You already may have asked your doctor, "What should I eat?" or "Are any foods definitely good or bad for me?" Even though there is *no definite proof* that a healthy diet will help fight your cancer, there are other benefits. At a minimum it can help you feel better, give you more strength and energy, and enable you to cope with some of the side effects caused by your treatment. It also can lessen the need for medications that cause side effects and could interfere with your cancer treatment. The bottom line is good nutrition *can* improve your quality of life and *may* help you in your battle against prostate cancer.

The importance of finding out whether alternative therapies are beneficial has greatly increased because of the growing interest in active surveillance of prostate cancer. Currently, more than 60% of men diagnosed today have low-risk prostate cancer and, as explained in earlier chapters, most of them will not benefit from aggressive treatment. However, active surveillance is hard to accept for many men and their families because they view it as "doing nothing." Active surveillance might become more acceptable if any of these "alternative" interventions can show a long-term benefit. Men would then feel that they are "doing something."

Medical journals contain many studies aimed at finding out whether dietary and lifestyle changes are good for men with this disease. One well-done trial included 93 men with low-risk prostate cancer. They all chose to have active surveillance rather than immediate treatment and were assigned to no intervention (control group) or to a "lifestyle program" consisting of the following:

- A vegan diet supplemented with soy, fish oil, vitamin E, selenium, and vitamin C

- Moderate exercise (walking 30 minutes 6 days a week)

- Stress management techniques (yoga, stretching, breathing, imagery, and relaxation for 60 minutes per day)

- A one-hour weekly support group meeting to encourage them to follow the program.

The vegan diet was mostly fruits, vegetables, whole grains, legumes, and soy. Only 10% of calories were from fat. The results are shown in the table.

Table 39.1 Effect of Lifestyle Changes in Men with Prostate Cancer

	Control Group	Experimental Group
PSA at start of study	6.4 ng/ml	6.2 ng/ml
PSA after one year	6.7 ng/ml	6.0 ng/ml
Percentage of men getting surgery, radiation, or hormones within one year	14%	0%
Average weight lost after one year	0 lbs	10 lbs

The study found that the group following the lifestyle changes had a slightly lower average prostate-specific antigen (PSA) level after one year. Also, fewer men went off active surveillance. Usually, active surveillance is stopped when the PSA rises or if other changes suggest the cancer is growing. That happened to six men in the control group but none in the experimental group.

Despite these early encouraging results, using PSA to assess response has many problems because it is not a reliable predictor of long-term outcomes. Many questions still need to be answered such as:

- Will this intervention continue to prevent the disease from progressing?

- Will it help men avoid suffering from their cancer in the future?

- Is the entire program really needed or will some portion of it be enough to get the same benefit?

Regarding the last question, good studies have shown that vitamin E and selenium do not prevent prostate cancer. That might mean they are not helping these men and can be excluded from this program. Although it is far too early to draw any conclusions, the results with this program are encouraging and worth further investigation. If nothing else, men who make such changes seem to have a better quality of life and are not being harmed (Group II).

Every five years, two government agencies publish *The Dietary Guidelines for Americans*, which contains general suggestions about diet for the general public. The last edition was in 2010 and the next one will appear in 2015. You can access this guideline and the new edition on the Internet for free at www .health.gov/dietary guidelines/. The two main ideas of the current guideline are:

- **Maintain calorie balance over time to achieve and sustain a healthy weight.**

  - Consume enough calories from foods and beverages to meet daily needs and increase the calories expended through physical activity.

- **Focus on consuming nutrient-dense foods and beverages.**

  - Limit intake of sodium, solid fats, added sugars, and refined grains. Emphasize nutrient-dense foods and beverages; vegetables, fruits, whole grains, fat-free or low-fat milk and milk products; seafood, lean meats, and poultry; eggs, beans and peas, and nuts and seeds.

The current guideline provides details about "do's and don'ts."

Some of the current recommendations listed in the guideline include:

- Increase vegetable and fruit intake.

- Eat a variety of vegetables, especially dark-green, red, and orange colored ones.

- Consume at least half of all grains as whole grains. Increase whole-grain intake and decrease refined grains.

- Increase intake of fat-free or low-fat milk and milk products, such as milk, yogurt, cheese, or fortified soy beverages.

- Choose a variety of protein foods, which include seafood, lean meat and poultry, eggs, beans and peas, soy products, and unsalted nuts and seeds.

- Increase the amount and variety of seafood consumed by choosing seafood in place of some meat and poultry.

- Replace protein foods that are higher in solid fats with choices that are lower in solid fats and calories and/or are sources of oils.

- Use oils to replace solid fats where possible.

A smart approach for concerned men is to review their current diet with a certified dietitian to see what changes may be needed. Although the Internet is full of "recommendations," the truth is that no diet has been shown to improve the outcome for men with prostate cancer. Even so, following a healthy diet is the best way to maximize one's health (Group I).

Many of the food recommendations appearing on Internet sites are made because they contain ingredients that are active against prostate cancer in laboratory studies. A partial list includes fish oils, soy, tomatoes, broccoli, berries, pomegranate juice, cauliflower, watercress, cabbage, and other cruciferous vegetables. The studies have mostly been uncontrolled and often show inconsistent results. Some studies showed men had less aggressive cancers from increased intake of these items and others showed no effect. Studies of prostate cancer cells growing in the laboratory found that *extracts* from these foods stop or slow down the growth of prostate cancer cells. However, no well-done studies have been done to know which of these food products will help men with the disease or the amount to consume. The good news is they are not harmful when taken in moderation and are part of a healthy diet (Group II).

In laboratory studies, soy contains several chemicals that are active against prostate cancer. Some people believe soy intake is one reason Asian men have lower rates of prostate cancer than Americans. Soy extracts sold in health food stores are often promoted for men with this disease. Here too, uncontrolled studies show conflicting results. In one report, 20 men with recurrent prostate cancer drank soymilk three times a day for one year. Their PSA increased more slowly than men not taking it, but a recent randomized study was stopped because the soy did not affect PSA. Foods containing soy do not appear to be harmful so incorporating them into your diet is quite reasonable. This may not be true for soy supplements (soy containing foods—Group II, soy supplements—Group III).

Garlic contains several ingredients including sulfur, arginine (an amino acid), isoflavones, and selenium. Consuming garlic has been recommended as a way to reduce the risk of some cancers, including prostate cancer. Several uncontrolled epidemiological studies (chapter 4) looked at whether garlic intake prevented prostate cancer, and the conclusions were mixed. Studies will be difficult to do in men with prostate cancer because of the varied ways garlic is prepared. Although laboratory studies suggest that one of the ingredients in garlic blocks the growth of prostate cancer cells, no prospective studies have been done treating men with this disease. It does have minor potential risks including heartburn and nausea, and it may be a blood thinner (food—Group II, supplements—Group III).

Brazil nuts have been recommended because they contain high amounts of selenium. However, a government study in 2010 found that selenium did not prevent prostate cancer. No proper studies have been done in men with prostate cancer to know its effect. The only real downside to eating Brazil nuts is the high calorie content (Group II).

Herbs and Other Dietary Supplements

Herbs are substances from plants that are used for medicines or for flavoring foods. Since many drugs in use today have come from this source, it seems logical that other untested herbs also might be helpful to treat disease. Some of them have been shown to affect prostate cancer cells in laboratory experiments but it is unknown whether they would have a similar effect in men with the disease. This has not stopped them from being promoted by health books or websites. Because of the challenge of doing proper studies, companies sometimes "overstate" their case and promote a supplement inappropriately.

In 1994, Congress passed a law called the *Dietary Supplement Health and Education Act*. It set certain rules about dietary supplements that include:

- They must be intended to supplement the diet.

- They can contain one or more herbs, vitamins, minerals, amino acids, or other botanical agents.

- They are to be taken by mouth as a tablet, powder, liquid, or capsule.

- They must be labeled as being a dietary supplement.

- They do not require proof that they are safe or effective.

- Companies are permitted to claim that a supplement supports health, can replace a deficiency, or can be related to a body function if research supports the claim.

- They cannot make false claims about the effect.

- They must state, "It is not intended to diagnose, treat, cure, or prevent any disease."

The last point is critical because many of the supplements on the market overstep this boundary. The FDA increasingly is sending out warnings to companies about their claims. Keep this in mind when you consider taking a supplement based on claims made in magazines or on the Internet. The problem with many of these supplements is that little is known about their interaction with traditional medications. The government does not have the money to check out every claim. For that reason, consult with your doctor before taking them. Be sure there is no added risk due to the other medications you are taking.

Two obstacles to finding out whether herbs and supplements are useful is the high cost of doing proper studies and the difficulty in making money after they are done. Valid studies could take many years to complete because prostate cancer usually grows very slowly. Some studies measure changes in the time it takes for the PSA to double in value (PSA doubling time) as a way to tell whether the cancer is being affected. Those with a long doubling time are thought to be less dangerous. A European study assigned 42 men with a rising PSA after radical prostatectomy or radiation to receive either a placebo or a supplement containing soy, isoflavones, lycopene, silymarin, and antioxidants. At the end of 10 weeks, the PSA doubling time in the group getting the supplements was 1150 days compared with only 445 days in the control group. As stated often in this book, the PSA doubling time is an unreliable indicator that is not recognized by the FDA when deciding about the effectiveness of new therapies. Although the results of this study are encouraging, several questions need answering.

- What dose and preparation are needed of each supplement?

- Are all of them needed or could some be eliminated?

- What are the side effects and how often do they occur?

- Do any of the supplements interfere with other medications?

Larger and longer studies are needed to determine whether this combination of supplements will improve survival or cause any side effects (Group III).

The government website (www.nutrition.gov) is a useful resource for many alternative therapies. Some information about herbs used for prostate cancer is included below. Only those agents most commonly used for this disease or cancer in general are included.

Aloe vera has been used as a topical gel to reduce burns to the skin from radiation treatments. No good scientific studies support this claim (Group III).

Astragalus has been used in Chinese medicine in combination with other herbs to boost the immune system. Almost all the available studies are from Chinese journals but their quality is difficult to evaluate. The herb is considered to be safe but little is known about its effect in prostate cancer patients (Group III).

Bitter almond (Pygeum africanum) often is combined with saw palmetto to treat urinary problems in men. Laboratory studies show it inhibits the growth of prostate cancer cells. Although it appears safe in humans for up to one year of use, there is no evidence that it has any effect on men with prostate cancer (Group II).

Black Cohosh has been used in women to treat hot flashes and other symptoms of menopause. It has also been suggested for men with hot flashes caused by hormone therapy. Well-done studies have failed to show any improvement in hot flashes in women and some severe side effects have occurred, such as liver failure (Group III).

Cat's claw has been used to help improve the immune system. It has not been well studied in men with prostate cancer. Little is known about its side effects or whether it interacts with other drugs (Group III).

Echinacea has been recommended to treat and prevent colds. Since the immune system of cancer patients often is weakened, there is an increased risk for infections. Randomized studies testing three preparations showed no ability to prevent or shorten the duration of the common cold. No studies have been done in men with prostate cancer (Group IV).

Ephedra has been used for weight loss, increased energy, and improved exercise performance. Although there is some evidence it can help men lose weight, the risk of stroke or heart attack is increased. In 2004, the FDA banned the sale of any supplement containing Ephedra (Group IV).

Evening primrose oil comes from the yellow flowers of a plant and contains an essential fatty acid. Normally, essential fatty acids must be obtained from our diet because our body can't make them. This supplement is made from the plant's seeds. It has been promoted for prostate health and to reduce inflammation but no studies are available to assess its true effect or identify side effects (Group III).

Flaxseed and flaxseed oil contain fiber, lignan, alpha linoleic acid, and omega-3 fatty acids. It is used as a laxative and to lower cholesterol and frequently recommended for men with prostate cancer. No long-term studies have been done. A short-term study assigned men with localized prostate cancer to:

- A low-fat diet supplemented with 30 g per day of flaxseed

- A low-fat diet alone

- A regular diet supplemented with flaxseed

- A control group

They all were followed for 21 days before having their prostate removed. The prostate glands were examined for the ability of the cancer cells to divide, which might be a crude measure of how well they grow. The study found that the cancer cells in the flaxseed-treated men did not divide as well as the controls or those following only a low-fat diet. No side effects were reported. Since studies show that flaxseed can reduce absorption of some drugs taken by mouth and limit their effectiveness, you should ask your doctor whether it is safe for you. Although no conclusion can be made, these early results support doing more extensive studies (Group II).

Genistein is one of the active ingredients in soy that is similar to human estrogen but much weaker. Estrogen is known to slow down the growth of prostate cancer; as per laboratory studies, genistein, too, slows down the growth of prostate cancer cells. A prospective study was done in men with prostate cancer. They were given genistein capsules three times a day for six months. Sixteen men were on active surveillance of which nine had a stable or slightly lower PSA at the end of the study. The genistein was stopped in 5% of the men due to diarrhea. The long-term benefits and side effects of genistein supplements are not known (Grade III).

Ginkgo biloba is commonly recommended to improve memory, mental function, and sexual function. Since these are concerns for men on hormone therapy, it could be helpful, but well-done studies failed to show any improvement in memory. Some Internet sites recommend ginkgo for prostate cancer patients, but they cite studies that do not really support that opinion. Side effects include an increased risk of bleeding and stomach problems. There are no prospective studies in men with prostate cancer (Group III).

Ginseng is often promoted to boost the immune system. Laboratory studies found that two ingredients in this herb inhibited the growth of prostate cancer cells in the laboratory. According to the National Institutes of Health (NIH), a government website, ginseng at recommended doses appears safe, although it may cause problems in diabetics. Its effect in men with prostate cancer is unknown (Group II).

Goldenseal (yellow root) is an herb used by Native Americans for several health conditions. One of its ingredients is *berberine*, which stopped the growth of prostate cancer cells in a laboratory experiment. Although promoted on the Internet for the symptoms of prostate cancer, no clinical studies support this claim. The NIH states there is little information available about the safety of its long-term use at higher doses (Group III).

Grape seed extract contains antioxidants. The NIH is funding studies to find out whether it will prevent prostate cancer. One major ingredient is called *gallic acid*, which stopped prostate cancer cells from growing in the laboratory. It is well tolerated in humans, but no studies have been done to determine its effect on men with prostate cancer (Group II).

Green tea is widely used in Asian countries and the United States. It is often promoted for men with prostate cancer. Two active chemicals present in green tea have the abbreviations EGCG and ECG. Laboratory experiments show that extracts of EGCG slow the growth of prostate cancer in mice. In 2009, a review of published studies was unable to conclude that green tea prevents cancer. Also, no controlled studies have been done to know its effect on men with prostate cancer. Drinking a few cups of green tea a day appears safe, but some cases of liver toxicity have been reported with green tea extracts. Since it contains caffeine, it may cause difficulty sleeping and more frequent urination. The safety of green tea extracts has not been well studied in men with prostate cancer (green tea—Group II, green tea extracts—Group III).

Licorice root extract contains ingredients that may slow down the growth of cancer. A prospective, randomized study was started to determine the effect of combining licorice root with docetaxel in men with androgen-independent prostate cancer. Unfortunately, the study closed because not enough patients enrolled. This extract was one of the ingredients in PC-SPES, an herbal mixture promoted years ago for prostate cancer patients. PC-SPES is no longer available because the company making it was sued and went out of business when the product was found to contain estrogen.

Licorice root extract combined with other herbs also has been tested in mice with prostate cancer and shown to slow down tumor growth. The safety of men taking it for more than a few weeks is unknown (Group III).

Milk thistle has been used to reduce the growth of several tumors including prostate cancer. Two of its active ingredients, *silymarin* and *silibinin*, were found to inhibit the growth of prostate cancer cells and tumors in several laboratory studies. This may lead to testing in men with the disease. It does not appear to have major side effects (Group II).

Mistletoe extract (Iscador) is widely used in Europe for cancer patients and many studies have been published, although none included men with prostate cancer. The randomized, studies found no benefit from the extract and many of the other studies were poorly done. The overall conclusion was that mistletoe extract might improve survival. Major side effects were not reported in the European studies and the NIH states it is safe when used in proper doses. Its role in men with prostate cancer is unknown (Group II).

Omega-3 fatty acids are widely recommended for their heart health benefits. In 2006, a government agency reviewed all studies related to cancer and found no clear proof it prevented cancer. Uncontrolled studies suggested that men consuming low amounts of omega-3 fatty acids had a higher chance of getting aggressive prostate cancer and dying from the disease. However, no valid conclusions can be made. Since it has few side effects and appears to lower the risk of dying from heart disease, it may be worth taking. The evidence is strongest for fish and fish oil (fish and fish oil—Group I, omega-3 supplements—Group II).

Pomegranate juice is a food source that contains many antioxidants. Some of its ingredients appear active against prostate cancer cells in laboratory experiments. That led to a prospective study in 46 men with a rising PSA level after being treated for prostate cancer. The PSA doubling time was determined before starting to drink eight ounces of pomegranate juice per day (made by POM Wonderful). A PSA test was repeated every three months and the juice was stopped if the PSA doubled or the cancer got worse. The PSA doubling time increased in 83% of the men during 56 months of treatment. Pomegranate juice did not reduce the testosterone level or cause any significant side effects.

What conclusion can be made from this study? Unfortunately, it does not prove pomegranate juice helps men with prostate cancer. In March 2010, the FDA warned POM Wonderful that its claim of slowing down the progress of prostate cancer was a violation of the Federal Food Act. If you have a rising PSA, taking eight ounces of pomegranate juice per day has some weak scientific support and many people love the taste (Group II).

Pomi-T® Polyphenols are chemicals that are active against prostate cancer cells in laboratory studies. They are present in pomegranate seeds, broccoli, green tea and turmeric. A randomized study is underway comparing a combination of extracts from these four substances called Pomi-T to a placebo in men on active surveillance or watchful waiting following a rise in their PSA after radical prostatectomy or radiation therapy. Men took their treatment twice a day for six months and the preliminary results showed that those taking the polyphenol mixture had a significantly smaller rise in their PSA and a higher percentage of men with a stable or lower PSA. The main side effects were gastro-intestinal complaints. The only problem was that the men getting Pomi-T had an average age that was almost five years lower than the placebo group. These are encouraging results but they do not yet prove a true benefit from these supplements. The combination does appear to be safe (Group II).

Red clover belongs to a family of plants called legumes. Like soy, it contains isoflavones, which are active against prostate cancer cells in laboratory studies. One uncontrolled study gave red clover extract to 20 men in Australia a few weeks before they had a radical prostatectomy. An examination of their prostate gland showed more cancer cells had died compared with a group of men not receiving the extract. No studies have been done to see whether red clover extract has any long-term benefit in men with this disease. It does appear safe when used for a short time (Grade II).

Saw palmetto (Serenoa repens) is a very popular herb promoted for treating symptoms of prostate enlargement. However, in 2006, a randomized study found it offered no improvement in men with moderate to severe urinary symptoms. In 2010, an extensive review of published studies also concluded that saw palmetto did not improve urinary symptoms. This herb also has no effect on PSA levels. Although it does not cause serious side effects, there is no evidence that it benefits men with prostate cancer (Group II).

Turmeric (Circumin) is an herb that is commonly used to season Indian and Asian food. Laboratory studies found it slowed down the growth of prostate cancers in mice. Although it is certainly safe to use, its effect in men with prostate cancer is unknown (Group II).

Yohimbe is an herb from the bark of the yohimbe tree. It contains a chemical called yohimbine, which is sold as a prescription drug to treat men with erection problems. The amount of yohimbine in over-the-counter supplements is variable, its effectiveness is unknown, and significant side effects may occur (Group III).

Zinc is an essential nutrient needed to make proteins and DNA. It is concentrated in the prostate gland and thought to help maintain a healthy prostate, but well-done studies have not been done. It can cause side effects at higher doses and can interact with some prescription drugs (Group III).

Antioxidants

One of the possible reasons that cancers occur is because of the effect of free radicals. They are unstable molecules that have the ability to alter normal cells, proteins, and DNA. Antioxidants are chemicals that stop free radicals from causing damage to cells. Vitamins A, C, and E, and selenium are antioxidants that have been tested in randomized studies as preventive agents for prostate cancer. So far, they have not shown any benefit. Even though they do not prevent prostate cancer, could they help men who already have the disease? The answer is possibly yes, but not one well-done study has found any benefit. There is no evidence they increase survival and they do not make any other treatments more effective. Without those studies, the impact of these antioxidants will remain unknown.

Despite the lack of any studies showing they help, another question is whether they are completely safe or whether taking them could harm some men? The table shows the known side effects from these agents. Vitamin E in particular may make chemotherapy less effective or may increase the side effects of ketoconazole.

Table 39.2 Side Effects of Antioxidant Vitamins and Minerals

Antioxidant	Side Effects
Vitamin A	Fatigue, irritability, mental changes, anorexia, stomach discomfort, nausea, vomiting, mild fever, excessive sweating, thinning of the bones
Vitamin C	Nausea, vomiting, heartburn, stomach cramps, headache, an increased risk of bleeding, and kidney stones
Vitamin E	Fatigue, intestinal cramping, inflammation in veins, acne, and diarrhea, increase in blood pressure in certain people, prolonged or increased risk of bleeding
Selenium	Nausea, vomiting, nail changes, loss of energy, irritability, loss of hair, inflammation of finger nails, fatigue, irritability, nausea, vomiting, garlic breath odor, a metallic taste, muscle tenderness, shaking, lightheadedness, facial flushing, blood clotting problems, damage to liver and kidney, increased risk of diabetes

Another concern about taking these agents is that no one knows what dose is best because no studies have done any comparison.

Higher amounts certainly increase the risk of side effects. The bottom line is that they have no proven benefit in men with prostate cancer. (Group II except vitamin E—Group III).

Lycopene is an antioxidant found in tomatoes, grapefruit, watermelon, and papaya. Lycopene is thought to reduce the risk of prostate cancer. In laboratory studies, it is active against prostate cancer cells. A small prospective, randomized study was done in men scheduled to have a radical prostatectomy. For three weeks before surgery, 15 men were given lycopene and 11 men received no supplement. Although the study found fewer men in the lycopene group had cancer growing outside the prostate, the study groups were not balanced. This means the results do not prove lycopene was helpful. On the positive side, no side effects were reported. Further studies are needed to know whether men with prostate cancer benefit from this supplement (food—Group II, supplements—Group II).

Vitamin D deficiency occurs in any adults, particularly those who do not get enough outdoor exposure. This is considered to be a factor in the development of colon and breast cancer. Uncontrolled studies suggest a health benefit from maintaining a vitamin D level of 40–60 ng/ml. Blood tests are available to check your level. An intake of 2000 International Units per day of vitamin D_3 is considered safe. No studies have shown a benefit from maintaining higher levels in men with prostate cancer, but it may be helpful for overall health (Group II).

Homeopathy or Naturopathic Medicine

The idea behind homeopathy is to give small amounts of substances that if taken in larger doses would cause the same symptoms as the disease being treated. This is supposed to result in patients "healing themselves." The FDA requires that homeopathic remedies can only be sold over the counter if they are promoted for minor health problems. If they are recommended to treat a more serious illness, like cancer, they must be sold by prescription. This whole field is controversial. Presently, there is no good evidence for a beneficial effect of homeopathy in men with prostate cancer and little is known about side effects (Grade III).

Mind–Body Medicine

The idea of this approach is to get the mind to help heal the body and lower stress. It includes meditation, yoga, hypnosis, and counseling. There is little evidence for any risks and they may reduce stress and improve quality of life. A study done in 10 men with a rising PSA level after radical prostatectomy looked at the effect of a stress reduction program and a low fat, plant-based diet on PSA levels over four months. The PSA doubling time increased in eight of them. It is unknown what role stress reduction played in this response or whether there is any long-term benefit. There is no evidence of any harm (Group II).

The Bottom Line on Complementary Therapies

By now, you realize that this is a very confusing topic. The fact is that little research has been done to know which, if any, interventions are truly good for men with prostate cancer. Until more is known, incorporating the items in Group I and Group II into your treatment plan is reasonable provided you first check with your doctor. Be aware that anyone who tells you interventions are completely safe is not giving you the whole story. Even without supporting evidence, you still might decide to take some of them because the risks are acceptable to you. As with everything else in this book, the goal is to help you make an informed choice.

Using the Internet

40

One of the most profound changes for anyone looking for information about health has been the explosion of information on the Internet. Putting the words "prostate cancer" in a search engine gave more than 70 million citations in April 2013. The abundance of information is a two-edged sword. It definitely can provide men with very valuable and useful information, but it can also be inaccurate and biased. The challenge is to separate the good from the bad, which is not easily done.

Today, anyone can create a website relatively easily without having to meet any specific requirements. Documents on the World Wide Web are unregulated and unmonitored. As yet, no certified regulators are responsible for verifying that a website contains accurate and unbiased information. One day a site will give you the right information and then something changes making the information incorrect. Knowledge about prostate cancer is changing quite rapidly and many sites are not updated in a timely manner. Even support group websites do not contain the most up-to-date information, so relying on them could give you the wrong information. Some websites may appear balanced, unbiased, and accurate, but the information they contain is several years old and no longer correct. The most important message here is to be very careful when using the Internet and make sure to check out the accuracy of the information.

A major concern about using the Internet is that many of the websites are really marketing tools promoting doctors, hospitals, or company products. The information they contain may appear to be very reliable, but often it is biased and very misleading.

So where does this leave you? Should you avoid the Internet or embrace it? Are there things you can do or questions you can ask that will help you find websites you can trust? The answer is yes. The place to begin is with sites that have been created by medical organizations or health agencies. Some examples include:

- **The National Cancer Institute** or NCI (www.cancer.gov): This site provides information about ongoing or completed research studies and general information about diagnosis and treatment of all cancers. It is reasonably up-to-date.

- **The Centers for Disease Control**, or CDC (http://cdc.gov): Provides a general overview of the treatment options for prostate cancer and other diseases.

- **The Agency for Healthcare Research and Quality**, or AHRQ (http://ahrq.gov): Critically reviews medical topics with summaries based on good scientific methods.

Questions to Ask about an Internet Site

Your goal for every web search is to find information that is accurate and up-to-date with little bias. Getting the answers to the following questions may help you decide whether the information is trustworthy:

- Was the site created to provide unbiased information or will it somehow benefit those involved bringing in more business?

- Is the author of the information identified with a description of their credentials, their education, or their experience, and is there a way to contact them?

- Is the date the information was created clearly indicated so you can tell whether it is current?

- Is the author in any way connected with or supported by a medical company that makes a product or treatment?

- Is the site promoting a doctor, hospital, clinic, or specific treatment, which could indicate a bias?

- Are ads visible on the website promoting the treatment that is the focus of the topic being discussed?

Prostate Videos

In response to the need for unbiased, up-to-date information, I have created a unique video website that can be accessed for free at www. ProstateVideos.com. Many men and their partners more easily understand information that is explained to them rather than having to read it; in other words, they are visual learners. This site contains information about every aspect of prostate cancer, which is presented as if I am sitting across from a patient, having a conversation. Although it has not been put together with input from multiple doctors, it strictly follows the principles of evidence-based medicine that are used throughout this book. It includes the pros and cons of all the options available for all stages of prostate cancer. A treatment will be recommended only if well-done studies clearly show it is better than the other options available. This website is an excellent supplement to reading this book and it is updated regularly when new information appears. Currently it contains over 130 videos with more being made and old ones being replaced if the information changes.

The Bottom Line on Using the Internet

Anyone reading this book clearly is interested in learning more about prostate cancer and the options for treating it that they heard from their doctor. The Internet can be a great aid but caution is needed because so much of the information is biased, inaccurate, and out-of-date. If you are aware of its limitations and use it cautiously, it can be helpful.

The Role of Support Groups and Counseling

41

Most doctors treating men with prostate cancer have focused their time and effort on the "medical" aspects of the disease. However, too often they haven't routinely addressed the mental and emotional effects it has on men and their families. Fortunately, this gap has been partly filled by counselors and support groups, which:

- Provide men and their significant others with information about treatments they were not told about or that were not adequately explained by their doctor.

- Act as a source of encouragement by the long-term survivors for those with a similar condition.

- Help people express their feelings and cope with any emotional difficulties caused by their disease or the side effects of treatment.

- Offer an opportunity to talk with men who have gone through the process of choosing a treatment and living with the results.

- Enable women to share their experiences of coping with their partner's disease and its effect on their relationship.

The number of support groups keeps growing and only a few are listed below with their URLs. Many more are available on the Internet.

- Us TOO, International – www.UsToo.org

- Malecare – http://malecare.org

- You Are Not Alone – www.yananow.org

- Women Against Prostate Cancer – www.womenagainstpros tatecancer.org

The History of Us TOO, International

One of the largest prostate cancer support groups in the United States is called Us TOO. It was started in 1990 in response to unmet needs by one of my own patients. He had been treated with a new type of radiation therapy that caused him very severe problems with his bowels and urinary control. Although every option was explored for treating those problems, he and his wife became anxious and depressed. They asked me, "Isn't anyone else having the same trouble? Aren't there other men and wives we can talk to about how they are dealing with these problems?"

After reading about the value of the breast cancer support group called Y-Me, it seemed to me that there was an unmet need for men with prostate cancer. A short time later, I invited my prostate cancer patients and their wives to a meeting I arranged at the University of Chicago. The executive director of the "Y-Me" group also was invited to talk about the purpose and benefits of patient support groups. Following that initial meeting, my patients organized themselves into the first chapter of Us TOO, International, and with financial support from a pharmaceutical company, they helped establish other chapters throughout the United States. It is now a tax-free corporation with an executive board, fundraising activities, and educational programs. Over 325 Us TOO chapters have been set up throughout the United States and several other countries. Most chapters have a monthly meeting where they invite a guest speaker to talk on some aspect of the diagnosis or management of prostate cancer. After each meeting, attendees talk with each other and provide support.

Is There Anything Negative about Support Groups?

Ideally, a support group should result in nothing but benefits to those who attend. But participating in a support group does have a potentially negative aspect. The people who attend often are very passionate about what they believe is the "right" thing or "best" thing to do for various aspects of the disease. Someone who had a good result from his treatment may strongly encourage a newly diagnosed individual to choose that same treatment. They may fail to recognize why a different treatment might be more appropriate for another patient. Keep in mind that members of a support group are patients, not physicians, and they may be quite biased in how they present information. Sometimes they move beyond providing support and counseling to outright "recommending" treatment without knowing all the facts. They also tend to encourage the use of unconventional approaches for treating the disease such as herbs, vitamins, and supplements without being aware of their limitations or risks.

The Bottom Line on Support Groups

Despite the potential limitations, support groups provide many important benefits. If you are aware of the possible biases then you'll find attending one or more meetings to be worth your time. Thousands of men and their significant others have benefitted from attending meetings. Although support groups may not be for everyone, you should know that they exist, they are free to attend, they make newcomers feel comfortable, and they have no specific requirements other than that you "tell your story." Surprisingly, many doctors still are not tuned in to the benefits to their patients of attending a support group meeting; they will not make you aware of them nor will they encourage you to attend. Generally, support groups can best be summed up by the Us TOO motto: "Learning to cope through knowledge and hope."

Is There a Role for Counseling?

A diagnosis of prostate cancer is accompanied by many negative emotions including fear, anger, panic, and depression. Perhaps you already had trouble coping with changes in your sexual function before your cancer was detected. Prostate cancer treatment brings another set of emotions depending on what was done to you and whether any side effects occurred. Confronting those feelings is something you may have not faced before and it can affect your quality of life and the relationship with your spouse or life partner.

If you are having any emotional or psychological difficulties, what should you do? The first and best advice is *don't despair*. Psychiatrists, psychologists, and social workers are trained to help you cope. The best advice you can get is to be open to the idea of seeking out one of them. There is nothing wrong with your deciding to get help with these emotions. Short-term depression and anxiety are common among men with prostate cancer yet few doctors will ask about it or suggest seeing a therapist. If needed, antidepressants and other medications can be very helpful, especially while you cope with your diagnosis and try to decide which treatment is right for you. Many men begin to feel better after they have been treated. The need for medication or counseling decreases or goes away unless someone is having severe side effects. Your partner also may be struggling because of worries about the possibility of your life getting cut short. They too can benefit from counseling. The best advice is to confront your feelings rather than avoid them and keep an open dialogue with your partner so you can help each other get through it. Following your recovery, you can resume living your life again. If you have specific concerns about your disease, make sure to discuss them with your doctor. Not uncommonly, men think they are in greater danger than is really the case. That certainly increases the level of anxiety. The bottom line is to realize that a diagnosis of prostate cancer can cause a lot of distress, but psychological support is available and beneficial.

What to Do When Therapy Is No Longer Effective

Despite all the advances in treating prostate cancer in the past few years, some men eventually will die from their disease. A difficult decision to make is when to stop receiving medications and other treatments that are not successfully fighting the cancer and accept what is going to happen. No one can tell you when that should be done because it is a very personal decision. But when it happens, the goals change from trying to live as long as possible to controlling pain, maintaining one's quality of life, and learning to accept one's impending mortality.

The Role of Hospice

Hospice is not so much a place to go for medical care as it is a concept. The word means "guesthouse" in Latin, but in the 1960s a British doctor started a team approach to delivering care that included modern pain control methods for people nearing death. In 1974, the first hospice began in the United States and today they provide invaluable services to people who are at the end stage of their lives. Hospice is composed of a team of professionals including physicians, nurses, aides, social workers, counselors, therapists, spiritual caregivers, and volunteers. Although patients can be cared for at an inpatient location, hospice mostly provides services at home. Two of its advantages are the ability to remain in the comfort of your own home and have family members and friends present at all times. For most people, this is far better than the impersonal environment of a hospital.

When someone enters hospice, they stop all the treatments aimed at trying to prolong their life and instead focus on feeling as good as possible for as long as possible. Without hospice, pain often is not adequately controlled. The drugs prescribed by many physicians may keep you comfortable for part of the time but not for all 24 hours in the day. The goal of hospice is to provide comfort and support while making sure that pain is completely eliminated or at least greatly reduced throughout the entire day and night. Hospice workers will train someone at home to make sure you get the drugs needed to achieve this goal. There is no reason for anyone to endure even one hour of pain when medications are available that can eliminate or greatly reduce it.

Controlling pain is not simply a matter of prescribing a pill. The best results come from titrating the pain medication, which means increasing the dose gradually or combining different drugs until the right amount is found. Narcotics often play a necessary role and you should not worry about taking them out of fear of becoming addicted. If those are the only drugs that make the pain tolerable then using them is the right thing to do.

Many men develop breakthrough pain, which means the drugs control the pain for a few hours but it returns before the next dose is due. A second drug is often very helpful in such cases. Adding a nonsteroidal anti-inflammatory drug (NSAID), can prevent pain from recurring before another narcotic is taken. It can also reduce the need to raise the dose of the narcotic being used. Examples of some of the more common over-the-counter NSAIDs include:

- Advil

- Motrin

- Naprosyn

- Aleve

- Aspirin

One mistake patients often make is waiting to take their medication until after their pain returns. A better approach is to take a drug before the pain develops because it helps keep a person pain-free for a greater part of the day and night. The bottom line is that no one should have to endure pain without making every effort to control it and hospice staff is very experienced at doing that.

When Should You Consult Hospice?

A good time to consult hospice is before it is needed. You can be receiving chemotherapy or other treatments and still be evaluated by a member of the hospice staff. The value of that approach is it will make for a smoother, more rapid transition when you decide the time is right. On average, men with prostate cancer spend the last six months of their lives in hospice.

What to Do When the End Is Near

In 1969, Elisabeth Kübler-Ross wrote a book called *On Death and Dying*. She suggested there were five stages of coping with grief that dying patients usually progressed through near the end of their lives. They are:

- Denial – People feel as if, "This can't be happening, not to me."

- Anger – "This is not fair, why is it happening to me?"

- Bargaining – "Just let me live a little longer so I can see my grandchildren graduate from school."

- Depression – "I'm so sad, why go on? I know I am dying so why delay it?

- Acceptance – "It's going to be OK. I can't fight it, I may as well prepare for it."

These stages do not always happen in the order listed and not everyone goes through each stage, but the last one is very important. When a man denies what is happening, it often will create a separation between him and his family. A healthier approach is to get to a point that one's feelings can be discussed with friends and family, which leads to achieving an inner comfort. Everyone must accept the inevitable limit to their lives, but reaching that end can be done peacefully and with dignity.

Glossary

active surveillance—Also known as *delayed therapy*. Patients are monitored at regular intervals by having a DRE, a PSA level test, and repeat prostate biopsies. Unlike watchful waiting, where no attempt is made to treat the cancer in the prostate, active surveillance takes a delayed approach to curing the disease. This occurs if, and only if, the cancer shows signs of getting worse.

adrenal glands—Located on top of the kidneys, these glands produce hormones such as adrenaline, but they also produce a small portion of a man's testosterone.

5-alpha reductase inhibitors (5-ARIs)—Group of drugs that prevent normal prostate cells from converting testosterone to dihydrotestosterone.

androgen ablation—General term for lowering or blocking the male hormone, testosterone.

androgen deprivation therapy (ADT)—Treatment aimed at reducing androgens, which stimulate prostate cancer cells to grow, in order to make prostate cancer grow more slowly. Also known as *hormone therapy*.

androgen-independent prostate cancer (AIPC)—Prostate cancer cells that grow despite castrate level of serum testosterone.

androstenediol—Chemical produced in the adrenal glands that can be converted by the body into testosterone.

androstenedione—Chemical produced in the adrenal gland that can be converted to testosterone.

androsterone—Male hormone made in the liver from the metabolism of testosterone.

Aneuploid cells—Cells with more than a normal amount of DNA.

antiandrogen—A drug that stops testosterone from stimulating cancer cells.

antiandrogen withdrawal (AAWD)—Unusual response in which tumor cell growth slows rather than increases when antiandrogen drugs are stopped.

antibodies—Protein produced by the body's immune system when it detects harmful substances, called *antigens*.

antigens—Any substance that your body thinks is foreign. The immune system tries to destroy antigens with antibodies.

artificial penile implant—Device implanted inside the penis to enable men to engage in sexual intercourse.

artificial urinary sphincter—A device inserted inside the body to stop or reduce leakage of urine.

benign prostate hypertrophy (BPH)—Enlargement of the prostate gland.

bilateral adrenalectomy—Surgical removal of both adrenal glands.

bilateral orchiectomy—Removal of both testicles. Another way of describing surgical castration.

biochemical disease-free survival (bDFS)—The time before PSA rises above a certain value.

bladder neck contracture—*See* Urethral stricture.

bone scan—Performed by first injecting a small amount of radioactive drug called technetium-99 into a vein. It circulates throughout the body. Abnormal bones take up the radioactivity and show up with a gamma counter as a dark area.

bound prostate-specific antigen (PSA)—Form of PSA that binds to proteins circulating in the bloodstream.

brachytherapy—A form of radiation therapy wherein a therapeutic radioisotrope is inserted into the body to irradiate the tissue.

cancer of the Prostate Risk Assessment (CAPRA) score—A method of determining whether cancer will return after a radical prostatectomy. It combines a patient's age, his PSA, clinical state, Gleason score, and the percentage of the biopsy cores that contain cancer. The lowest score is 0 and the highest score is 10.

capsular penetration—Cancer cells growing outside the capsule of the prostate.

capsule—Very thin layer of tissue surrounding the prostate.

castration-resistant prostate cancer (CRPC)—Growth of prostate cancer despite a low serum testosterone.

catheter—A thin tube used to drain urine from the bladder through the penis. Also known as a Foley catheter.

chemotherapy—The use of drugs to treat cancer.

clinical stage—The extent to which a cancer has spread.

colostomy—When there is damage to the rectum during surgery, the intestine must be brought to an opening created in the skin. A bag is worn over the opening to drain the bowel's contents.

combined androgen blockade (CAB)—ADT using two drugs. One of them lowers testosterone and the second one blocks the action of testosterone.

complementary and alternative medicine (CAM)—A wide variety of medical and healthcare systems, practices, and products not generally considered part of conventional medicine, including such things as the use of herbs, massage therapy, vitamins, homeopathic and naturopathic medicine, hypnosis, tai chi, and others.

corpus cavernosum—Pair of cylinder-shaped rods in the penis containing many blood vessels that fill with blood during an erection.

corpus spongiosum—Spongy tissue surrounding the male urethra within the penis that fills with blood during sexual stimulation.

corticosteroids—Steroids produced in the adrenal glands that are involved in body processes such as stress response and immune response. Those used with prostate cancer are prednisone, hydrocortisone, and dexamethasone.

cryotherapy—Also known as cryosurgery or cryoablation. A treatment in which very cold temperatures are delivered to the prostate.

CT scan—Computed tomography. Imaging technique that uses computer-processed x-rays to produce tomographic images that show "slices" of specific areas of the body. (In older literature, sometimes known as a CAT scan.)

cytotoxic chemotherapy—Uses drugs that kills cells.

D'Amico risk statification—A combination of the PSA level, the DRE results, and the Gleason score. Divides cancers into low-, intermediate-, and high-risk. The higher the risk group, the greater the odds that the cancer eventually will spread and cause harm if not treated aggressively.

delayed therapy—*See* Active surveillance.

digital rectal examination (DRE)—A doctor inserts a gloved, lubricated index finger into the rectum and presses it against the rectal wall to feel the prostate gland and determine size and texture.

dihydrotestosterone (DHT)—Potent male hormone formed from testosterone by the enzyme 5-alpha reductase.

DNA (deoxyribonucleic acid)—Molecule that includes the hereditary instructions used in the development and functioning of all known living organisms.

DRE—*See* Digital rectal examination.

ejaculatory duct—The tube through which fluid produced by the seminal vesicles passes into the urethra, along with fluid produced by the prostate and sperm produced by the testes.

EKG—*See* Electrocardiogram.

electrical muscle stimulation (EMS)—Produces electrical pulses that are able to stimulate the pelvic floor muscles to contract, which might strengthen them.

electrocardiogram (EKG)—Measurement of the electrical activity of the heart.

endorectal MRI—Imaging technique in which MRI is used together with a special probe placed into the rectum to obtain high-quality images of the prostate and the nearby structures.

evidence-based medicine (EBM)—EBM assesses the quality (i.e., risks and benefits) of medical studies that are used to advise patients of the best treatment for their disease, including no treatment at all.

external beam radiation therapy (EBRT)—An external source of radiation is pointed at a particular part of the body.

external urinary sphincter—One of two sets of muscles, along with the internal urinary sphincter that help keep control of urine in the bladder. The external urinary sphincter is a striated muscle, which means a person can exert voluntary control over contracting and relaxing it.

extracapsular—Outside the capsule of the prostate gland.

focal cryotherapy—Treating only a portion of the prostate with crytotherapy rather than the entire gland.

Foley catheter—*See* Catheter.

FRAX—A fracture risk assessment tool for determining the likelihood of getting a pelvic fracture due to osteoporosis or similar conditions.

free prostate-specific antigen (PSA)—Chemical forms of PSA that circulate in the bloodstream without binding to other proteins.

general anesthesia—The patient is put to sleep and usually a tube is placed down his windpipe through the mouth. A ventilator controls breathing and delivers a gas that keeps the patient asleep.

Gleason grading system—Prostate cancer grading system named after Donald Gleason, a pathologist, who developed it with other colleagues in the 1960s. The result is known as a *Gleason score*.

Gleason score—Score given to prostate cancer based on the appearance of cancer cells under a microscope.

gonadotropin-releasing hormone (GnRH) antagonist—Drug that stops the body from releasing hormones from the brain that normally play a role in sexual function, sperm production and stimulating prostate cancer cells without producing a temporary rise in testosterone.

gray (GY)—Unit of radiation energy.

HDR—High dose rate.

HDR brachytherapy—High dose rate brachytherapy. Also known as temporary brachytherapy.

high-grade prostatic intraepithelial neoplasia (HGPIN)—Abnormal prostate cells that have some features of cancer cells.

high-risk category—The PSA is over 20 ng/ml or the Gleason score is between 8–10 or the clinical stage is T2B or T3

homeopathy—Using small amounts of substances that if taken in larger doses would cause the same symptoms as the disease being treated.

hormone—Chemicals produced in certain organs that affect other parts of your body.

hormone deprivation—The process of taking away male hormones in the body.

hormone refractory prostate cancer—Prostate cancer that has progressed despite a reduction in the testosterone level in the body.

hormone therapy—See Androgen-deprivation therapy (ADT).

hospice—End-of-life care that focuses on easing pain and meeting patients' emotional needs as they face death.

hypothalamus—A part of the brain that helps to regulate the testosterone level in the body.

image-guided radiation therapy (IGRT)—The position of the prostate is constantly monitored during external radiation using a CT scan that is built into the radiation machine.

immune system—The body's defense system against things that may harm it such as bacteria, viruses, wounds, and even cancer.

immunotherapy—Using the immune system to fight disease.

intensity-modulated radiation therapy (IMRT)—A modification of 3D-CRT, the radiation is broken up into narrow beams rather than a single, wide beam. The intensity of each beam is adjusted according to the shape of the prostate, allowing greater control of the dose given to the prostate and the surrounding organs.

intermediate-risk category—Prostate examination shows a tumor on both sides of the prostate but not outside the gland; the Gleason score is less than 7 or the PSA is 10 to 20 ng/ml.

intermittent androgen deprivation therapy (IADT)—In IADT, men are given one or two drugs that interfere with testosterone production or its action for several months and then they are stopped after the PSA reaches a certain level. It is restarted either when the PSA rises to a certain number or after a set number of months. This process is repeated until the PSA no longer decreases when the treatment is restarted.

internal urinary sphincter—One of two sets of muscles, along with the external urinary sphincter that help keep control of urine in the bladder.

international prostate symptom score (IPSS)—A survey used to measure urinary symptoms. It has seven questions, each with five possible answers so the total score can range from 7 to 35.

Kattan nomogram—Tools for estimating odds of progression, survival or recurrence after treatment for prostate cancer.

laparoscopic radical prostatectomy—Minimally invasive method for removing the prostate using a telescope and surgical instruments that are inserted through the skin into the abdominal cavity.

local progression—The chance of developing problems due to enlargement of the tumor in the prostate gland.

localized prostate cancer—When cancer cells are contained inside the prostate.

locally advanced prostate cancer—When cancer cells are found outside the prostate capsule.

low-risk category—The prostate examination shows no cancer or only a lump on one side of the gland; the Gleason score is less than 7 and the PSA is less than 10 ng/ml.

luteinizing hormone (LH)—A protein released by the pituitary gland. It enters the blood stream and goes to the testicles where it stimulates the production of testosterone.

luteinizing hormone-releasing hormone (LHRH)—Hormone produced in a region of the brain called the hypothalamus, which plays a role in controlling testosterone in the body.

luteinizing hormone-releasing hormone (LHRH) agonist—A drug that stops the testicles from producing testosterone.

luteinizing hormone-releasing hormone (LHRH) antagonist—A drug that prevents the release of luteinizing hormone from the brain leading to a reduction in the production of testosterone without causing a rise in testosterone.

luteinizing hormone-releasing hormone (LHRH) receptors—Area in the pituitary where luteinizing hormone-releasing hormone binds leading to the release of luteinizing hormone.

lymph nodes—Small glands scattered throughout the body that help fight infection.

lymphocele—After lymph nodes are removed, sometimes lymph fluid leaks into the surrounding tissues and forms a fluid collection, which can cause pain and fever.

maximum androgen blockade (MAB)—Type of prostate cancer hormone therapy that combines lowering the testosterone and blocking male hormones from the adrenal gland.

medicated urethral system for erection (MUSE)—A small suppository containing alprostadil that is placed inside the urethra at the tip of the penis to produce an erection.

meta-analysis—A way of combining the results of several studies that have already been performed. It is not a formal study that enrolls patients.

metastasized—When cancer cells are found in other parts of the body.

mind-body medicine—The idea is to get the mind to help heal the body and lower stress. It includes meditation, yoga, hypnosis, and counseling.

MRI—Magnetic resonance imaging. Uses a strong magnetic field to give detailed images of your body.

nadir—In men with prostate cancer, usually refers to the lowest PSA level or testosterone level attained in response to treatment.

nerve-sparing radical prostatectomy—A radical prostatectomy where the prostate is removed but the pelvic nerves that enable men to have erections are spared from removal or damage.

nonsteroidal anti-inflammatory drugs (NSAIDs)—Drugs such as aspirin, Motrin, Advil, Aleve, and Celebrex used for mild pain relief to treat inflammation.

Partin tables—A statistical model that uses PSA, clinical stage, and Gleason score from a prostate biopsy to show the probability that cancer is growing outside the prostate, into the seminal vesicles and into the lymph nodes.

pelvic lymph node dissection (PLND)—Removal of the lymph nodes from the pelvic area.

pelvic nerves—Two nerves located between the prostate gland and rectum. They control a man's ability to achieve an erection and thus are an important aspect of any surgery to the prostate.

penile implant—Artificial devices placed inside the penis that creates erections.

penis—The main external sexual organ or a man. Also conveys the urethra through which urine is disposed from the body from the bladder.

perineum—Area located around the rectal area of the body.

PET scan—Positive emission tomography. Nuclear imaging technique that produces a three-dimensional image of the area of the body scanned.

placebo—A medically inert treatment, used in some randomized studies to test the actual therapeutic effectiveness of a new treatment.

ploidy analysis—Technique that measures the amount of genetic material, called DNA, contained in the cells harvested from a biopsy.

posterior lobe—One of five regions that compose the prostate gland. Prostate cancer usually manifests in the posterior lobe.

priapism—Erection that persists for several hours and requires medical intervention for it to be resolved.

ProstaScint® scan—Test that uses antibodies and a small amount of radioactive material, which are injected into a vein and then attach to a protein on the surface of prostate cancer cells. The ProstaScint scan can find prostate cancer cells anywhere in the body.

prostate bed—Tissue in front of the rectum where the prostate gland originally was located prior to surgical removal.

prostate gland—The normal adult prostate is approximately the size of a walnut and weighs about 20 grams. The prostate sits in your lower pelvis, tucked behind your pubic bone and just beneath your bladder. It has five regions or lobes. The prostate secretes fluid during ejaculation that combines with fluid from the seminal vesicles to make up semen.

prostatic acid phosphatase—Enzyme produced by the prostate, sometimes used to determine the extent of prostate cancer.

prostate-specific antigen (PSA)—A protein produced in the prostate by normal cells and cancer cells.

protein-specific antigen (PSA) bounce—The PSA level goes above 0.2 ng/ml usually within the first two years after radiation to the prostate.

protein-specific antigen (PSA) density—Determined by dividing the PSA level by the size of the prostate as determined from a prostate ultrasound.

protein-specific antigen (PSA) doubling time—A measure of how long it takes for the PSA to double in value.

protein-specific antigen velocity (PSAV)—Speed at which the PSA level is rising in the bloodstream.

proton beam therapy (PBR)—Radiation therapy using protons.

radiation absorbed dose (RAD)—Metric term used for measuring the amount of radiation absorbed by the body.

radical perineal prostatectomy—Performed through an incision made in the skin underneath the scrotum in front of the rectum.

radical prostatectomy—An operation to remove the prostate gland and some of the tissue around it, including the seminal vesicles and often including the vas deferens.

radical retropubic prostatectomy (RRP)—A radical prostatectomy performed through a cut made in the skin extending from below the belly button to the public bone.

radiopharmaceuticals—Drugs that contain a radioactive compound.

robot-assisted laparoscopic radical prostatectomy (RALP)—A laparoscopic radical prostatectomy performed using a robotic instrument called a DaVinci, which is guided by a surgeon sitting several feet away from the operating table.

salvage radiation—Radiation given to a man with recurrent disease after his prostate has been removed.

salvage radical prostatectomy—Removal of the prostate after a man has been treated with radiation therapy that did not eliminate the cancer.

seed implantation—Also known as permanent brachytherapy, when radioactive material is left in the body, and as temporary brachytherapy, when radioactive material is left in the body for a short time and then is removed.

SEER—Surveillance, Epidemiology, and End Results national cancer registry.

seminal vesicles—A pair of small organs behind the bladder and prostate gland that secrete much of the fluid that makes up semen during ejaculation.

skeletal-related events (SREs)—Consequence of bone metastases including fractures, pain and spinal cord compression.

"sling operation"—Operation used to reduce urinary incontinence using a synthetic mesh that increases the resistance in the urethra.

smooth muscle—Muscle that operates automatically, beyond a person's control, such as the muscle in the heart.

sodium flouride PET/CT bone scan—*See* PET scan.

sound—A dilator or a metal instrument, that is passed into the penis and through a scar that may form in the urinary tract to stretch it so that urine may pass unobstructed.

spot radiation—External radiation to the selective bones.

stereotactic body radiation therapy (SBRT)—A special type of external beam radiation therapy using focused radiation beams that target a tumor using detailed imaging scans.

steroids—Chemicals produced in the body (e.g., testosterone, cholesterol) that control many bodily functions.

striated muscle—Muscle that is under a person's voluntary control to contract and relax, such as the biceps in the arm.

surgical castration—Removal of the testicles with the aim of lowering testosterone in the body, since the hormone can stimulate cancer growth. See Bilateral orchiectomy.

surgical drain—A thin tube that is placed near a surgical site that allows fluids to drain outside the body.

testicles—Two egg-shaped glands located in the scrotal sac beneath the penis. Their two main functions are to produce sperm, thus making a man fertile, and to produce a hormone called testosterone.

testosterone—A male hormone responsible for your male characteristics such as hair growth, muscle development, sex drive, and the growth of the prostate gland.

testosterone escape—Increase in the testosterone level above the castrate range of 50 ng/dL.

testosterone gel—A treatment for raising testosterone in the body. It is applied to the skin of the arm or shoulder once a day.

three-dimensional conformal radiation (3D-CRT)—Radiation using computers, which plan the treatment from different angles to the body according to the shape of the prostate.

TNM system—A system for staging cancers; T is the extent of cancer within an organ, N is the presence of cancer in the lymph nodes, and M is for metastases or the presence of cancer in other parts of the body.

total androgen blockade—Therapy used to eliminate or block the male sex hormones in the body coming from the testicles and adrenal glands.

transperineal biopsy—Prostate biopsy that is performed by passing needles through the skin in the perineal area and directing them into the prostate.

transrectal biopsy—Prostate biopsy performed by passing needles through the rectal wall and directing them into the prostate.

transrectal prostate ultrasound—Imaging technique that uses sound waves to help direct the prostate biopsy needle into specific locations in the prostate gland. Often used to stage prostate cancer.

transurethral resection of the prostate (TURP)—An operation performed through the penis to remove prostate tissue to improve symptoms from an enlarged prostate.

tumor—An abnormal growth of cells. May be malignant (cancerous) or nonmalignant (benign).

tumor grade—How cancer cells look under a microscope. It is a measure of how fast a cancer might grow or spread.

tumor stage—A way of expressing the location of cancer in the body.

ultrasensitive prostate-specific androgen (PSA)—Test to detect every amount of PSA in a blood sample.

ureter—Tube that carries urine from the kidney to the bladder.

urethra—The tube that carries urine from the bladder out through the tip of the penis.

urethral stricture—A narrowing of the urethra following surgery or trauma resulting in slow urinary flow or complete blockage. Also known as *bladder neck contracture.*

urinary bladder—*See* Bladder

vacuum erection device (VED)—A hollow plastic cylinder that fits over the penis. Air is pumped out of the chamber by a battery-operated motor. This creates a vacuum, which draws the blood into the penis, resulting in an erection.

vas deferens—Long, thin, musuclar tubes through which sperm from each testicle is released during an orgasm. The end of each vas deferens joins with a seminal vesicle to form the ejaculator duct.

vasectomy—Surgical procedure in which the vas deferens are cut, thus making it impossible for a man to eject sperm in his semen during orgasm.

volume study—A method for assessing the size of the prostate gland.

watchful waiting—A treatment in which no therapy is given to the prostate gland and no attempt is made to cure the cancer. Instead, the patient is treated only if the cancer causes symptoms or if it spreads to other parts of the body.

Whitmore-Jewett system—One of two well-know schemes commonly used to stage prostate cancer.

XRT—*See* External beam radiation therapy.

Bibliography

Chapter 2

1. Beyersdorff D, Taymoorian K, Knösel T, et al. MRI of prostate cancer at 1.5 and 3.0 T: Comparison of image quality in tumor detection and staging. *Am J Roentgenol.* 2005;185:1214–1220.

2. Smith JA Jr, Scardino PT, Resnick MI, et al. Transrectal ultrasound versus digital rectal examination for the staging of carcinoma of the prostate: Results of a prospective, multi-institutional trial. J Urol. 1997;157(3):902–906.

Chapter 3

1. Epstein JI, Allsbrook WC Jr, Amin MB, Egevad LL. Update on the Gleason grading system for prostate cancer: Results of an international consensus conference of urologic pathologists. *Adv Anat Pathol.* 2006;13(1):57–59.

2. Ohori M, Wheeler TM, Scardino PT. The new American joint committee on cancer and international union against cancer TNM classification of prostate cancer. *Cancer.* 1994;74(1):104–114.

3. Even-Sapir E, Metser U, Mishani E, et al. The detection of bone metastases in patients with high-risk prostate cancer: 99mTc-MDP planar bone scintigraphy, single- and multi-field-of-view SPECT, 18F-fluoride PET, and 18F-fluoride PET/CT. J Nucl Med. 2006;47(2):287–297.

4. Eifler JB, Feng Z, Lin BM., et al. An updated prostate cancer staging nomogram (Partin tables) based on cases from 2006 to 2011. *BJU Int.* 2013;111(1):22–29.

Chapter 4

1. Owens D, Lohr K, Atkins D, et al. AHRQ series paper 5: Grading the strength of a body of evidence when comparing medical interventions: AHRQ and the effective health-care program. J Clin Epidemiol. 2010; 63(5):513–523.

Chapter 5

1. D'Amico AV, Chen MH, Roehl KA, et al Preoperative PSA velocity and the risk of death from prostate cancer after radical prostatectomy. N Engl J Med. 2004;351:125–135.

2. May M, Knoll N, Siegsmund M, et al. Validity of the CAPRA score to predict biochemical recurrence-free survival after radical prostatectomy. Results from a European multicenter survey of 1,296 patients. J Urol. 2007;178(5):1957–1962.

3. Zhao KH, Hernandez DJ, Han M, et al. External validation of University of California, San Francisco, Cancer of the Prostate Risk Assessment score. Urology. 2008;72(2):396–400.

4. Cooperberg MR, Freedland SJ, Pasta DJ, et al. Multiinstitutional validation of the UCSF cancer of the prostate risk assessment for prediction of recurrence after radical prostatectomy. Cancer. 2006;15:107(10):2384–2391.

5. Cuzick J, Swanson GP, Fisher G, et al. Prognostic value of an RNA expression signature derived from cell cycle proliferation genes in patients with prostate cancer: A retrospective study. Lancet Oncol. 2011 Mar;12(3):245–255.

Chapter 7

1. Lu-Yao GL, Albertsen PC, Moore DF, et al. Outcomes of localized prostate cancer following conservative management. JAMA. 2009;302(11): 1202–1209.

2. Bill-Axelson A, Holmberg L, Ruutu M, et al. Radical prostatectomy versus watchful waiting in early prostate cancer. N Engl J Med. 2005;352(19): 1977–1984.

3. Albertsen PC, Hanley JA, Fine J. 20-year outcomes following conservative management of clinically localized prostate cancer. JAMA. 2005;293(17):2095–2101.

4. Bill-Axelson A, Holmberg L, Filén FJ, et al. Radical prostatectomy versus watchful waiting in localized prostate cancer: The Scandinavian prostate cancer group-4 randomized trial. J Natl Cancer Inst. 2008;100(16): 1144–1154.

5. Wilt TJ, Michael KB, Karen M, et al. Radical prostatectomy versus observation for localized prostate cancer. N Engl J Med. 2012;367:203–213.

Chapter 8

1. Bastian PJ, Carter BH, Bjartell A, et al. Insignificant prostate cancer and active surveillance: From definition to clinical implications. Eur Urol. 2009;55:1321–1330.

2. Shappley WV III, Kenfield SA, Kasperzyk JL, et al. Prospective study of determinants and outcomes of deferred treatment or watchful waiting among men with prostate cancer in a nationwide cohort. J Clin Oncol. 2009;27(30):4980–4985.

3. Klotz L, Zhang L, Lam A, Nam R, Mamedov A, Loblaw A. Clinical results of long-term follow-up of a large, active surveillance cohort with localized prostate cancer. J Clin Oncol. 2010;28(1):126–131.

4. Klotz L. Strengthening evidence for active surveillance for prostate cancer. Eur Urol. 2013;63(1):e1–e14.

5. Godtman, RA, Holmberg E, Khatami A, et al. Outcome following active surveillance of men with screen-detected prostate cancer. Results from the Göteborg randomised population-based prostate cancer screening trial. Eur Urol. 2013;63(1):e1–e14.

6. Cooperberg MR, Cowan JE, Hilton JF, et al. Outcomes of active surveillance for men with intermediate-risk prostate cancer. JCO. 2011;29(2):228–234.

7. Klotz L, Zhang L, Lam A, et al. Clinical results of long-term follow-up of a large, active surveillance cohort with localized prostate cancer. JCO. 2010;28(1):126–131.

8. Loblaw A, Zhang L, Lam A, et al. Comparing prostate specific antigen triggers for intervention in men with stable prostate cancer on active surveillance. J Urol. 2010;184(5):1942–1946.

9. Thomas RJ, Williams MMA, Sharma H, et al. A double-blind, placebo RCT evaluating the effect of a polyphenol-rich whole food supplement on PSA progression in men with prostate cancer: The U.K. National Cancer Research Network (NCRN) Pomi-T study. J Clin Oncol. 2013;31 (suppl; abstr 5008).

Chapter 9

1. Potosky AL, Davis WW, Hoffman RM, et al. Five-year outcomes after prostatectomy or radiotherapy for prostate cancer: The prostate cancer outcomes study. J Natl Cancer Inst. 2004;96(18):1358–1367.

2. Hoffman RM, Hunt WC, Gilliland FD, Stephenson RA, Potosky AL. Patient satisfaction with treatment decisions for clinically localized prostate carcinoma. Results from the prostate cancer outcomes study. Cancer. 2003;97(7):1653–1662.

3. Han M, Partin AW, Zahurak M, Piantadosi S, Epstein JI, Walsh PC. Biochemical (prostate-specific antigen) recurrence probability following radical prostatectomy for clinically localized prostate cancer. J Urol. 2003;169(2):517–523.

4. Wilt TJ, Macdonald R, Rutks I, Shamliyan TA, Taylor BC, Kane RL. Systematic review: Comparative effectiveness and harms of treatments for clinically localized prostate cancer. Ann Intern Med. 2008;148(6):435–448.

5. Hu JC, Gu X, Lipsitz SR, et al. Comparative effectiveness of minimally invasive vs open radical prostatectomy. JAMA. 2009;302(14):1557–1564.

6. Alibhai SM, Leach M, Tomlinson G, et al. 30-day mortality and major complications after radical prostatectomy: Influence of age and comorbidity. J Natl Cancer Inst. 2005;97(20):1525–1532.

7. Thompson IM, Tangen CM, Paradelo J, et al. Adjuvant radiotherapy for pathological T3N0M0 prostate cancer significantly reduces risk of metastases and improves survival: Long-term follow-up of a randomized clinical trial. J Urol. 2009;181(3):956–962.

8. Engel JD, Sutherland DE, Williams SB, et al. Changes in penile length after robot-assisted laparoscopic radical prostatectomy. J Endourol. 2011;25(1):65–69.

9. Stephenson AJ, Kattan MW, Eastham JA, et al. Prostate cancer–specific mortality after radical prostatectomy for patients treated in the prostate-specific antigen era. J Clin Oncol. 2009;27(26):4300–4305.

Chapter 10

1. Heidenreich A, Ohlmann CH, Polyakov S. Anatomical extent of pelvic lymphadenectomy in patients undergoing radical prostatectomy. Eur Urol. 2007;52(1):29–37.

2. Messing EM, Manola J, Yao J, et al. Immediate versus deferred androgen deprivation treatment in patients with node-positive prostate cancer after radical prostatectomy and pelvic lymphadenectomy. *Lancet Oncol.* 2006;7(6):472–479.

Chapter 11

1. Kumar S, Shelley M, Harrison C, Coles B, Wilt TJ, Mason MD. Neo-adjuvant and adjuvant hormone therapy for localised and locally advanced prostate cancer. *Cochrane Database Syst Rev.* 2006;(4):CD006019.

2. Pilepich MV, Caplan R, Byhardt RW, et al. Phase III trial of androgen suppression using goserelin in unfavorable-prognosis carcinoma of the prostate treated with definitive radiotherapy: Report of radiation therapy oncology group protocol 85–31. *J Clin Oncol.* 1997;15(3):1013–1021.

3. Viani GA, Stefano EJ, Afonso SL. Higher-than-conventional radiation doses in localized prostate cancer treatment: A meta-analysis of randomized, controlled trials. *Int J Radiat Oncol Biol Phys.* 2009;74(5):1405–1418.

4. Agency for Healthcare Research and Quality. Comparative evaluation of radiation treatments for clinically localized prostate cancer: An update. Aug 2010. Available at http://www.cms.gov/coveragegeninfo/downloads/id69ta.pdf

5. Jones CU, Hunt, D, McGown DG, et al. Radiotherapy and short-term androgen deprivation for localized prostate cancer. *NEJM.* 2011;365:107–118.

6. D'Amico AV, Manola J, Loffredo M, et al. 6-Month androgen suppression plus radiation therapy vs radiation therapy alone for patients with clinically localized prostate cancer. A randomized controlled trial. *JAMA.* 2004;292(7):821–827.

7. D'Amico AV, Chen M-H, Renshaw AA, et al. Androgen suppression and radiation vs radiation alone for prostate cancer. A randomized trial. *JAMA.* 2008;299(3):289–295.

8. Sullivan JF, Stember DS, Deveci S, et al. Ejaculation profiles of men following radiation therapy for prostate cancer. *J Sexual Med.* 2013;10(5):1410–1416.

Chapter 12

1. Agency for Healthcare Research and Quality. Comparative effectiveness of therapies for clinically localized prostate cancer. Available at: http://effectivehealthcare.ahrq.gov/healthInfo.cfm?infotype=rr&ProcessID=9&DocID=79. Accessed October 2010.

2. Frank SJ, Grimm PD, Sylvester JE, et al. Interstitial implant alone or in combination with external beam radiation therapy for intermediate-risk prostate cancer: A survey of practice patterns in the United States. Brachytherapy. 2007;6(1):2–8.

3. Herstein A, Wallner K, Merrick G, et al. I-125 versus Pd-103 for low-risk prostate cancer: Long-term morbidity outcomes from a prospective randomized multicenter controlled trial. Cancer. 2005;11(5):385–389.

4. Zelefsky MJ, Zaider M. Low-dose-rate brachytherapy for prostate cancer: Preplanning vs intraoperative planning—intraoperative planning is best. Brachytherapy. 2006;5(3):143–144.

5. Ragde H, Korb LJ, Elgamal AA, Grado GL, Nadir BS. Modern prostate brachytherapy. Prostate-specific antigen results in 219 patients with up to 12 years of observed follow-up. Cancer. 2000;89(1):135–141.

6. Miller DC, Sanda MG, Dunn RL, et al. Long-term outcomes among localized prostate cancer survivors: Health-related quality-of-life changes after radical prostatectomy, external radiation, and brachytherapy. J Clin Oncol. 2005;23(12):2772–2780.

7. Filocamo MT, Li Marzi V, Del Popolo G, et al. Effectiveness of early pelvic floor rehabilitation treatment for post-prostatectomy incontinence. Eur Urol. 2005;48(5):734–738.

8. Ragde H, Elgamal AA, Snow PB, et al. Ten-year disease-free survival after transperineal sonography-guided iodine-125 brachytherapy with or without 45-gray external beam irradiation in the treatment of patients with clinically localized, low to high Gleason grade prostate carcinoma. Cancer. 1998;83:989–1001.

9. Beyer DC, McKeough T, Thomas T. Impact of short-course hormonal therapy on overall and cancer-specific survival after permanent prostate brachytherapy. Int J Rad Oncol Biol Phys. 2005;61(5):1299–1305.

10. Herstein A, Wallner K, Merrick G, et al. I-125 versus Pd-103 for low-risk prostate cancer: Long-term morbidity outcomes from a prospective randomized multicenter controlled trial. Cancer J. 2005 11(5):385–389.

11. Shen X, Keith SC, Mishra MV, et al. The impact of brachytherapy on prostate cancer–specific mortality for definitive radiation therapy of high-grade prostate cancer: A population-based analysis. Int J Rad Oncol Biol Phys. 2012;83(4):1154–1159.

12. Giberti C, Chiono L, Gallo F, et al. Radical retropubic prostatectomy versus brachytherapy for low-risk prostatic cancer: A prospective study. *World J Urol.* 2009;27(5):607–612.

Chapter 13

1. Thompson I, Thrasher JB, Aus G, et al. Guideline for the management of clinically localized prostate cancer. *J Urol.* 2007;177(6):2106–2131.

2. Babaian RJ, Donnelly B, Bahn D, et al. Best practice statement on cryo-surgery for the treatment of localized prostate cancer. *J Urol.* 2008;180(5):1993–2004.

3. Ellis DS, Manny TB Jr, Rewcastle JC. Cryoablation as a primary treatment for localized prostate cancer followed by penile rehabilitation. *Urology.* 2007;69(2):306–310.

4. Prepelica KL, Okeke Z, Murphy A, Katz AE. Cryosurgical ablation of the prostate: High-risk patient outcomes. *Cancer.* 2005;103(8):1625–1630.

5. Hubosky SG, Fabrizio MD, Schellhammer PF, Barone BB, Tepera CM, Given RW. Single-center experience with third-generation cryosurgery for management of organ-confined prostate cancer: Critical evaluation of short-term outcomes, complications, and patient quality-of-life. *J Endourol.* 2007;21(12):1521–1531.

6. Bahn DK, Lee F, Badalament R, Kumar A, Greski J, Chernick M. Targeted cryoablation of the prostate: Seven-year outcomes in the primary treatment of prostate cancer. *Urology.* 2002;60(2 suppl 1):3–11.

7. American Urological Association Education and Research, Inc. Best Practice Policy Statement on Cryosurgery for the Treatment of Localized Prostate Cancer. 2008. http://www.auanet.org/common/pdf/education/clinicalguidance/Cryosurgery.pdf

8. Porter MP, Ahaghotu CA, Loening SA, See WA/Disease-free and overall survival after cryosurgical monotherapy for clinical stages B and C carcinoma of the prostate: A 20-year follow-up. *J Urology.* 1997;158:1466–1469.

9. Shelley M, Wilt TJ, Coles B, et al. Cryotherapy for localised prostate cancer. *Cochrane Database Syst Rev.* 2007;(3):CD005010. Cochrane Library 2012, Issue 2.

10. Bahn D, de Castro Abreu AL, Gill IS, et al. Focal cryotherapy for clinically unilateral, low-intermediate risk prostate cancer in 73 men with a median follow-up of 3.7 years. Eur Urol. 2012;62(1):55–63.

11. Chin JL, Ng CK, Touma NJ, et al. Randomized trial comparing cryoablation and external beam radiotherapy for T2C–T3B prostate cancer. *Prostate Cancer Prostatic Dis.* 2007;11(1):40–45.

Chapter 14

1. Levine GN, D'Amico AV, Berger P, et al. Androgen-deprivation therapy in prostate cancer and cardiovascular risk: A science advisory from the American Heart Association, American Cancer Society, and American Urological Association. *CA Cancer J Clin.* 2010;60(3):194–201.

2. Studer UE, Collette L, Whelan P, et al. Using PSA to guide timing of androgen deprivation in patients with T0-4 N0-2 M0 prostate cancer not suitable for local curative treatment (EORTC 30891). Eur Urol. 2008;53(5):941–949.

3. Braga-Basaria M, Dobs AS, Muller DC, et al. Metabolic syndrome in men with prostate cancer undergoing long-term androgen-deprivation therapy. J Clin Oncol. 2006;24(24):3979–3983.

4. Salminen EK, Portin RI, Koskinen A, Helenius H, Nurmi M. Associations between serum testosterone fall and cognitive function in prostate cancer patients. *Clin Cancer Res.* 2004;10(22):7575–7582.

5. The Medical Research Council Prostate Cancer Working Party Investigators Group. Immediate versus deferred treatment for advanced prostatic cancer: Initial results of the medical research council trial. Br J Urol. 1997;79(2):235–246.

6. Smith MR, Mortin RA, Barnette KG, et al. Toremifene to reduce fracture risk in men receiving androgen deprivation therapy for prostate cancer. J Urol. 2013;189(1):S45–S50.

7. Studer UE, Whelan P, Albrecht W, et al. Immediate or deferred androgen deprivation for patients with prostate cancer not suitable for local treatment with curative intent: European Organisation for Research and Treatment of Cancer (EORTC) Trial 30891. J Clin Oncol. 2006;24(12): 1868–1876.

8. Kawakami J, Cowan JE, Elkin EP, et al. Androgen-deprivation therapy as primary treatment for localized prostate cancer: Data from Cancer of the Prostate Strategic Urologic Research Endeavor (CaPSURE). *Cancer.* 2006;106(8):1708–1714.

9. Sharif N, Gulley JL, Dahut WL. Androgen deprivation therapy for prostate cancer. *JAMA.* 2005;294(2):238–244.

10. Brawer, MK. Hormonal therapy for prostate cancer. *Rev Urol.* 2006; 8(suppl 2):S35–S47.

11. Warde P, Mason M, Ding K, et al. Combined androgen deprivation therapy and radiation therapy for locally advanced prostate cancer: A randomised, phase 3 trial. *The Lancet.* 2011;378(9809):2104–2111.

12. Vasudeva P, Goel A, Dalela D. Survival following primary androgen deprivation therapy among men with localized prostate cancer. *Indian J Urol.* 2008;24(4):590–591.

13. Lu-Yao GL, Albertsen PC, Moore DF, et al. Outcome of localized prostate cancer treatment following conservative management. *JAMA.* 2009;302(11):1202–1209.

14. Moinpour C, Berry DL, Ely B, et al. Preliminary quality-of-life outcomes for SWOG-9346: Intermittent androgen deprivation in patients with hormone-sensitive metastatic prostate cancer (HSM1PC)—Phase III. *J Clin Oncol.* 2012;30(suppl; abstr 4571).

15. Saad F, Gleason DM, Murray R, et al. Long-term efficacy of zoledronic acid for the prevention of skeletal complications in patients with metastatic hormone-refractory prostate cancer. *J Natl Cancer Inst.* 2004; 96(11):879–882.

Chapter 15

1. Colombel M, Poissonnier L, Martin X, Gelet A. Clinical results of the prostate HIFU project. *Eur Urol Supplements.* 2006;5(6):491–494.

2. Poissonnier L, Chapelon JY, Rouvière O, et al. Control of prostate cancer by transrectal HIFU in 227 patients. *Eur Urol.* 2007;51(2):381–387.

3. Ganzer R, Fritsche HM, Brandtner A, et al. Fourteen-year oncological and functional outcomes of high-intensity focused ultrasound in localized prostate cancer. BJUI 2013; http://www.ncbi.nlm.nih.gov/pubmed/23356910

Chapter 16

1. Chen RC, Clark JA, Manola J, Talcott JA. Treatment "mismatch" in early prostate cancer: Do treatment choices take patient quality-of-life into account? *Cancer.* 2008;112(1):61–68.

2. Penson DF, Feng Z, Kuniyuki A, et al. General quality-of-life 2 years following treatment for prostate cancer: What influences outcomes? Results from the prostate cancer outcomes study. *J Clin Oncol.* 2003;21(6):1147–1154.

3. Gore JL, Kwan L, Lee SP, Reiter RE, Litwin MS. Survivorship beyond convalescence: 48-month quality-of-life outcomes after treatment for localized prostate cancer. *J Natl Cancer Inst.* 2009;101(12):888–892.

4. Miller DC, Sanda MG, Dunn RL, et al. Long-term outcomes among localized prostate cancer survivors: Health-related quality-of-life changes after radical prostatectomy, external radiation, and brachytherapy. *J Clin Oncol.* 2005;23(12):2772–2780.

5. Steineck G, Helgesen F, Adolfsson J, et al. Quality-of-life after radical prostatectomy or watchful waiting. *N Engl J Med.* 2002;347(11): 790–796.

6. Sanda MG, Dunn RL, Michalski J, et al. Quality of life and satisfaction with outcome among prostate-cancer survivors. *N Engl J Med.* 2008;358:1250–1261.

7. Smith DP,King MT, Egger S, et al. Quality of life three years after diagnosis of localised prostate cancer: Population-based cohort study. *BMJ.* 2009;339:b4817.

8. Zini C, Hipp E, Thomas S, et al. Ultrasound- and MR-guided focused ultrasound surgery for prostate cancer. *World J Radiol.* 2012;4(6): 247–252.

9. Maestroni U, Dinale F, Minari R, et al. High-intensity focused ultrasound for prostate cancer: Long-term follow up and complications rate. *Adv Urol.* 2012;2012(article ID 960835):4.

10. Resnick MJ, Koyama T, Fan KH, et al. Long-term functional outcomes after treatment for localized prostate cancer. *N Engl J Med.* 2013;368: 436–445.

11. Potosky AL, Davis WW, Hoffman RM, et al. Five-year outcomes after prostatectomy or radiotherapy for prostate cancer: The prostate cancer outcomes study. *J Natl Cancer Inst.* 2004;96(18):1358–1367.

12. Steineck G, Helgesen F, Adolfsson J, et al. Quality of life after radical prostatectomy or watchful waiting. *N Engl J Med.* 2002;347:790–796.

Chapter 18

1. Goldstein I, Lue TF, Padma-Nathan H, et al. Oral sildenafil in the treatment of erectile dysfunction. 1998. *J Urol.* 2002;167(2 pt 2):1197–1203.

2. Masson P, Lampert SM, Brown M, Shabsigh R. PDE-5 inhibitors: Current status and future trends. *Urol Clin North Am.* 2005;32(4):511–525.

3. Mulhall JP, Ahmed A, Branch J, Parker M. Serial assessment of efficacy and satisfaction profiles following penile prosthesis surgery. *J Urol.* 2003;169(4):1429–1433.

4. Haab F, Trockman BA, Zimmern PE, Leach GE. Quality-of-life and continence assessment of the artificial urinary sphincter in men with minimum 3.5 years of follow-up. *J Urol.* 1997;158(2):435–439.

5. Guimarães M, Oliveira R, Pinto R, et al. Intermediate-term results, up to 4 years, of a bone-anchored male perineal sling for treating male stress urinary incontinence after prostate surgery. *BJU Int.* 2009; 103(4):500–504.

6. Carmel M, Hage B, Hanna S, et al. Long-term efficacy of the bone-anchored male sling for moderate and severe stress urinary incontinence. *BJU Int.* 2010;106(7):1012–1016.

7. Montague DK. Artificial urinary sphincter: Long-term results and patient satisfaction. *Adv Urol.* 2012:2012(article ID 835290):4.

8. Cornu JN, Merlet B, Ciofu C, et al. Duloxetine for mild to moderate postprostatectomy incontinence: Preliminary results of a randomised, placebo-controlled trial. *Eur Urol.* 2011;59(1):148–154.

9. Montorsi F, Guazzoni G, Strambi LF, et al. Recovery of spontaneous erectile function after nerve-sparing radical retropubic prostatectomy with and without early intracavernous injections of alprostadil: Results of a prospective, randomized trial. *J Urol.* 1997;158(4):1408–1410.

10. Montorsi F, Nathan HP, McCullough A, et al. Tadalafil in the treatment of erectile dysfunction following bilateral nerve sparing radical retropubic prostatectomy: A randomized, double-blind, placebo controlled trial. J Urol. 2004;172(3):1036–1041.

11. Köhler TS, Pedro R, Hendlin K, et al. A pilot study on the early use of the vacuum erection device after radical retropubic prostatectomy. BJU Int. 2007;100(4):858–862.

12. Raina R, Agarwal A, Ausmundson S, et al. Early use of vacuum constriction device following radical prostatectomy facilitates early sexual activity and potentially earlier return of erectile function. Int J Impot Res. 2006;18(1):77–81.

13. Padma-Nathan H., McCullough AR, Giuliano F, et al. Postoperative nightly administration of sildenafil citrate significantly improved the return of normal spontaneous erectile function after bilateral nerve-sparing radical retropubic prostatectomy with and without early intracavernous injections of alprostadil: Results of a prospective, randomized trial. J Urol. 2003;169(4):375–376.

14. Centemero A, Rigatti L, Giraudo D, et al. Preoperative pelvic floor muscle exercise for early continence after radical prostatectomy: A randomised controlled study. Eur Urol. 2010;57(6):1039–1043.

Chapter 19

1. Caloglu M, Ciezki J. Prostate-specific antigen bounce after prostate brachytherapy: Review of a confusing phenomenon. Urology. 2009; 74(6):1183–1190.

2. Freedland SJ, Humphreys EB, Mangold LA, et al. Risk of prostate cancer-specific mortality following biochemical recurrence after radical prostatectomy. JAMA. 2005;294(4):433–439.

3. Roach M III, Hanks G, Thames H, Jr, et al. Defining biochemical failure following radiotherapy with or without hormonal therapy in men with clinically localized prostate cancer: Recommendations of the RTOG-ASTRO Phoenix Consensus Conference. Int J Radiat Oncol Biol Phys. 2006;65(4):965–974.

4. Jhaveri FM, Zippe CD, Klein EA, Kupelian PA. Biochemical failure does not predict overall survival after radical prostatectomy for localized prostate cancer: 10-year results. Urology. 1999;54(5):884–890.

5. Eifler JB, Feng Z, Lin BM, et al. An updated prostate cancer staging nomogram (Partin tables) based on cases from 2006 to 2011. BJU Int. 2013;111(1):22–29.

6. Critz FA, Williams WH, Levinson AK, et al. Prostate-specific antigen bounce after simultaneous irradiation for prostate cancer: The relationship to patient age. J Urol. 2003;170(5):1864–1867.

7. Babaian RJ, Donnelly B, Bahn D, et al. AUA best practice statement on cryosurgery for the treatment of localized prostate cancer. J Urol. 2008;180:1993–2004.

8. Ismail M, Ahmed S, Kastner C, et al. Salvage cryotherapy for recurrent prostate cancer after radiation failure: A prospective case series of the first 100 patients. BJU Int. 2007;100(4):760–764.

9. Robinson JW, Donnelly BJ, Coupland K, et al. Quality of life 2 years after salvage cryosurgery for the treatment of local recurrence of prostate cancer after radiotherapy. Urol Oncol. 2006;24(6):472–486.

10. Uddin Ahmed H, Cathcart P, Chalasani V, et al. Whole-gland salvage high-intensity focused ultrasound therapy for localized prostate cancer recurrence after external beam radiation therapy. Cancer. 2012; 118(12):3071–3078.

11. Crook JM, O'Callaghan CJ, Duncan G, et al. Intermittent androgen suppression for rising PSA level after radiotherapy. N Engl J Med. 2012;367(10):895–903.

Chapter 21

1. Freedland SJ, Partin AW, Humphreys EB, Mangold LA, Walsh PC. Radical prostatectomy for clinical stage T3a disease. Cancer. 2007;109(7): 1273–1278.

2. Hsu CY, Wildhagen MF, van Poppel H, Bangma CH. Prognostic factors for and outcome of locally advanced prostate cancer after radical prostatectomy. BJU Int. 2010;105(11):1536–1540.

3. Gerber GS, Thisted RA, Chodak GW, et al. Results of radical prostatectomy in men with locally advanced prostate cancer: Multi-institutional pooled analysis. Eur Urol. 1997;32(4):385–390.

4. Akakura K, Isaka S, Akimoto S, et al. Long-term results of a randomized trial for the treatment of stages B2 and C prostate cancer: Radical prostatectomy versus external beam radiation therapy with a common endocrine therapy in both modalities. Urology. 1999;54(2):313–318.

5. Thompson IM, Tangen CM, Paradelo J, et al. Adjuvant radiotherapy for pathological T3N0M0 prostate cancer significantly reduces risk of metastases and improves survival: Long-term follow up of a randomized clinical trial. J Urol. 2009;181(3):956–962.

6. Bolla M, Van Poppel H, Tombal B, et al. 10-year results of adjuvant radiotherapy after radical prostatectomy in pT3N0 prostate cancer (EORTC 22911). Int J Rad Oncol Biol Phys. 2010;78(3), Supplement:S29.

Chapter 22

1. Roach M III, Bae K, Speight J, et al. Short-term neoadjuvant androgen deprivation therapy and external-beam radiotherapy for locally advanced prostate cancer: Long-term results of RTOG 8610. J Clin Oncol. 2008;26(4):585–591.

2. Pilepich MV, Winter K, Lawton CA, et al. Androgen suppression adjuvant to definitive radiotherapy in prostate carcinoma—long-term results of phase III RTOG 85–31. Int J Radiat Oncol Biol Phys. 2005;61(5):1285–1290.

3. Bolla M, Gonzalez D, Warde P, et al. Improved survival in patients with locally advanced prostate cancer treated with radiotherapy and goserelin. N Engl J Med. 1997;337(5):295–300.

4. Quon JL, Yu JB, Soulos PR, et al. The relation between age and androgen deprivation therapy use among men in the Medicare population receiving radiation therapy for prostate cancer. J Geriatr Oncol. 2013;4(1):9–18.

5. Nabid A, Carrier N, Martin A-G, et al. High-risk prostate cancer treated with pelvic radiotherapy and 36 versus 18 months of androgen blockade: Results of a phase III randomized study. J Clin Oncol. 2013;31(suppl 6; abstr 3).

6. Mottet N, Peneau M, Mazeron JJ, et al. Addition of radiotherapy to long-term androgen deprivation in locally advanced prostate cancer: An open randomised phase 3 trial. Eur Urol. 2012;62(2):213–219.

7. Zelefsky MJ, Leibel SA, Gauldin PB, et al. Dose escalation with three-dimensional conformal radiation therapy affects the outcome in prostate cancer. *Int J Rad Oncol Biol Phys.* 1998;41(3):491–500.

8. Lawton CA, Yan Y, Lee WR, et al. Long-term results of an RTOG Phase II trial (00-19) of external-beam radiation therapy combined with permanent source brachytherapy for intermediate-risk clinically localized adenocarcinoma of the prostate. *Int J Radiat Oncol Biol Phys.* 2012;82(5):e795–801.

9. Sathya JR, Davis IR, Julian JA, et al. Randomized trial comparing iridium implant plus external-beam radiation therapy with external-beam radiation therapy alone in node-negative locally advanced cancer of the prostate. *J Clin Oncol.* 2005;23(6):1192–1199.

Chapter 23

1. Medical Research Council Prostate Cancer Working Party. Immediate versus deferred treatment for advanced prostatic cancer: Initial results of the medical research council trial. *Br J Urol.* 1997;79(2):235–246.

2. Nguyen PL, Je Y, Schutz FAB, et al. Association of androgen deprivation therapy with cardiovascular death in patients with prostate cancer. A meta-analysis of randomized trials. *JAMA.* 2011;306(21):2359–2366.

3. Levine GN, D'Amico AV, Berger P, et al. Androgen-deprivation therapy in prostate cancer and cardiovascular risk: A science advisory from the American Heart Association, American Cancer Society, and American Urological Association: Endorsed by the American Society for Radiation Oncology. *CA: Cancer J Clin.* 2010;60(3):194–201.

4. Crook JM, O'Callaghan CJ, Duncan G, et al. Intermittent androgen suppression for rising PSA level after radiotherapy. *N Engl J Med.* 2012; 367:895–903.

Chapter 26

1. Oefelein MG, Feng A, Scolieri MJ, Ricchiutti D, Resnick MI. Reassessment of the definition of castrate levels of testosterone: Implications for clinical decision making. *Urology.* 2000;56(6):1021–1024.

2. Loprinzi CL, Michalak JC, Quella SK, et al. Megestrol acetate for the prevention of hot flashes. *N Engl J Med.* 1994;331(6):347–352.

3. Segal RJ, Reid RD, Courneya KS, et al. Resistance exercise in men receiving androgen deprivation therapy for prostate cancer. J Clin Oncol. 2003;21(9):1653–1659.

4. Perachino M, Cavalli V, Bravi F. Testosterone levels in patients with metastatic prostate cancer treated with luteinizing hormone-releasing hormone therapy: Prognostic significance? BJU Int. 2010;105(5):648–651.

5. Salminen EK, Portin RI, Koskinen A, Helenius H, Nurmi M. Associations between serum testosterone fall and cognitive function in prostate cancer patients. Clin Cancer Res. 2004;10(22):7575–7582.

6. Tombal B. Appropriate castration with luteinizing hormone-releasing hormone (LHRH) agonists: What is the optimal level of testosterone? Eur Urol Suppl. 2005;4(5):14–19.

7. Kaisary AV, Tyrrell CJ, Peeling WB, Griffiths K. Comparison of LHRH analogue (Zoladex) with orchiectomy in patients with metastatic prostatic carcinoma. Br J Urol. 1991;67(5):502–508.

8. Eisenberger MA, Blumenstein BA, Crawford ED, et al. Bilateral orchiectomy with or without flutamide for metastatic prostate cancer. N Engl J Med. 1998;339:1036–1042.

Chapter 28

1. Ornstein DK, Rao GS, Johnson B, Charlton ET, Andriole GL. Combined finasteride and flutamide therapy in men with advanced prostate cancer. Urology. 1996;48(6):901–905.

2. Crawford ED, Eisenberger MA, McLeod DG, et al. A controlled trial of leuprolide with and without flutamide in prostatic carcinoma. N Engl J Med. 1989;321(7):419–424.

3. Leibowitz RL, Tucker SJ. Treatment of localized prostate cancer with intermittent triple androgen blockade: Preliminary results in 110 consecutive patients. Oncologist. 2001;6(2):177–182.

4. Presti JC Jr, Fair WR, Andriole G, et al. Multicenter, randomized, double-blind, placebo-controlled study to investigate the effect of finasteride (MK-906) on stage D prostate cancer. J Urol. 1992;148(4):1201–1204.

5. Eisenberger MA, Blumenstein BA, Crawford ED, et al. Bilateral orchiectomy with or without flutamide for metastatic prostate cancer. N Engl J Med. 1998;339(15):1036–1042.

Chapter 29

1. Paes FM, Serafini AN. Systemic metabolic radiopharmaceutical therapy in the treatment of metastatic bone pain. *Semin Nucl Med*. 2010;40(2): 89–104.

2. Saad F, Gleason DM, Murray R, et al. A randomized, placebo-controlled trial of zoledronic acid in patients with hormone-refractory metastatic prostate carcinoma. *J Natl Cancer Inst*. 2002;94(19):1458–1468.

3. Bamias A, Kastritis E, Bamia C, et al. Osteonecrosis of the jaw in cancer after treatment with bisphosphonates: Incidence and risk factors. *J Clin Oncol*. 2005;23(34):8580–8587.

4. Fizazi K, Carducci M, Smith M, et al. Denosumab versus zoledronic acid for treatment of bone metastases in men with castration-resistant prostate cancer: A randomised, double-blind study. *Lancet*. 2011;377:813–822.

5. van den Hout WB, van der Linden YM, Steenland E, et al. Single- versus multiple-fraction radiotherapy in patients with painful bone metastases: Cost-utility analysis based on a randomized trial. *J Natl Cancer Inst*. 2003;3(95):222–229.

Chapter 31

1. Kantoff PW, Higano CS, Shore ND, et al. Sipuleucel-T immunotherapy for castration-resistant prostate cancer. *N Eng J Med*. 2010;363(5):411–422.

2. Higano CS, Schellhammer PF, Small EJ, et al. Integrated data from 2 randomized, double-blind, placebo-controlled, phase 3 trials of active cellular immunotherapy with sipuleucel-T in advanced prostate cancer. *Cancer*. 2009;115(16):3670–3679.

3. Schellhammer PF, Chodak G, Whitmore JB, et al. Lower baseline prostate-specific antigen is associated with a greater overall survival benefit from sipuleucel-T in the immunotherapy for prostate adenocarcinoma treatment (IMPACT) trial. *Urology*. 2013;S0090-4295(13):00225-2.

Chapter 32

1. DeBono JS, Logothetis CJ, Molina A, et al. Abiraterone and increased survival in metastatic prostate cancer. *N Engl J Med*. 2011;364:1995–2005.

Chapter 33

1. Tindall DJ, Rittmaster RS. The rationale for inhibiting 5a-reductase isoenzymes in the prevention and treatment of prostate cancer. J Urol. 2008;179(4):1235–1242.

2. Hedlund PO, Henriksson P. Parenteral estrogen versus total androgen ablation in the treatment of advanced prostate carcinoma: Effects on overall survival and cardiovascular mortality. The Scandinavian Prostatic Cancer Group (SPCG)-5 Trial Study. Urology. 2000;55(3): 328–333.

Chapter 34

1. Petrylak DP, Tangen CM, Hussain MH, et al. Docetaxel and estramustine compared with mitoxantrone and prednisone for advanced refractory prostate cancer. N Engl J Med. 2004;351(15):1513–1520.

2. Tannock IF, Osoba D, Stockler MR, et al. Chemotherapy with mitoxantrone plus prednisone or prednisone alone for symptomatic hormone-resistant prostate cancer: A Canadian randomized trial with palliative end points. J Clin Oncol. 1996;14(6):1756–1764.

3. Tannock IF, de Wit R, Berry WR, et al. Docetaxel plus prednisone or mitoxantrone plus prednisone for advanced prostate cancer. N Engl J Med. 2004;351(15):1502–1512.

Chapter 35

1. Scher HI, Fizazi K, Saad F, et al. Increased survival with enzalutamide in prostate cancer after chemotherapy. N Engl J Med. 2012;367:1187–1197.

2. de Bono JS, Logithetis CJ, Molina A, et al. Abiraterone and increased survival in metastatic prostate cancer. N Engl J Med. 2011;364:1995–2005.

3. Fizazi K, Scher HI, Molina A, et al. Abiraterone acetate for treatment of metastatic castration-resistant prostate cancer: Final overall survival analysis of the COU-AA-301 randomised, double-blind, placebo-controlled phase 3 study. Lancet Oncol. 2012;13(10):983–992.

Chapter 36

1. Ernst DS, Tannock IF, Winquist EW, et al. Randomized, double-blind, controlled trial of mitoxantrone/prednisone and clodronate versus mitoxantrone/prednisone and placebo in patients with hormone-refractory prostate cancer and pain. J Clin Oncol. 2003;21(17):3335–3342.

2. Kantoff PW, Halabi S, Conaway M, et al. Hydrocortisone with or without mitoxantrone in men with hormone-refractory prostate cancer: Results of the cancer and leukemia group B 9182 study. J Clin Oncol. 1999;17(8):2506–2513.

3. De Bono JS, Oudard M, Ozguroglu S, et al. Cabazitaxel or mitoxantrone with prednisone in patients with metastatic castration-resistant prostate cancer (mCRPC) previously treated with docetaxel: Final results of a multinational phase III trial (TROPIC). Journal of Clinical Oncology, 2010 ASCO Annual Meeting Proceedings (Post-Meeting Edition). 2010;28(15_Suppl):4508.

Chapter 37

1. Ryan CJ, Smith MR, de Bono JS, et al. Abiraterone in metastatic prostate cancer without previous chemotherapy. N Engl J Med. 2013;368:138–148.

Chapter 38

1. US National Institutes of Health clinical trials website: Available at: www.clinicaltrials.gov

Chapter 39

1. Chan JM, Elkin EP, Silva SJ, Broering JM, Latini DM, Carroll PR. Total and specific complementary and alternative medicine use in a large cohort of men with prostate cancer. Urology. 2005;66(6):1223–1228.

2. Perabo FG, von Low EC, Ellinger J, von Rücker A, Müller SC, Bastian PJ. Soy isoflavone genistein in prevention and treatment of prostate cancer. Prostate Cancer Prostatic Dis. 2008;11:6–12.

3. Sonn GA, Aronson W, Litwin MS. Impact of diet on prostate cancer: A review. *Prostate Cancer Prostatic Dis.* 2005;8(4):304–310.

4. Thomas RJ, Williams MMA, Sharma H, et al. A double-blind, placebo RCT evaluating the effect of a polyphenol-rich whole food supplement on PSA progression in men with prostate cancer: The U.K. National Cancer Research Network (NCRN) Pomi-T study. *J Clin Oncol.* 2013:31 (suppl; abstr 5008).

Chapter 42

1. Peters L, Sellick K. Quality-of-life of cancer patients receiving inpatient and home-based palliative care. *J Adv Nurs.* 2006;53(5):524–533.

Index